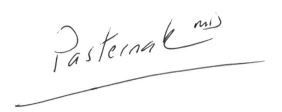

Headache

OTHER TITLES IN THE ACP KEY DISEASES SERIES

ASTHMA
Edited by Raymond G. Slavin and Robert E. Reisman

DEPRESSION
Edited by James L. Levenson

DYSPEPSIA
Edited by David A. Johnson, Philip O. Katz, and Donald O. Castell

LYME DISEASE
Edited by Daniel W. Rahn and Janine Evans

OBESITY
Edited by Barry Gumbiner

For a catalogue of publications available from ACP, contact:

Customer Service Center
American College of Physicians
190 N. Independence Mall West
Philadelphia, PA 19106-1572
215-351-2600
800-523-1546, ext. 2600

Visit our Web site at www.acponline.org

Headache

A Guide for the Primary Care Physician

Elizabeth W. Loder, MD, FACP

Spaulding Rehabilitation Hospital and
Harvard Medical School

Vincent T. Martin, MD

Cincinnati Headache Center and
University of Cincinnati

EDITORS

AMERICAN COLLEGE OF PHYSICIANS

PHILADELPHIA

Clinical Consultant: David R. Goldmann, MD, FACP
Manager, Book Publishing: Diane McCabe
Developmental Editor: Victoria Hoenigke
Production Supervisor: Allan S. Kleinberg
Senior Production Editor: Karen C. Nolan
Interior Design: Kate Nichols
Cover Design: Elizabeth Swartz
Index: Nelle Garrecht

Printed in the United States of America
Printed by Versa Press
Composition by UB Communications

Library of Congress Cataloging-in-Publication Data

Headache / edited by Elizabeth Loder, Vince Martin.
        p ; cm.—(Key diseases series)
    Includes bibliographical references.
    ISBN: 1-930513-38-0
        1. Headache. I. Loder, Elizabeth. II. Martin, Vince, 1958- III. ACP key diseases series.
    [DNLM: 1. Headache—diagnosis. 2. Headache—therapy. WL 342 H43156 2004]
    RC392.H4122 2004
    616.8'491—dc22

                                                                    2004052993

The authors and publisher have exerted every effort to ensure that drug selection and dosage set forth in this book are in accordance with current recommendations and practice at the time of publication. In view of ongoing research, occasional changes in government regulations, and the constant flow of information relating to drug therapy and drug reactions, the reader is urged to check the package insert for each drug for any change in indications and dosage and for added warnings and precautions. This care is particularly important when the recommended agent is a new or infrequently used drug.

04 05 06 07 08 / 9 8 7 6 5 4 3 2 1

To my husband, John, and my sons,
Thomas and Stephen — EWL

To my mother, Frances Swift; my father,
Thomas B. Martin; and my wife, Vickie
A. Martin — VTM

Contributors

Roger K. Cady, MD
Director
Headache Care Center and
    Primary Care Network
Springfield, Missouri

Anne H. Calhoun, MD
Associate Professor of Neurology
University of North Carolina
Chapel Hill, North Carolina;
Director of Women's Medicine
Headache Wellness Center
Greensboro, North Carolina

Kathleen Farmer, PsyD
Headache Care Center & Primary
    Care Network
Springfield, Missouri

Frederick G. Freitag, DO
Assistant Director
Diamond Headache Clinic
Chicago, Illinois;
Affiliate Instructor
Department of Family Medicine
Chicago College of Osteopathic
    Medicine
Downers Grove, Illinois;
Clinical Associate Professor
Department of Family Medicine
Rosalind Franklin Medical
    School
Chicago, Illinois

C. David Gordon, MD
Director
Internal Medicine Services
Michigan Head-Pain &
    Neurological Institute
Ann Arbor, Michigan

Susan Hutchinson, MD
Director
Headache Center
Women's Medical Group
    of Irvine
Irvine, California

Elizabeth W. Loder, MD, FACP
Director
Headache Management Program
Spaulding Rehabilitation Hospital
Assistant Professor of Medicine
Harvard Medical School
Boston, Massachusetts

Morris Maizels, MD
Department of Medicine
Kaiser Permanente
Woodland Hills, California

Vincent T. Martin, MD
Co-Director
Cincinnati Headache Center
Professor of Internal Medicine
University of Cincinnati
Cincinnati, Ohio

Eric M. Pearlman, MD, PhD
Assistant Professor of Pediatrics
Georgia Neurological Institute
Assistant Professor of Pediatrics
Mercer University School of
    Medicine
Savannah Campus
Savannah, Georgia

Curtis P. Schreiber, MD
Director of Medical Programs
Primary Care Network
Springfield, Missouri

Robert Smith, MD
Professor Emeritus and Founding
    Director
Department of Family Medicine
University of Cincinnati
Cincinnati Headache Center
Cincinnati, Ohio

Timothy R. Smith, MD, RPh
Mercy Health Research and Ryan
    Headache Center
St. Louis, Missouri

Glen D. Solomon, MD, FACP
Chairman
Department of Medicine
Advocate Lutheran General
    Hospital
Park Ridge, Illinois;
Associate Professor of Medicine
The Ohio State University
    College of Medicine
Columbus, Ohio

Frederick R. Taylor, MD
Headache Specialist
Park Nicollet Clinic;
Director
Comprehensive Multidisciplinary
    Headache Center
Minneapolis, Minnesota

Timothy Wallace, PhD
Staff Psychologist
Headache and Pain Program
Spaulding Rehabilitation Hospital
Instructor of Psychology
    (Psychiatry)
Harvard Medical School
Boston, Massachusetts

Preface

Headache is among the most common complaints encountered in primary care practice. A seemingly endless list of disorders, some of them serious, can be associated with headache; consequently, the chief concern of most physicians and patients is to assess the likelihood of a dangerous secondary headache. Upon evaluation, though, most patients presenting with the *symptom* of headache will turn out to have one of the primary headache *syndromes*—migraine, tension-type, or cluster headache. These are conditions of long duration that require ongoing management and treatment reassessment. For most patients, this is best provided in the context of primary care.

The latest volume in the ACP Key Diseases series, *Headache* was written to enable physicians, nurse practitioners, and physician assistants to manage the spectrum of headache disorders encountered within primary care. Authors were selected for their primary care backgrounds because we felt they best understood the issues of primary care physicians in the management of headache patients. We recognize that "time is of the essence" for all primary care physicians; therefore we have tried to streamline the diagnosis and treatment of headache disorders when possible.

The organization of this book reflects the step-wise, methodical approach that seasoned primary care practitioners have always applied to evaluation of a clinical complaint. Chapter 1 gives an overview of the headache disorders encountered by primary care physicians. Chapter 2 discusses a general approach to headache diagnosis, and Chapter 3 presents a systematic method to distinguish dangerous secondary causes of headache from the primary headache disorders. Common forms of secondary headache that are particularly likely to be encountered in primary care practice are reviewed in greater detail in later chapters.

Chapter 4 discusses migraine headache and provides an abbreviated approach to its diagnosis and treatment. Detailed, evidence-based recommendations are provided, with reference to treatment guidelines where they exist. The dosages and suggested titration schedules given for these medications should allow for ease of use within primary care.

Tension-type and cluster headaches are discussed in Chapters 5 and 6 respectively. Patients infrequently present with tension-type headaches because they are not particularly disabling. Cluster headaches are differentiated from other primary headache disorders by their strict unilaterality, ipsilateral autonomic symptoms, and severe pain. Treatment algorithms demonstrate straightforward management of these disorders by primary care physicians.

Subjects of particular importance in treating special populations are examined in Chapters 7 to 13. These include headache in children and adolescents, women, and the elderly. Management of the patient with daily or frequent headaches, the clinical situation most commonly identified as challenging by primary care physicians, is reviewed thoroughly. Medication overuse and misuse, and the evidence base for popular complementary and alternative headache treatments, are also examined. Finally, the management of the "difficult" patient is given sensitive consideration.

An important goal of this book is to help the primary care physician gain confidence in identifying and managing patients with primary headache disorders, especially migraine. It is now clear that some of these patients are at risk of developing chronic and difficult-to-treat headaches over time; structural brain changes associated with long-duration migraine have also been identified. Early identification and scrupulous management of a host of other chronic disorders – among them hypertension, diabetes, and asthma – is known to prevent later morbidity in many patients. So, too, it seems with migraine and other chronic headache problems.

When patients present to specialty headache clinics after years of intractable headache and treatment failures, they can only be offered limited help. In contrast, patients who present in primary care with headache that is not yet chronic have potentially treatable disease and the most to gain from timely therapy. The principles of successful headache management are not complex, and an effort to incorporate them into one's practice will be regularly rewarded by improved patient results. We hope this book leaves you excited about the unique opportunity that primary care practitioners have to make a difference in the lives of headache patients.

Elizabeth W. Loder, MD, FACP
Vincent T. Martin, MD

ACKNOWLEDGMENTS—We extend our gratitude to the International Headache Society (IHS), who have kindly given us permission to reprint, in various tables, relevant headache diagnostic criteria. For reader convenience, these tables have been shaded. Appendix I gives the Society's 2004 Diagnostic Classification; again, our thanks to the IHS for allowing its reproduction.

Foreword

reatment of the patient with headache has always been a feature of primary care practice, but in recent years something fresh and important has been happening. Headache in primary care is evolving as a discrete area of practice, with its own educational and research focus. These efforts are being led by a new cadre of primary care headache experts, who are well represented among the contributors to this volume.

Headache treatment in primary care necessarily owes a great deal to the work of specialists and researchers. But scientific interest in headache is a relatively new phenomenon; indeed, headache specialists were few and far between when I first started in practice. Primary care practitioners were on their own, doing the best they could for their many headache patients. Most treatments and medications from years gone by have now been cast aside, but some are well worth remembering. In fact, much of what we take for granted today was first recognized, tested, and tried by primary care physicians.

Well over a century ago, in 1873, Edward Liveing, a generalist physician, as most physicians then were, detailed his observations on 50 patients in the first major treatise on migraine, *On Megrum, Sick-Headache and Some Allied Disorders: A Contribution to the Pathology of Nerve-Storms.* Oliver Sacks, in his introduction to a recent reprint of this classic work (1), writes that Liveing saw migraine as "an array of symptoms, of phenomena hanging together in loose relatively stable constellations, capable of abrupt reorganizations, permutations and transformations."

Liveing elevated the field of headache to a new professional level. His listings of symptoms, patient characteristics, and family features are an object lesson in clinical recording. His caring attitude towards his patients, and his clinical honesty, are best reflected in the words of helplessness he wrote when faced with a patient having an acute migraine attack: "There is scarcely anything to be done; patients so afraid of noise, motion, or anything approaching them, prefer to be left perfectly alone, than to be tormented by useless measures."

And it was mainly so in my early practice days. The only treatments I had available were narcotic analgesics to relieve the pain and barbiturates to help patients relax and sleep. But things were beginning to change. Among a handful of pioneers addressing the problem seriously were Harold Wolff, John Graham, and Arnold Friedman in the United States; Russell Brain and Macdonald Critchley in the United Kingdom; and Federigo Sicuteri in Italy.

In 1945, Harold Wolff had made the first great treatment breakthrough when he demonstrated the vasoconstrictive effect of ergotamine tartrate on the temporal artery, associated with the relief of migraine (2). The impact of this discovery on general practice, however, was at first negligible. Some patients found that the treatment increased their nausea, and isolated reports of peripheral gangrene were discouraging. Soon after entering practice, however, I began using Cafergot cautiously. This combination of ergotamine tartrate and caffeine worked well in spite of its limitations, and this was exciting. There was now something specific physicians could do for headache patients. I wanted to learn more.

There was, unfortunately, no systematized approach to headache diagnosis at that time. This had to wait some years, for Arnold Friedman and an *ad hoc* committee appointed by the National Institutes of Health, who published the first comprehensive headache classification in the *Journal of the American Medical Association* in 1962 (3).

Studying in England gave me the opportunity to attend the occasional headache lectures given by Russell Brain or Macdonald Critchley, the leading neurologists in that country. These were superbly delivered, filled with finer neurological points, but unfortunately of little value to a busy practitioner now seeing an increasing number of headache patients. Eventually I found help nearer at hand.

A practitioner colleague, Denis Craddock, a pioneer in primary care education and editor of *An Introduction to General Practice,* devoted an entire chapter in that work to headache, one which today presents a picture of what good primary headache practice was like in the early 1950s (4). It also provides a baseline to measure the enormous advances made since then. And, as with Liveing's treatise 80 years earlier, there remain nuggets of sound headache practice in Craddock's work.

Craddock emphasized the importance of taking a careful headache history. He realized that stress could be an important factor. Patients should be allowed time to express their feelings; this could be therapeutic and provide valuable counseling opportunities. Migraine is the commonest disabling headache occurring in general practice, where it may present without classic features. Late-onset migraine should raise the fear of serious underlying disease. Craddock decried useless tests such as sinus X-rays. All of this he claimed he had learnt *after* leaving medical school by carefully observing his patients.

Some of Craddock's views are clearly erroneous. He attributed milder headaches to constipation, eyestrain, tight hats, and stuffy atmosphere. Reflecting the gender bias of those days, no reference was made to the higher prevalence of migraine in women and throughout the chapter the patient is always referred to as male.

Scientific studies in general practice began with work on infectious diseases by William Pickles, a Yorkshire general practitioner and first president of the College of General Practitioners. His meticulous epidemiological observations showed how much valuable information could be gained from studying the diseases encountered in routine practice (5). For Pickles, every practice was a potential research laboratory.

At the same time, Michael Balint, a Hungarian psychoanalyst and bio-chemist then living in England, recognized the crucial role the family doctor played in the National Health System (6). He stressed the importance of the doctor-patient relationship and how the attitude of the physician can deter-mine what help the patient receives. How significant this was in the care of headache patients! Pickles and Balint together had helped to create the new discipline of academic general practice.

Encouraged by their work, I started a general practice teaching and re-search unit at Guy's Hospital Medical School at the University of London. Because of my interest in headache, a patient support group, the British Migraine Association, sought my help. Its members complained that the medical profession largely ignored their problem. In 1964, I helped them or-ganize the first migraine meeting for general practitioners, with Macdonald Critchley as the main speaker.

Encouraged by the interest these events occasioned, the Migraine Trust was established to raise funds for headache education and research. The first Migraine Trust symposium was held in 1966 in London at the National Hospital, Queen Square, leading to a series which continues to this day. As secretary of the Trust, I had the honor of coordinating the first two sym-posia and to edit their proceedings (7,8). Under Critchley's leadership, the search for the underlying mechanisms of headache had begun in earnest.

In 1968 I accepted an invitation to start a department of family medi-cine at the University of North Carolina at Chapel Hill. During this period of personal change and professional adjustment, I continued to see headache patients. I was learning a great deal, patient by patient. As time progressed, the number of these patients increased, my local colleagues being only too eager to pass on their "headache problems". Patient education and headache diaries became essential tools. I began seeing headache patients separately from other patients. I was evolving into a primary care headache specialist, realizing that headache is quintessentially a primary care problem (9).

It was also a time of accelerating growth in headache research. Mike Moskowitz was unraveling the mysteries of the trigemino-vascular system (10); Pat Humphrey discovered the first triptan (11); and Jes Olesen and his colleagues produced in 1988 the first International Headache Society (IHS) classification, now the standard diagnostic criteria and of particular impor-tance in headache research and clinical trials (12). The second edition of the criteria, published 16 years later, added many new headache subtypes (13).

There can be no doubt that the IHS criteria are invaluable to re-searchers and scientists. Yet a headache diagnostic classification *designed for use in primary care* remains an urgent need. Under-diagnosis and inad-equate treatment of migraine, especially, are major problems.

Important steps are being taken, however, to raise headache practice standards in primary care. Roger Cady in the United States has developed a nation-wide educational network (13) that reaches many thousands of prac-titioners. Andrew Dowson in the United Kingdom leads a new international primary care educational organization, Headache Care for Practicing Physicians. Its journal focuses on the needs of primary care practitioners and is a welcome addition to the present array of excellent specialist journals.

Primary care is the only setting in which millions of patients receive headache treatment, and this is likely to remain so. Dowson summed up the problem: "How may we transfer the major advances in headache research and management that have occurred over the past 15 years into the primary care arena?" (14).

The present volume makes a major contribution towards answering this question. Loder and Martin's *Headache* takes its place on my bookshelf alongside the seminal works of Liveing and Craddock. Together they represent some of the milestones marking the long journey made by primary care physicians in their increasingly successful efforts to diagnosis and treat the various types of headache.

Robert Smith, MD

REFERENCES

1. **Sacks O.** Introduction to On Megrum by Edward Liveing. Nijmegen: Arts & Boeve; 1997 [reprint of 1873 edition].
2. **Wolff HG.** Headache and Other Head Pain. New York: Oxford University Press; 1948.
3. **National Institutes of Health.** Ad Hoc Committee on Classification of Headache (Arnold Friedman, chairman). JAMA. 1962;179:718-9.
4. **Craddock D.** The patient with a headache. In: Craddock D, ed. An Introduction to General Practice. London: Lewis; 1953.
5. **Pemberton J.** Will Pickles of Wensleydale. Royal College of General Practitioners. London; 1984 [reprint].
6. **Balint M.** The Doctor, His Patient and Illness. London: Churchill Livingstone; 1964.
7. **Smith R.** Background to migraine. In: Proceedings of First Migraine Symposium. London: Heinemann; 1967.
8. **Smith R.** Background to migraine. In: Proceedings of Second Migraine Symposium. London: Heinemann; 1969.
9. **Smith R.** The evolution of headache management in primary care. Headache Care. 2004;1:3-6.
10. **Moskowitz MA.** The trigemino-vascular system and pain mechanisms: pain research and clinical management. Proceedings of Fifth World Congress on Pain, vol 3; 1988.
11. **Humphrey PP, Feniuk W, Marriott AS, et al.** Preclinical studies on the anti-migraine drug, sumatriptan. Eur Neurol. 1991;31:282-90.
12. **International Headache Society.** Classification and diagnostic criteria for headache disorders, cranial neuralgias and facial pain. Cephalalgia. 1988;8(Suppl 7):1-96.
13. **International Headache Society.** The International Classification of Headache Disorders, 2nd ed. Cephalalgia. 2004;24(Suppl 1):9-160.
14. **Dowson AJ, Tepper SJ, Cady RK.** New initiatives for the management of headache in primary care. Headache Care. 2004;1:7-13.

Contents

1

Headache in the Primary Care Setting

Elizabeth W. Loder, MD

eadache is a principal complaint in 2% of primary care appointments and 2.6% of emergency department visits (1). Its ubiquity and variety make it a particularly difficult symptom to sort out. Because mild, physiologically unimportant headache is a normal part of life, experienced on occasion by essentially everyone, some complaints of headache may have no medical implications and require little or no treatment. However, headache can also be an important symptom of other medical disorders; a seemingly endless, sometimes confusing, and occasionally dangerous array of illnesses can involve or present with headache. Finally, the primary headache syndromes, especially migraine, are increasingly recognized as illnesses in their own right, with new evidence suggesting that a subset of patients have progressive disease. These patients benefit from early detection and management to forestall the development of chronic, treatment-refractory headache.

All of these forms of headache—from the benign and medically unimportant to the disabling or dangerous—are most often reported to, and managed by, a primary care physician (PCP). This suggests that familiarity with the epidemiology of headache, along with a clearly formulated strategy for headache evaluation and management, will be of value to all clinicians. This chapter aims to put the primary headache disorders in context among other problems seen and managed in that setting. It reviews the prevalence and distribution of common causes and forms of headache, the medical, social, and economic burden they pose for sufferers, and barriers to serious-headache recognition and management. The chapter closes with an overview of "best practices" in the management of primary headache disorders in primary care.

Epidemiology of Headache

Accurate perceptions about the prevalence of various causes of headache are important. The frequency with which various causes of headache occur depends to some extent on the population in question. Secondary causes of headache, such as central nervous system infections or tumors, will be relatively common in a population of patients with human immunodeficiency virus, for example, and relatively rare in a college health service. Nonetheless, in almost all medical settings, both physicians and the general public greatly overestimate the likelihood that a chief complaint of headache is due to a serious underlying medical problem. The vast majority of headaches are not secondary to underlying illness but are in fact one of a trio of primary headache disorders. These "Big Three" are tension-type headache, migraine, and cluster headache, with migraine being by far the most common headache seen in a primary care setting. A diary study of 377 patients with a chief complaint of headache in a primary care setting showed that 94% had a diagnosis of either migraine (76%) or migrainous headache (headache missing only one diagnostic feature of migraine) (18%). Few patients consulted for tension-type headache (2).

The following review of the epidemiology of primary headache disorders helps put them in proper perspective among other causes of headache.

Tension-Type Headache

The most common headache disorder in the general population is episodic tension-type headache, which affects 40% of the population at some time over the course of a year. These are the bilateral, pressing or squeezing headaches of everyday life that do not have many accompanying features. Because tension-type headache is so prevalent, however, the aggregate social impact is high. Chronic forms of the disorder are very disabling on an individual level but have little social impact because they are relatively uncommon (3). Physicians may understandably, but incorrectly, assume that because tension-type headache is the most common type of headache in the general population, it is also the most common type seen in a medical setting. In fact, tension-type headache is relatively *uncommon* in medical settings. This seeming paradox actually reflects the fact that tension-type headache, because it is usually mild, infrequent, and causes little disability, rarely prompts medical consultation.

Over-diagnosis of tension-type headache is common. This is supported by a large study that prospectively assessed the prevalence and diagnosis of headaches defined according to International Headache Society criteria among 1203 patients consulting their PCP with a complaint of headache. The initial diagnosis was recorded, and patients with a new diagnosis of migraine (n = 272) or a nonmigraine diagnosis (n = 105) completed detailed headache diaries over a period of 6 months. These diaries were examined by a panel of experts, blinded to the initial PCP diagnosis, who then categorized patients as having migraine without aura, migraine with aura, migrainous headache, episodic tension-type headache, or "headache not classifiable". Upon expert review, an initial PCP diagnosis of migraine was confirmed in 98% of patients, but an initial PCP diagnosis of nonmigraine headache turned out to be incorrect in 79% of cases, almost entirely because those patients turned out to have migraine rather than tension-type headache (2). These data suggest that clinicians should think carefully before making a diagnosis of tension-type headache.

Migraine

Migraine is also a common primary headache disorder, with a 1-year prevalence of 18% in women and 6% in men. Migraine is a chronic, frequently incapacitating neurovascular disorder, often of very long duration, characterized by attacks of severe headache, autonomic nervous system dysfunction, and in some patients an aura involving neurologic symptoms (4). The World Health Organization places migraine among the top 20 causes of disability worldwide and considers a day with migraine to be as disabling as a day of schizophrenia or paraplegia.

Although not as common as tension-type headache in the general population, migraine is the most common headache disorder encountered in most medical settings. Medical providers may not realize that migraine is more prevalent than other conditions commonly encountered in primary care, such as rheumatoid arthritis (affecting 2.1 million people in the United States), asthma (14.6 million, with a lifetime prevalence of 10.5%), diabetes (17 million, or 6.2% of the population), and osteoarthritis (20.7 million) (5-7). Because migraine prevalence peaks between the ages of 25 and 55, typically a period of life with significant occupational and family responsibility, the burden of migraine is amplified.

Data from a recently completed study illustrate the extent of the problem. The American Migraine Study II was conducted in 1999 with the object of describing the prevalence, sociodemographic profile, and burden of migraine in the United States, and of comparing these results with the first AMS study done in 1989. A validated, self-administered questionnaire was sent to 20,000 households to identify migraine sufferers 12 years of age or older, based on modified International Headache Society criteria for the disorder. Of 43,527 age-eligible individuals, 29,727 responded to the questionnaire, for a 68.3% response rate. Twenty-three percent, or nearly one in every four, of respondent households contained at least one person with migraine. The overall 1-year prevalence of migraine in this study was 13% (18.2% in females and 6.5% in males). When extrapolated to the population as a whole, these figures suggest there are 28 million migraine sufferers age 12 or over in the United States: 21 million females and 7 million males (4).

In both males and females, the prevalence distribution of migraine is an inverted U-shaped curve. Prevalence rises through early adult life and then falls after midlife. At all ages beyond puberty, migraine is substantially more common in women than in men.

Before puberty, migraine is somewhat more common in boys than in girls. The incidence (new cases) of migraine without aura peaks around age 12 in boys and age 15 in girls. Although half of all migraine onsets begin before the age of 20, migraine can begin at any age (8,9).

The Burden of Migraine
It is useful to distinguish between the individual burden of migraine and the burden it imposes on society. The burden to an individual with the disorder is caused by symptoms during attacks, by anticipation of symptoms between attacks, by the reductions in quality of life that can be demonstrated in people with migraine when compared with the general population, and in lost work time. Frequent attacks of migraine have been demonstrated to reduce family, social, and recreational activities. Societal burden is usually studied and described in economic terms, with a distinction between direct costs and indirect costs. Direct costs are those associated with medical care for migraine, while indirect costs are measured by lost work time, decreased work productivity, and reduced function in other domains. For work statistics, it is useful to distinguish absenteeism from reduced effectiveness.

Indirect costs for migraine are higher than direct costs. Individuals with migraine require on average 3.8 days of bed rest for men and 5.6 days of bed rest for women per year. When these figures are extrapolated to the entire American population, estimates are that migraine is responsible for about 112 million bedridden days per year. Missed work and reduced effectiveness at work are estimated to cost employers about $13 billion per year. By way of comparison, the annual productivity loss due to non-insulin-dependent diabetes mellitus (NIDDM) has been estimated at $2.6 million (10). Patients between the ages of 30 and 49 incur greater indirect costs than younger and older workers, reinforcing the disproportionate impact of this disease on people during their most economically and personally productive years. During this time, the prevalence of migraine in women is threefold higher than in men. This difference decreases later in life but does not disappear; prevalence remains substantially higher in women even at age 70.

Direct costs for migraine, however, are also substantial. One study determined that, excluding the cost of diagnostic tests and medications, the average patient used about $817 in health care resources annually to treat migraine. Patients for the study were selected from participants in a clinical trial evaluating the efficacy of a migraine medication. Of 929 patients, over two thirds (648) responded to a survey request for information about their use of health care services during the previous 12 months. Table 1-1 highlights some of the personal and economic costs of migraine.

It is particularly important to recognize that the suffering, lost economic opportunities, and medical costs of migraine are not evenly shared between sufferers. In fact, a relatively small number of sufferers who miss the equivalent of 6 or more days of work per year account for the bulk of the lost work time attributable to migraine. Fifty-one percent of women miss the equivalent of 6 or more days of work per year due to migraine, but they account for 93% of all work lost due to migraine. Similarly, 38% of men with migraine lose that same amount of time (6 days/year), but they account for 85% of total work loss because of migraine. This "compression of disability" suggests that at least some highly disabled migraine sufferers are good targets for intervention (11-13).

Under-Diagnosis of Migraine

In 1989, only 39% of people with migraine (as identified by questionnaire) reported having received a diagnosis of migraine from a medical practitioner. Ten years later, the proportion of medically diagnosed migraine sufferers had increased to 48%. Unfortunately, however, the majority of migraine sufferers remain undiagnosed. One explanation for this may be that patients receive other, incorrect, headache diagnoses. In AMS II, 32% of undiagnosed migraineurs, according to their report, received a physician diagnosis of tension headache, whereas 42% of undiagnosed migraine sufferers reported a diagnosis of "sinus headache". Other factors also appeared to contribute to the chance that migraine would not be recognized: low income, youth, and male sex were associated with a decreased probability of reporting a physician diagnosis of migraine.

Table 1-1   Migraine by the Numbers

One-year general population prevalence of migraine	
Males	6%
Females	18%
Combined	13%
Days of bed rest per year per individual due to migraine	
Males	3.8
Females	5.6
Cost of lost work time and decreased productivity attributable to migraine	$13 billion/year
Annual costs for emergency department visits for migraine	$646 million – $1.94 billion*

*Source: Barron R, Carlsen J, Duff SB, Burk C. Estimating the cost of an emergency room visit for migraine headache. Journal of Drug Assessment. 2001;4(3). Accessed online at PJB Publications Web site on 27 April 2004.

Failure to seek medical consultation for headache is another factor contributing to under-diagnosis. In 1989 and 1999, this group of "never consulters" accounted for about one third of undiagnosed migraine sufferers. The percentage of "lapsed consulters" (i.e., those who have previously seen a doctor for headache but not within the past year) decreased from 50% to 21% of all migraine sufferers. The percentage of "current consulters" (i.e., those who have seen a doctor for headache in the last year) tripled from 1989 to 1999, to almost 47%. This increase, while encouraging, should not obscure the fact that over half of migraine sufferers are not seeking care, and that many people with migraine who do consult a doctor do not receive a specific diagnosis or therapy (2,14).

Many people who suffer with severe headache continue to receive care on an episodic basis in emergency departments. In 1999, there were 102.7 million emergency department visits. Of these, 2.8 million were for headache, representing nearly 3% of total visits for the period (3). Despite the availability of cost-effective migraine-specific agents like DHE and the triptans, most headache sufferers diagnosed with migraine in the emergency department received IV opioids and an antiemetic as their only treatment (4).

Cluster Headache

Cluster headache is a highly distinct and recognizable, but rare, cause of benign recurrent headache. It is a short, strictly unilateral headache with pronounced autonomic accompaniments. Because of its rarity, cluster headache is under-recognized; symptoms are often misattributed to migraine or dental or sinus problems. The prevalence of cluster headache is difficult to determine because it is so rare. Of the handful of epidemiologic studies that exist, prevalence estimates range from 0.03 to 0.092%. Peak incidence occurs in men between the ages of 40 and 49, with a male to female ratio of 4-5:1. This disorder is associated with smoking and alcohol exposure, although causality has not been demonstrated (15,16).

Frequent Headache

Headaches occurring 15 or more days per month affect 5% of women and 2.8% of men. The two most common headache disorders that occur with this frequency are chronic tension-type headache and transformed or chronic migraine, which will be discussed together as "chronic daily headache" (17). It is this group of patients who are most disabled by headache and who incur and create much of the cost of headache care. Targeting these patients for intensive treatment, in the form of "disease management" or other integrated care strategies, is likely to prove highly effective in reducing these problems, because even modest reductions in the frequency of disabling headaches will translate into fewer emergency department visits and decreased absence from work and social roles (18).

A Primary Care Perspective

Because the primary headache disorders are such common conditions, what is the appropriate perspective on their management in primary care? To begin with, it is important to recognize that most patients with primary headache do seek care in this setting. Of the migraine sufferers who consult a doctor, about two thirds consult primary care physicians, a group which includes general practitioners, family practitioners, internists, and pediatricians; only 16% consulted neurologists or headache specialists (18). In the primary care setting, the approach to diagnosis and headache classification has traditionally centered on distinguishing between primary and secondary headaches. Ongoing management of primary headache disorders such as migraine may or may not be viewed as a role appropriate for the primary care clinician. However, migraine is increasingly viewed as a chronic illness, because sufferers experience high rates of symptom recurrence and sustained functional impairment (19).

Evidence is mounting that in some patients migraine can be a progressive disorder (20). Recent imaging studies demonstrate that migraine sufferers have elevated risks compared with controls for subclinical infarctions, especially in the region of the posterior circulation, an area implicated in other studies of stroke in migraineurs (21). These findings, and those of diffuse white matter lesions on MR scanning, correlated with migraine frequency. It has been suggested that these lesions reflect "cumulative brain insults due to repeated migraine attacks" (22). Another study has shown increased levels of iron deposition in areas of the brainstem (e.g., the periaqueductal gray matter) that are important in modulating pain. In this study, too, findings correlated with attack frequency (23).

Conclusion

The primary headache disorders are common in patients seen in the primary care setting. Headaches are a common cause of disability, and severely symptomatic patients have multiple attacks of headache per year. From a public health perspective, therefore, improved detection and treatment of headaches in this setting could have major impact.

One of the biggest challenges in contemporary health care is how to shift from episode-driven treatment of illness toward more comprehensive, preventive treatment. The management of primary headache disorders— migraine, in particular—has undergone a revolution in the past decade, reflecting a growing assortment of treatments and a shift in treatment strategies from nonspecific, symptomatic medications to those that target underlying neural mechanisms in the hope of decreasing the likelihood of future attacks. Prompt disease control is increasingly a goal of treatment, one which will necessarily involve primary care providers in the detection and ongoing management of illness.

Referral for consultation should occur in situations where the physician is uncertain of the diagnosis, the headache does not respond to treatment, or medical or psychiatric comorbidity limits treatment.

Key Points

- All forms of headache, from benign to disabling or dangerous, are most often managed by a primary care physician.
- Both physicians and patients greatly overestimate the likelihood that headache is due to a serious disorder.
- Migraine is more prevalent than many other conditions commonly seen in primary care settings (e.g., rheumatoid arthritis, asthma, diabetes, osteoarthritis).
- Tension-type headaches, although the most common headache disorder in the general population, are *uncommon* in medical settings. Tension-type headache is over-diagnosed.
- Migraine is the most common headache disorder seen in medical settings but remains under-diagnosed.

REFERENCES

1. 2001 National Hospital Ambulatory Medical Care Survey.
2. **Tepper SJ, Dahlof C, Dawson A, Newman L.** Prevalence and diagnosis of migraine in patients consulting their primary care physician with a complaint of headache: data from the Landmark Study. Headache. In press.
3. **Schwartz B, Stewart WF, Simon D, Lipton RB.** Epidemiology of tension-type headache. JAMA. 1998;279:381-3.
4. **Lipton RB, Stewart WF, Diamond S, et al.** Prevalence and burden of migraine in the United States: data from the American Migraine Study II. Headache. 2001;41:646-57.
5. www.cdc.gov/nedss/.
6. www.arthritis.org.
7. www.census.gov.
8. **Lipton RB, Stewart WF.** Migraine in the United States: a review of epidemiology and health care use. Neurology. 1993;43(suppl 3):S6-10.

9. **Stewart WF, Linet MS, Celantano DD, et al.** Age- and sex-specific incidence rates of migraine with and without visual aura. Am J Epidemiol. 1991;134:1111-20.

10. **Huse DM, Oster G, Killen AR, et al.** The economic costs of non-insulin-dependent diabetes mellitus. JAMA. 1989;262:2708-13.

11. **Silberstein SD, Lipton RB.** Epidemiology of migraine. Neuroepidemiology. 1993;12:179-94.

12. **Hu HX, Markson LE, Lipton RB, et al.** Burden of migraine in the United States: disability and economic costs. Arch Intern Med. 1999;159:813-8.

13. **Stewart WF, Lipton RB, Simon D.** Work-related disability: results from the American Migraine Study. Cephalalgia. 1996;16:231-8.

14. **Lipton RB, Diamond S, Reed M, et al.** Migraine diagnosis and treatment: results from the American Migraine Study II. Headache. 2001;41:638-45.

15. **Ekbom K, Ahlborg B, Schele R.** Prevalence of migraine and cluster headache in Swedish men of 18. Headache. 1978;18:9-12.

16. **Finkel AG.** Epidemiology of cluster headache. Curr Pain Headache Rep. 2003;7: 144-9.

17. **Scher AI, Stewart WF, Liberman J, Lipton RB.** Prevalence of frequent headache in a population sample. Headache. 1998;38:497-506.

18. **Lipton RB, Stewart WF, Simon D.** Medical consultation for migraine: results from the American Migraine Study. Headache. 1998;38:87-96.

19. **Loder E, Biondi D.** Disease modification in migraine: a concept that has come of age? Headache. 2003;43:135-43.

20. **Scher AI, Stewart WF, Ricci JA, Lipton RB.** Factors associated with the onset and remission of chronic daily headache in a population-based study. Pain. 2003;106: 81-9.

21. **Kruit MC, van Buchem MA, Hofman PAM, et al.** Migraine as a risk factor for subclinical brain lesions. JAMA. 2004;291:427-34.

22. **Lipton RB.** Is migraine a progressive brain disease? JAMA. 2004;291:493-4.

23. **Welch KMA, Nagesh V, Aurora SK, Gelman N.** Periaqueductal gray matter dysfunction in migraine: cause or the burden of illness? Headache. 2001;41:629-37.

2

What Kind of Headache is It?

Morris Maizels, MD

Elizabeth W. Loder, MD

t is possible to distinguish serious from benign headaches, and to accurately classify most primary headache disorders, within the limited time available for most primary care visits. A systematic approach to headache diagnosis consists of efficient history-taking and physical examination, determination of whether the headache is benign or worrisome, and recognition of the five benign headache patterns commonly seen in primary care.

Diagnosis

Headache diagnosis is clinical; no "gold standard" tests or biological markers exist. The International Headache Society (IHS) first published a complete classification of headache disorders in 1988. Its revised, 2004 criteria are given in Appendix I. These criteria describe the classic presentation of each headache type and enable researchers to study homogeneous populations of headache sufferers.

Two features of the new classification system are important: 1) the older terms "classic" and "common" migraine have been replaced by the descriptive terms "migraine with aura" and "migraine without aura", and 2) the term "tension-type headache" replaces older terms such as "tension headache" or "muscle contraction headache". This is because neither muscle tension nor psychological tension is reliably associated with these moderate, nondescript headaches.

Separating Benign from Serious Headache

Secondary headaches are the result of another illness, such as infection or tumor. Benign, or *primary,* headache disorders are those in which the headache condition, by itself, is the problem and not attributable to some other illness. Secondary headaches are much less common than primary headaches. However, because of the potential seriousness of these underlying disorders, secondary causes need to be considered before the more common diagnoses are explored.

A mnemonic that is useful in recalling some (though not all) of the features predictive of dangerous headaches is **SNOOP** (1):

S ystemic symptoms (fever, weight loss) or systemic cancer/HIV
N eurological symptoms or signs (confusion, altered consciousness)
O nset sudden, abrupt, or split-second
O lder patient with new onset or progressive headache
P revious headache history not reassuring (first, worst, or different headache)

Other headache patterns and features that increase the possibility of a serious secondary headache are listed in Table 2-1.

What About Brain Tumors?

Brain tumor and aneurysm are uncommon but catastrophic causes of headache that both doctors and patients fear missing. Isolated headache without other neurological signs or symptoms is an unusual presentation of brain tumor, however, in one series occurring in only 8% of patients (2). Vasquez-Barquero and co-authors concluded that "isolated headache for longer than 10 weeks will only exceptionally be secondary to an intracranial neoplasm".

The "classic" profile of a brain tumor headache (i.e., severe, worse in the morning, associated with nausea or vomiting) was found in only in 17% of patients. The most typical pattern was headache with tension-type features (77%). Migraine-like headaches occurred in 9% of patients. Headaches were worse when bending forward in 32% of patients, and nausea or vomiting occurred with headache in 40%. Of the 32% of patients with previous history of headache, 78% had headache with their tumor, a headache always more severe or frequent and associated with other symptoms (e.g., seizure, confusion, prolonged nausea, hemiparesis) or abnormal signs. Vasquez-Barquero and co-authors concluded that nausea, vomiting, abnormal neurological examination, or significant changes in previous headache pattern suggest the possibility of an underlying tumor.

The temporal pattern of headache can also suggest diagnostic possibilities (Table 2-2).

Recognizing Common Headache Patterns

Although red flags indicating secondary causes need to be watched for, most patients (>90%) with headaches troublesome enough to seek medical

Table 2-1   Headache Patterns and Features That Increase the Possibility of a Serious Secondary Headache

Headache Pattern or Feature Characteristic of a Serious Disorder	Comment
• First, worst, or different headache	• Careful follow-up necessary to document benign evolution
• Sudden onset and peak intensity within seconds ("thunderclap" headache) or "worst headache ever"	• Consider evaluation for subarachnoid hemorrhage (plain CT with LP if negative)
• Progressive, unresponsive to treatment attempts	• Patient may have treatment-resistant form of primary headache, but secondary headache must be considered
• Abnormal neurological signs or symptoms, including altered personality or cognition	• Suggestive of central nervous system lesion or other secondary headache
• Unexplained fever and/or neck stiffness	• Suggestive of infectious cause
• Recent onset in patient with cancer, HIV, anticoagulation, or >50 y/o	• Secondary cause of headache more likely
• Onset during pregnancy	• Headache can be initial sign of preeclampsia, occurring before proteinuria and hypertension develop; cerebral venous thrombosis is another possibility

Table 2-2   Headache Pattern and Diagnostic Possibilities

Acute Single Headache

- First attack of migraine
- Subarachnoid hemorrhage
- Meningitis/encephalitis
- Systemic infection
- Optic neuritis
- Glaucoma
- Post-traumatic headache
- Pressor reaction

Acute Recurrent Headache

- Migraine
- Cerebrovascular insufficiency
- Intermittent hydrocephalus
- Cerebral tumor
- Pseudotumor cerebri
- Subarachnoid hemorrhage
- Cluster headache
- Trigeminal neuralgia
- Pheochromocytoma

Subacute Headache (days to weeks)

- Subdural hematoma
- Tumor
- Brain abscess
- Pseudotumor cerebri
- Temporal arteritis

Chronic Daily Headache (months to years)

- Tumor
- Pseudotumor cerebri
- Chronic tension-type headache
- Transformed migraine

Adapted from Silberstein SD, Lipton RB, Goadsby PJ. Headache in Clinical Practice, 2nd ed. London: Martin Dunitz; 2002.

evaluation have a primary headache disorder. The "Big Three" primary headache disorders are migraine, tension-type, and cluster headache.

- Migraine is the most common headache problem that causes patients to seek medical help. *Unless you have an unusual practice, most of the patients you see complaining of headache have some form of migraine.*

- Tension-type headache is the most common headache disorder, but it is usually mild and self-limited. Tension-type headache rarely prompts medical consultation.

- Cluster headache, the most severe of the three conditions, is uncommon.

Just as we correctly recognize that for a 68-year-old man complaining of chest pain the most likely diagnosis is coronary artery disease and not Tietze's syndrome, so it is important to recognize the likelihood of various headache diagnoses. In a 32-year-old woman complaining of recurrent, disabling headaches the most likely diagnosis is migraine, not tension-type headache or brain tumor.

Taking a Headache History

Most of the information needed to develop a headache diagnosis comes from the history; physical examination and laboratory tests are principally useful to exclude specific, dangerous causes of headache.

Practice Management Tips

Effective headache management requires time. The amount of time the physician spends with the patient, especially at the initial visit, is more highly correlated with patient outcome than any other variable. There are several practical ways to be as thorough as possible while remaining efficient.

- *Scheduling*—Some patients who have suffered significant disability from headache have a strong desire to "tell" their story. If necessary, suggest that a separate visit be set up and devoted solely to discussion of the headache problem. While awaiting that visit, the patient can be asked to keep a detailed record of the headaches using, for example, one of the diaries in Appendix III. Most patients respond positively to the suggestion that the headache problem is important enough to warrant thorough evaluation and appreciate the suggestion that the detailed information written in the headache diary will be useful in developing a treatment plan.

- *Telephone Calls*—Important issues such as medication changes and treatment discussions should be handled in face-to-face office visits, not over the telephone. Review your telephone policy with patients at the first visit. Office visits are used to develop a treatment plan or strategy for both acute and chronic headache problems; if this is not working, a return office visit is the appropriate next step.

  • *Billing*—If more than 50% of a visit is devoted to counseling, reimbursement will be based on time. Document the total visit time, the fact that more than 50% was devoted to counseling, and provide details about the nature of the counseling (e.g., "trigger, lifestyle factors and treatment options for headache").

The patient interview should elicit basic information about

- Headache location
- Headache duration
- Quality of the pain
- Severity of the pain
- Frequency of headaches
- Associated features (nausea and/or vomiting, light or noise sensitivity)
- Aura, neurological symptoms, aggravation with Valsalva
- Headache triggers (aggravating and precipitating factors), relievers, patterns (hormonal, diurnal)
- Relevant medical and family history
- Medication history

Questions and techniques used by headache experts to efficiently and accurately elicit information about important headache features are given below. Questions that do not suggest a correct answer are best: "Do you have any other symptoms with your headaches?" provides more reliable information than the leading question "Do you have nausea or vomiting with your headaches?"

Questions

"Tell me about your headaches."

  A. Observe verbal and non-verbal communication (clues to axis I and II psychiatric diagnoses).
  B. Attend to your own feelings about the patient (clues to axis I and II diagnoses).

"Do you have more than one headache type?"

Obtain history of each headache type of concern to patient.

"What do you think is causing your headaches?"

Listening without interruption and asking open-ended questions will reveal ideas regarding headache causation and other concerns and priorities, and may provide clues to the presence of psychiatric problems such as personality disorders, anxiety, somatization, and even delusions.

"What were your headaches like when they first began?"

This is the single best question to ask patients with confusing or chronic headaches. Often the patient will describe an early pattern of intermittent, severe headaches (usually migraine) that eventually became chronic. If headache has changed over time, determine whether the change was sudden or gradual and if it was associated with physical or emotional trauma or life changes.

"What do your headaches keep you from doing?"

Frequent absence from work or school because of headache usually indicates severe disability. These obligations are often the last part of the patient's life to be affected; family or social activities may be sacrificed first.

"How do you know it's a [headache 1] headache and not a [headache 2] headache?"

Physicians sometimes feel frustrated by patients who report multiple types of headache. Often, each headache is given a label: "my 'migraine', my 'tension' headache, my 'sinus' headache". Although these "different" kinds of headache are usually variable presentations of a single disorder (usually migraine), it helps to hear the description of each.

Techniques

Observe discrepancies between history and behavior.

A carefully groomed, smiling patient who reports having a "10/10" headache during the interview may be using the physical complaint of headache to express emotional pain. Such an observation has important diagnostic and treatment implications.

Screen for co-morbidities

A. Psychiatric
1. Depressive disorders
2. Anxiety disorders
3. Chemical dependency
4. Personality disorders
5. History of abuse or trauma

B. Other pain conditions
1. Fibromyalgia
2. Chronic
3. Other chronic pain

Five Common Headache Patterns

As previously mentioned, headache diagnosis has been systematized by the International Headache Society. Unfortunately, the IHS criteria were developed for research purposes and perform less well in the clinical setting. Primary care clinicians will find a focus on pattern recognition, not memorization of the individual criteria, most useful in identifying individual headache syndromes that require treatment.

The major characteristics of five common headache patterns (migraine, tension-type headache, cluster headache, other primary headache syndromes, chronic daily headache) are listed below, followed by a more thorough description of each.

Migraine

Key characteristics

- Throbbing, unilateral or bilateral
- Nausea, vomiting, and sensitivity to light or noise are common
- Only 20% of migraine patients have aura
- Episodic disabling headaches but often with a spectrum of milder headaches that are also migraine
- Often misdiagnosed as tension headache or sinus or neck problem
- Complicated forms of migraine exist but are rare

The IHS criteria for migraine with and without aura are listed in Tables 2-3 and 2-4. A useful mnemonic for the diagnosis of migraine, based on the IHS criteria, is **SULTANS:**

S evere
U ni -
L ateral
T hrobbing
A ctivity worsens headache
N ausea
S ensitivity to light and sound

The pain of migraine is often unilateral, over the temple, but may also be bilateral and involve any area of the head, including the occiput or neck, face, and cheek. Unilateral head pain that varies sides is *strongly suggestive* of migraine. Patients often characterize the headache as both throbbing and pressure-like, or starting with one and evolving into the other (see Table 2-3). Migraine is often accompanied by nausea, vomiting, or profound sensitivity to sensory stimuli such as light, sound, and smell. It is generally made worse by routine physical activity such as climbing stairs or bending over. Complaints of poor concentration or memory difficulties are common.

Migraine most commonly begins early in life; onset after age 40 is not common. Eighty percent of patients seeking migraine treatment are women. Twenty-four million Americans have migraine, and most of these sufferers experience some degree of disability. In its pure form, migraine is an

---

Table 2-3   International Headache Society Diagnostic Criteria for Migraine without Aura

A. At least 5 attacks fulfilling criteria B-D
B. Headache attacks lasting 4-72 hours (untreated or unsuccessfully treated)
C. Headache has at least 2 of the following characteristics:
   1. Unilateral location
   2. Pulsating quality
   3. Moderate or severe pain intensity
   4. Aggravation by, or causing avoidance of, routine physical activity (e.g., walking or climbing stairs)
D. During headache at least one of the following:
   1. Nausea and/or vomiting
   2. Photophobia and phonophobia
E. Not attributed to another disorder

From International Headache Society. The International Classification of Headache Disorders, 2nd ed. Cephalalgia. 2004;24(Suppl 1):9-160; with permission.

Table 2-4   International Headache Society Diagnostic Criteria for Migraine with Aura*

A. At least 2 attacks fulfilling criteria B-D
B. Aura must be fully reversible and consist of at least one of the following symptoms:
   1. Visual
   2. Sensory
   3. Dysphasic speech
C. At least 2 of the following:
   1. Homonymous visual symptoms and/or unilateral sensory symptoms
   2. Aura symptoms develop gradually over >5 minutes and/or different aura symptoms occur in succession over 5 minutes
   3. Each aura symptom lasts >5 minutes and <24 hours
D. Headache begins during the aura or follows the onset of aura within 60 minutes
E. Not attributed to another disorder

From International Headache Society. The International Classification of Headache Disorders, 2nd ed. Cephalalgia. 2004;24(Suppl 1):9-160; with permission.
*These criteria are termed "typical aura with migraine headache" under new (2004) IHS diagnostic criteria. If the patient has hemiplegia as the aura symptom, the headaches are termed "hemiplegic migraine".

---

episodic disorder, and patients are well between attacks. Frequency can vary from one attack once every few years to one or more attacks per week; the term "chronic migraine" is used when attacks occur more than 15 days per month. Although rare, organic causes of headache such as glaucoma, hypertensive crises, or early subarachnoid hemorrhage sometimes mimic migraine in their early stages. For this reason, a history of at least five similar headaches should be obtained before making a definite diagnosis of migraine.

An episode of migraine can last for 24 to 72 hours. Patients may also experience "aura", focal neurological symptoms that precede the onset of headache, fading away after 30 to 60 minutes. Such migraines were formerly called "classic migraine". However, *aura is not required for the diagnosis of migraine;* in fact, only 15% to 30% of patients with migraine experience aura. The most common aura involves visual disturbances such as bright flashing lights (photpsia) or an area of lost or depressed vision (scotoma). The visual disturbances associated with aura can be remarkably varied. Some are colorful, others monochromatic. "Fortification spectra" may occur, so-called because the curved, saw-tooth line of the visual illusion resembles the fortifications of medieval walled cities. Other neurological events (e.g., weakness, numbness, confusion, alteration in consciousness) are rare.

Aura symptoms usually evolve gradually, whereas the deficit in transient ischemic neurological events or stroke is often maximal at onset. Aura is usually experienced 15 to 30 minutes before headache but can sometimes last into or beyond the headache. Aura may also occur without subsequent headache. Conversely, patients who do tend to have aura with migraine may not always have aura with every headache. Although pain may be maximal at migraine onset in some patients, especially those with early morning attacks that awaken them, more often it begins at a mild-to-moderate level and builds over a period of hours to maximal severity. After the pain has faded, many patients experience postdromal symptoms of irritability, changes in mood, appetite or gastrointestinal function. fatigue, and motion sensitivity.

In addition to severe, disabling headaches that are easily recognized as migraine, most migraineurs also have mild, "forme fruste" versions of their headache. In these headaches, the typical features of migraine may not always develop, either because the patient aborts the headache with early treatment or because the headache simply does not fully evolve. Most of these milder headaches are in fact the early stages of migraine. Caution should be exercised in making an additional diagnosis of tension-type headache in patients whose severe headaches are clearly migraine.

Uncommon or "variant" presentations of migraine are easily misdiagnosed. Patients with migraine who describe their headache pain as bilateral, located in the occipital or cervical area, or who report being under stress are especially likely to be inaccurately diagnosed with tension-type headache. Patients with migraine who have previously received a diagnosis of "sinus headache" are also at high risk of misdiagnosis.

"Is It My Neck? Is It My Sinuses?"

The pain of migraine can be felt over the bridge of the nose, the cheeks, or the retro-orbital area. Over-the-counter "sinus headache" medications frequently contain vasoconstrictive decongestants or analgesics such as acetaminophen that can be effective in migraine attacks. This seeming response to "specific" medication reinforces in the patient's mind the idea that the headache is sinus in origin. In addition, if antibiotics are prescribed, when the migraine headache improves in a day or so patients may credit the antibiotic rather than the passage of time. Avoiding over-diagnosis of "sinus headache" is important to avoid unnecessary and potentially dangerous overuse of antibiotics.

True sinus-caused headache is rare and generally accompanies only severe cases of acute sinus inflammation. This should be easily recognizable because of associated signs and symptoms such as purulent nasal drainage and fever. Headache as a feature of chronic sinus infection is not common.

A recent evaluation of 24 patients with self-identified sinus headaches found that 23 (96%) satisfied criteria for migraine (3). All of these patients had nasal congestion as part of their headache syndrome, which probably led them to attribute their symptoms to sinus problems. However, the sinus headaches in these patients were relieved with sumatriptan.

Neck pain is also common in migraine. In a survey of 144 patients with migraine, 108 (75%) complained of associated neck pain. Migraine can begin with, or be preceded by, a sensation of tightness or tension in the neck; alternatively, neck pain may develop during the headache and last beyond it. Patients who complain of neck pain as part of their headache are commonly diagnosed as having tension headaches. Many undergo physical therapy or chiropractic manipulation, often with benefit. However, neck pain due to migraine resolves along with the headache when patients are treated with specific anti-migraine medication (4). Patients with migraine whose neck complaints resolve with migraine-specific therapy are unlikely to have associated cervical pathology.

Tension-Type Headache

Key characteristics

- Headaches lasting 30 minutes to 7 days
- Bilateral, mild-to-moderate in intensity, pressing or squeezing
- Not worse with physical activity
- No associated nausea, vomiting, photophobia, or phonophobia, or just one
- Not reliably caused by muscular or psychological factors

The IHS criteria for the diagnosis of tension-type headache are listed in Table 2-5. Tension-type headache is subclassified as *episodic* (attacks occurring less than 15 days per month) or *chronic* (attacks occurring 15 or more days per month for at least 6 months).

The pain of tension-type headache is typically bilateral and lasts from 15 minutes to 7 days. The pain is described as pressure or vise-like, often beginning in the occipital/neck region. The patient with chronic tension-type headache may occasionally experience migraine-like symptoms (nausea

---

Table 2-5 International Headache Society Diagnostic Criteria for Tension-Type Headache

A. At least 10 previous headache episodes fulfilling criteria B-D
B. Headache lasting from 30 minutes to 7 days
C. At least 2 of the following pain characteristics:
  1. Pressing/tightening (non-pulsating quality)
  2. Mild or moderate intensity (may inhibit but does not prohibit activities)
  3. Bilateral location
  4. No aggravation by walking stairs or similar routine physical activity
D. Both of the following:
  1. No nausea or vomiting (anorexia may occur)
  2. Photophobia and phonophobia are absent, or one but not the other is present
E. Not attributed to another disorder
  At least one of the following:
    Subdivision Diagnosis
    1. Infrequent episodic tension-type headache (<1 day/month on average, a total of <12 days/year)
    2. Frequent episodic tension-type headache (≥1 day/month but <15 days/month for at least 3 months)
    3. Chronic tension-type headaches (≥15 days/month on average for >3 months)
The criteria also allow subdivisions based on presence or absence of pericranial muscle tenderness on manual palpation.

From International Headache Society. The International Classification of Headache Disorders, 2nd ed. Cephalalgia. 2004;24(Suppl 1):9-160; with permission.

---

or sensitivity to light or noise) but not to the extent of fulfilling most criteria for migraine.

Tension-type headache is over-diagnosed; remember that, by definition, it is *not* a disabling or severe headache. Most patients with intermittent tension-type headache self-treat using over-the-counter medications with good results. A patient whose headache is severe enough to consult a physician is unlikely to have tension-type headache. A recent study showed that over 80% of patients diagnosed as having tension-type headache in fact have migraine upon more careful evaluation. Thus caution should be exercised in making a diagnosis of tension-type headache.

Cluster Headache

Key characteristics

- One headache every other day up to 8 headaches per day, lasting 15 minutes to 3 hours untreated or unsuccessfully treated
- Always unilateral, behind eye

Table 2-6   International Headache Society Diagnostic Criteria for Cluster Headache

A. At least 5 attacks fulfilling criteria B-D
B. Severe or very severe unilateral orbital, supraorbital, and/or temporal pain lasting 15-180 minutes if untreated
C. Headache is accompanied by at least one of the following:
  1. Ipsilateral conjunctival injection and/or lacrimation
  2. Ipsilateral nasal congestion and/or rhinorrhoea
  3. Ipsilateral eyelid oedema
  4. Iipsilateral forehead and facial sweating
  5. Ipsilateral miosis and/or ptosis
  6. Restlessness or agitation
D. Attack frequency from one every other day to 8 per day
E. Not attributed to another disorder

From International Headache Society. The International Classification of Headache Disorders, 2nd ed. Cephalalgia. 2004;24(Suppl 1):9-160; with permission.

- Steady, severe pain
- Must have at least one associated autonomic sign on side of pain (e.g., conjunctival injection, lacrimation, rhinorrhea, ptosis, miosis)

The IHS criteria for the diagnosis of cluster headache are listed in Table 2-6. Like tension-type headache, cluster headache is subclassified as either episodic or chronic. In *episodic* cluster headache, attacks generally occur one to eight times daily in "cluster" cycles lasting from 7 days to 1 year, then remit for a month or longer. In *chronic* cluster headache, there are no headache-free periods or, if so, they are less than 1 month in duration.

Other names for cluster headache include "suicide headache" and "alarm clock headache". The latter refers to the peculiar tendency of cluster headache attacks to occur at specific times, especially in association with the first rapid-eye movement period of sleep, which occurs about 90 minutes after sleep onset.

Cluster headache, although rare, is the most stereotyped of the primary headache disorders and thus easily recognized. Most primary care physicians will see only 2 or 3 cases over their career. However, treatment for cluster headache differs in several important ways from that for migraine headache, and accurate diagnosis will spare a patient months or years of ineffective or dangerous treatment.

Many patients with migraine mistakenly believe that they have cluster headache. This confusion is understandable in view of the tendency for migraine attacks to occur in flurries over several weeks and then to decrease in frequency. This natural waxing and waning of migraine, however, should not be confused with the more characteristic complete remissions and exacerbations of true cluster headache.

Other Primary Headache Syndromes

Other primary headache syndromes are less common than migraine, tension-type, or cluster headache and are often misdiagnosed. In general, patients correctly diagnosed with these syndromes should be referred for specialty consultation.

Several brief headache syndromes are often referred to as the trigeminal autonomic cephalgias (TACs); cluster headache is also a TAC but is considered separately because of its importance. Other TACs include short-lasting, unilateral neuralgiform headache attacks with conjunctival injection, tearing, sweating, and rhinorrhea (SUNCT syndrome); chronic and episodic paroxysmal hemicrania; and hemicrania continua.

Chronic and episodic paroxysmal hemicranias are severe burning or throbbing pains located unilaterally in the distribution of the first division of the trigeminal nerve and are generally associated with autornomic features. The duration of the attacks are longer than SUNCT but shorter than cluster headache (on average 5 to 10 minutes); they can recur up to 40 times daily. The paroxysmal hemicranias are uniquely sensitive to indomethacin, to the extent that diagnosis depends on a therapeutic response to the drug. A therapeutic trial of indomethacin 25 mg PO tid confirms diagnosis.

Hemicrania continua is also responsive to indomethacin treatment. Attacks are unilateral, with no side shift. They are moderate-to-severe in intensity and are generally associated with mild or no autonomic features. Hemicrania continua can resemble chronic tension-type headache except for its unilaterality. Some patients have superimposed attacks of migraine. Thus, in any unremitting headache disorder, a trial of indomethacin is worth trying in refractory patients.

Some short-lasting headaches can have an underlying organic cause. Headaches triggered by cough, strain, or exertion require careful evaluation that may include diagnostic testing. The headaches may be dull, throbbing, or explosive, and may last seconds to minutes or persist for days. Space-occupying lesions and Arnold-Chiari malformation type I are the most commonly reported structural abnormalities.

Less-common primary headache syndromes, excluding TACs, are given in Table 2-7.

**Table 2-7   Less-Common Primary Headache Syndromes
(Excluding Trigeminal Autonomic Cephalgias)**

- Primary stabbing headache
- Hypnic headache
- Primary headache associated with sexual activity
- Primary cough headache

Chronic Daily Headache

Key characteristics

- Not a single diagnosis but a syndrome of frequent headache that can evolve from a variety of headache syndromes.
- Most patients have mixed features of migraine and tension-type headache.
- Daily headaches are worrisome.
- The evolution of the headache over time is important in diagnosis.
- The possibility of medication overuse should be considered in all patients with daily headache.

Four to five percent of the population has chronic daily headache, arbitrarily defined as headache occurring more than 15 days a month and lasting at least 4 hours. Chronic daily headache is not a single diagnostic entity. It includes patients with a variety of headache syndromes, including transformed migraine, chronic tension-type headache, and new-onset daily persistent headache. One study interviewed 230 patients about the initial characteristics of their headaches; 22% had daily headaches from onset. In those whose daily headaches had initially been episodic, 19% reported an abrupt, rather than gradual, change to a daily headache pattern (5).

Patients with chronic daily headache account for the majority of referrals to tertiary headache centers; 50% to 82% of these patients overuse abortive headache medications, with paradoxical worsening of headache. Medication-induced, or drug-rebound, headache remains an unrecognized epidemic.

Daily headache is always worrisome. Even when not due to an underlying, secondary problem, it is associated with significant personal and occupational disability. A substantial number of these patients require evaluation and management in a specialty headache or pain clinic. Primary care providers can help prevent headache worsening by identifying and referring these patients for such evaluation and treatment in a timely fashion. As with other chronic illnesses, comprehensive treatment is most effective when employed early, before the development of counter-productive behavior patterns or disability.

Chronic Daily Headache: Different Paths Lead to the Same Disorder

Transformed Migraine

Patients with headaches that at times fulfill criteria for migraine and at other times for tension-type headache have in the past been labeled as having "mixed headache". The 1988 IHS criteria suggested that these patients be labeled as having two headache types. However, an additional diagnostic category of "chronic migraine" (CM) has been added to the current (2004) criteria. This diagnosis requires occurrence of headaches with migraine-like features at least 15 days/month (see Appendix I). Many patients, though, still require two diagnoses because, although they have frequent headache, it does not meet the criterion for migraine of at least 15 days/month. Headache specialists have long recognized that episodic migraine may, over time, evolve into a near-daily headache pattern that is sufficiently characteristic to warrant its own label, whether "transformed migraine" (TM) or "chronic migraine". Patients with TM experience headaches on a daily or near-daily basis, often tension-type in nature, but have intermittent, superimposed headaches that fulfill criteria for migraine. TM and CM are often, but not always, associated with medication overuse, defined as the use of abortive headache medications ≥15 days/month.

Chronic Tension-Type Headache

Chronic tension-type headache occurring in isolation is a rare disorder. Most of these patients also have intermittent episodes of migraine. However, a small subset of patients exists in whom the initial headache disorder is an episodic tension-type headache that becomes chronic over time.

New Daily Persistent Headache

New daily persistent headache (NDPH) is daily from onset. Patients often have no previous headache history. A precipitating event is noted in over half of patients, most commonly a febrile or viral illness, general surgery, or a stressful life event (5). These headaches are often refractory to therapy and may persist indefinitely.

Medication Overuse

Recognition of medication overuse is important because in 75% of headache patients regular use of pain relievers is causing or aggravating the headache. Aggravation of a pre-existing headache problem by drug rebound is the most common cause of transformed migraine, and some experts believe it is important in other daily headache syndromes, including post-concussive headache. Patients with drug-rebound headache are typically refractory to usual acute and prophylactic care and thus, if not properly diagnosed, are particularly frustrating to the PCP. The patient who repeatedly visits the emergency department for narcotics for headache relief most commonly has drug-rebound headache.

Patients overuse medication for a variety of reasons. These range from addiction and dependence to desperate attempts to obtain relief from inadequate or ineffective medications. Even in tertiary headache centers, about one third of patients with medication overuse do not improve following an adequate trial of medication withdrawal. Patients often experience exacerbation of headache in the first two weeks following analgesic withdrawal and may require 4 to 12 weeks (occasionally longer) to demonstrate benefit.

Physical and Neurological Examination

The patient presenting with headache should undergo a screening physical and neurological examination. This can be conducted in about 3 minutes.

1. Observe patient (this can be done while taking the history) to assess for gross disorders of movement, thought, and cognition
   A. Speech and language
   B. Thinking and memory
   C. Appearance, mood, behavior
   D. Obvious motor deficits, movement disorder
2. Funduscopic examination to assess papilledema and check for venous pulsations
3. Cranial nerve examination (abnormalities suggest intracranial pathology)
   A. Pupils (II, III), visual fields (II), extraocular movements (III, IV, VI)
   B. Facial movement and symmetry/speech (VII, VIII)
4. Upper and lower extremity examination (motor, cerebellar)
   A. Arm drift
   B. Arm and leg strength
   C. Wrist and thumb extension
5. Cerebellar
   A. Finger-to-nose, heel-to-shin
   B. Rapid alternating movements (finger tapping/rapid hand opening and closing)
6. Cortical function (abnormalities suggest organic brain syndrome or frontal lobe dysfunction)
   A. Stereognosis (identify coins/graphesthesia)
   B. Three-step command crossing midline. "Touch your right ear with your left little finger. Then close your eyes and stick your tongue out to the left."
   C. Three-step sequential hand movement. "I'm going to show you three movements with my hand. I want you to repeat the same movements." Demonstrate as follows: Hold left palm out upwards parallel to the floor. First the side of the right hand strikes the open left palm (chopping gesture), then right fist strikes palm, then right palm slaps palm.
7. Deep tendon reflexes
8. Babinski response
9. Check blood pressure and pulse (to assess for hypertension).
10. Place your fingers over the temporomandibular joints and ask the patient to open wide. Palpate the joints. Crepitus is not unusual, but significant

pain with either maneuver should prompt referral to a dentist for evaluation of temporomandibular joint problems.

11. Palpate the head and neck and observe neck range of motion. Crepitus on neck motion is not worrisome, but significant pain on palpation or motion should focus attention on cervical spine. Do not ignore this aspect of the examination. Patients, rightly or wrongly, expect thorough examination of the body part that hurts, in this case the head.

12. Check for carotid and ophthalmic bruits to assess for presence of vascular disease.

The American Academy of Neurology does not recommend diagnostic imaging studies in patients who meet criteria for migraine and have a normal neurological examination. This recommendation was based on a review of the scientific evidence, demonstrating a diagnostic yield of only 0.4% for imaging in such cases. The evidence was less clear for non-migraine headache: 2.4% of such patients had important abnormalities on imaging studies. Indications for imaging or laboratory studies are discussed in Chapter 3.

Key Points

- Separate benign from worrisome headaches. Most patients have benign headaches.
- Recognize common headache patterns and variations on these themes.
- Migraine is the most common headache presenting to the physician.
- Perform an efficient screening physical examination. Few patients require imaging or laboratory studies.
- Avoid common diagnostic pitfalls. Missing migraine or an incorrect diagnosis of sinus, tension, or cervical headache is a mistake often made.

REFERENCES

1. **Dodick DW.** Clinical clues and clinical rules: primary versus secondary headache. Adv Stud Med. 2003;3:S550-5.

2. **Vasquez-Barquero A, Ibanez FJ, Herrera S, et al.** Isolated headache as the presenting clinical manifestation of intracranial tumors: a prospective study. Cephalalgia. 1994;14:270-2.

3. **Schreiber CP, Cady RK, Billings C.** Subjects with self-described "sinus" headache meet IHS diagnostic criteria for migraine [Abstract]. Cephalalgia. 2001;21:298.

4. **Kaniecki RG, Totten J.** Cervicalgia in migraine: prevalence, clinical characteristics, and response to treatment [Abstract]. Cephalalgia. 2001;21:296-7.

5. **Li D, Rozen TD.** The clinical characteristics of new daily persistent headache. Cephalalgia. 2002;22:66-9.

3

Dangerous Secondary Causes
of Headache

Elizabeth W. Loder, MD

Frederick G. Freitag, DO

Vincent T. Martin, MD

Evaluating Possible Secondary Headache

An important clinical goal in any patient with a complaint of headache is to identify warning signs of secondary headache. The International Headache Society (IHS) diagnostic criteria for all primary headache disorders include the statement that "history, physical, and neurological examination do not suggest" a secondary headache or, if they do so, that "it is ruled out by appropriate investigations. . . ." In the majority of patients with a chief complaint of headache, a thorough history will reveal the presence of recurrent headaches meeting IHS criteria for one of the primary headache disorders. When such headaches have been occurring over a period of years and are separated by intervals without headache, further diagnostic investigations are rarely necessary and attention can be turned to finding effective treatment.

However, when the history does *not* follow typical patterns for migraine or other primary headaches, further evaluation for a possible dangerous or secondary cause of the headache is necessary. Table 3-1 lists historical or examination features that should prompt consideration of a dangerous or secondary cause of headache. Formulating a differential diagnosis in these cases requires a review of many of the conditions that can present with headache. A systematic approach helps the physician to avoid overlooking important secondary headache causes and includes a more detailed history, physical examination, and selected use of laboratory and radiological evaluation.

**Table 3-1   Some Clinical Presentations That Should Prompt Evaluation
for Secondary Headache**

- New headache
- Significant change in a previously stable headache pattern
- Headache described as the "worst" headache ever
- Headache in an older person, particularly in the absence of a previous history of similar headaches
- Headache associated with an abnormal neurological examination
- Headache associated with systemic signs or symptoms

History

In general, a history of previous identical headaches is reassuring. Occasionally, however, chronic headaches may have an ominous source, which is suspected only after careful evaluation. All new, changing, or progressive headaches, and headaches occurring in the elderly or those associated with systemic signs and symptoms, are potentially worrisome and require careful evaluation.

The IHS criteria specify that at least five attacks meeting migraine criteria must occur before a diagnosis of migraine can be made. A first occurrence of what seems to be migraine does not necessarily require testing or imaging studies but does warrant careful follow-up to ensure that the subsequent course of headache is benign. A good response of headache pain to migraine-specific therapy such as the triptans does not constitute proof of a migraine diagnosis, because some case reports demonstrate at least temporary improvement of secondary headaches to such treatment.

In patients with established headaches, the question "Has there been any important change in your headaches?" is useful, because a patient with a stable pattern of headache for 6 months has no more likelihood of an underlying tumor than does a patient without headache.

Physical Examination

The careful physical examination, particularly of the head and neck, is an essential component of a comprehensive headache evaluation, because it can identify conditions that may mimic or coexist with a primary headache disorder. There are several key steps in the headache physical examination:

- Evaluate blood pressure and pulse. Significant, uncontrolled hypertension can aggravate or occasionally cause headache. Hypertension, even if controlled, is a cardiac risk factor, and if poorly controlled is a contraindication to the use of potentially vasoconstrictive medications such as the ergots or triptans.

- Examine the heart and lungs. A new heart murmur or a gallop on cardiac examination or rales on pulmonary examination could suggest occult cardiac or pulmonary disease that may be related to the underlying headache disorder.

- Examine the patient's eyes. Abnormalities of extraocular movements could indicate a paresis or palsy of the third, fourth, or sixth cranial nerves. The pupillary size and response to light and accommodation should be evaluated. Miosis and ptosis ipsilateral to the headache could represent Horner's syndrome, which can be seen with cluster headache and tumors, as well as other disorders of the head and neck. The optic discs should be assessed for sharpness, and venous pulsations should be noted. Blurring of the optic disc margins can be benign but may also indicate increased intracranial pressure from a tumor or idiopathic intracranial hypertension; it generally warrants an imaging study.

- Check for signs of head trauma or injury, which may signal acute or chronic post-traumatic headache or, if very recent, raise suspicion for subdural hematoma.

- Palpate and check range of motion of the patient's head, neck, and temporomandibular joints (TMJ). Scalp or temple nodules or necrotic lesions can be seen in giant-cell arteritis. Muscle tenderness or neck pain is usually a trigger or consequence of headache, not a cause of it. Clicking of the TMJ is common and, in the absence of pain, does not need evaluation, but significant limitation of jaw opening or pain with palpation may deserve further attention.

- Test the other cranial nerves by having the patient smile, stick out tongue, wrinkle forehead, and show teeth. Check for weakness or asymmetry of facial muscle strength. Abnormal findings may signal central nervous system problems such as tumors.

- Evaluate balance when patient puts both feet together, extends arms, and spreads fingers with eyes closed. Problems maintaining balance may indicate a problem in the cerebellum or posterior fossa.

- Informally assess patient's demeanor, thought processes, and affect. When these do not correlate with pain reports, a psychiatric disorder should be considered (1,2).

Laboratory and Radiological Evaluation

When the headache history or physical examination suggests the possibility of a secondary cause of headache, diagnostic tests can be useful to exclude or confirm various organic causes of headache. There is, however, no test that proves someone has a benign cause of headaches. Testing may also be

---

Table 3-2   Some Secondary Causes of Headache That Can Be Detected by Lumbar Puncture

- Fungal meningitis
- Inflammation due to conditions such as vasculitis
- Meningeal carcinomatosis or lymphomatosis
- Subarachnoid hemorrhage
- Idiopathic intracranial hypertension
- Intracranial hypotension associated with CSF leaks

---

useful to 1) assess for co-morbid diseases that could complicate headache treatment, 2) establish a baseline for, and exclude contraindications to, drug treatment, and 3) measure drug levels to determine compliance, absorption, or medication overuse.

Lumbar Puncture

A diagnostic evaluation of spinal fluid pressure or composition is important in patients who present with sudden onset of severe headache ("thunderclap" headache), a situation in which subarachnoid hemorrhage must be ruled out. If a plain CT of the head is negative, a lumbar puncture *must* be performed to exclude the possibility of subarachnoid hemorrhage. Lumbar puncture is also useful in patients with progressive headache syndromes to detect, for example, fungal meningitis, vasculitis, or abnormal intracranial pressure. Table 3-2 lists conditions causing headache in which lumbar puncture is useful for diagnosis.

Imaging Studies

WHEN SHOULD AN IMAGING STUDY BE CONDUCTED?

Based on a review of published studies, the American Academy of Neurology (AAN) has recommended that

> [I]n adult patients with recurrent headaches that have been defined as migraine – including those with visual aura – with no recent change in pattern, no history of seizures, and no other focal neurological signs or symptoms, the routine use of neuroimaging is not warranted. In patients with atypical headache patterns, a history of seizures, or focal neurological signs or symptoms, CT or MRI may be indicated. (3)

The AAN identified 897 patients with headaches conforming to IHS criteria for migraine headache who had been imaged. In this group, three brain tumors were found, one considered incidental (and the patient's headaches persisted after surgery), one in a patient with a history of seizures and a recent change in the chronic headache pattern. One arteriovenous malformation (AVM) was discovered, also in a patient with seizures. The case-finding rate was 0.4%. The evidence was less clear for headaches that did not meet IHS criteria for migraine. A higher case-finding rate of 2.4% was

Table 3-3   Some Conditions Detected by Magnetic Resonance Imaging But Not by Computed Tomography

- Cerebrovascular
  - —Arterial dissection (MRA)
  - —Cerebral venous sinus thrombosis (MRV)
  - —CNS vasculitis
  - —Herpes encephalitis
- High and low intracranial pressure syndromes
- Tumors
  - —Posterior fossa abnormalities
  - —Pituitary lesions
  - —Leptomeningeal enhancement

found in this group of patients, leading to an AAN statement that: "At this time, there is insufficient evidence to define the role of CT and MRI in the evaluation of patients with headaches that are not consistent with migraine."

WHICH IMAGING STUDY?

A plain CT scan of the head without intravenous contrast is appropriate for a patient with acute or subacute headache where a recent subarachnoid hemorrhage or subdural hematoma is the main consideration. In almost every other case, consensus-based standards recommend use of MRI, usually performed with gadolinium enhancement (3). MRI is preferred because the added cost compared with CT is minimal and because it identifies a number of important secondary causes of headache that CT scans may fail to detect. Table 3-3 lists some of these conditions, which include certain tumors, aneurysms, and posterior fossa abnormalities such as Arnold-Chiari malformations (4). MR angiography is indicated when arterial dissection or intracranial aneurysm is suspected, and MR venography is indicated when cerebral venous sinus thrombosis is suspected.

Selected Dangerous Causes of Secondary Headache

Brain Tumor Headache

Many patients with headache fear they have a brain tumor. In fact, however, headache without other neurological symptoms was the presenting feature in only 8% of patients with brain tumor (5). Even physician views about the typical headache pattern in patients with brain tumor may be inaccurate.

One study of 111 patients with primary or metastatic brain tumors identified the "classic" profile of a brain tumor headache (severe, worse in the morning, associated with nausea or vomiting) in 17% (6). A pattern resembling tension-type headache was found in 77%, migraine-like headaches in 9%, and other headache patterns in the remaining 14%. Not unexpectedly, headache occurring with brain tumor may be more likely to occur in patients with a previous history of a benign cause of headache. Of the 32% of patients with a previous history of headache, 78% had headache with their tumor, but in every instance the headache was more severe or frequent and was associated with other symptoms (seizure, confusion, prolonged nausea, hemiparesis) or abnormal signs. These findings underscore the importance of careful evaluation when previously stable patients report a significant change in prior headache pattern.

Meningiomas are the most common type of benign brain tumor in adults, found in 3% of the general population in autopsy studies. They are slow growing and when found on an imaging study performed because of headache are often only an incidental finding.

In adults, pituitary adenomas constitute 5% of brain tumors. Headache is a common symptom, occurring in 33% to 72% of cases. The pain is usually mild, often described as continuous. The degree of headache does not correlate with pituitary tumor size, invasion of the cavernous sinus, or hypopituitarism, but three quarters of headaches improve after surgery. Pituitary apoplexy may be signaled by the abrupt onset in association with altered consciousness, cranial nerve palsies, and adrenal crisis, but headache is found in only 57% of patients with this diagnosis. Pituitary adenomas can cause hypersecretion, hyposecretion, or no change in anterior pituitary hormone release. When the tumor is over 1 cm in size, about one half of patients will have symptoms of hypothyroidism, adrenal insufficiency, or other syndromes associated with pituitary hormone insufficiency. Bitemporal hemianopsia is a characteristic visual disturbance, related to tumor pressure on the optic chiasm (7-10).

Cerebral Venous Sinus Thrombosis

Cerebral venous sinus thrombosis (CVST) is a cause of cerebral infarction. CVST can be caused by infections (especially sinusitis or mastoiditis), dehydration, and hypercoagulable states (these are especially common in the post-partum period, after miscarriage, with oral contraceptives, or with thrombophilic coagulopathies.) In many cases, the cause of CVST is never identified. CVST accounts for up to 80% of pregnancy-related cerebral ischemic events, with the majority of cases occurring in the second or third post-partum week.

Most patients with CVST do report headaches. The headache may be subacute and slowly progressive or of sudden onset like a "thunderclap" headache. Neurological deficits may be caused by hemorrhagic venous infarction of brain parenchyma or increased cerebrospinal fluid (CSF) pressure with a resultant mass effect. Symptoms such as weakness, changes in consciousness, or seizures may be present. Diagnostic criteria require the presence of seizures, focal neurological deficit, or increased intracranial pressure, but these characteristics are not always present. Magnetic resonance venography (MRV) is the most successful neuroimaging technique for identifying CVST.

Cerebrovascular Accident

Cerebrovascular accidents (CVAs), both ischemic and hemorrhagic, and transient ischemic attacks (TIAs) have been associated with the development of headaches. Headaches occur in 11% to 34% of large cerebral infarctions, 3% to 23% of lacunar infarctions, and 33% to 57% of intracerebral hematomas. Patients with TIAs experience headaches in 4% to 44% of cases. The headaches have no distinguishing clinical characteristics but begin in close temporal relationship to the onset of the focal neurological signs (11).

The neurological symptoms of stroke and TIA may be difficult to distinguish from those of migraine aura, particularly early in their onset. Neurological symptoms, however, tend to occur suddenly in those with stroke and progress more gradually in those with aura.

For unclear reasons, migraineurs may be at elevated risk for infarctions of the posterior circulation. A recent study identified a higher incidence of asymptomatic cerebellar infarcts in migraine patients with more than one attack than in controls, with an odds ratio of 9.3 (95% confidence interval, 1.1-76). An accompanying editorial suggested that, at least in a subset of patients, migraine may be a cause of progressive damage to the brain (12).

A diagnosis of migrainous infarction can be made only when the resulting neurological deficit is characteristic of the patient's previous auras and is accompanied by radiological evidence of a lesion in the corresponding region of the brain. Figure 3-1 shows an occipital infarct such as might be seen in a patient whose typical visual aura does not remit.

Subarachnoid Hemorrhage

Subarachnoid hemorrhage (SAH) is a leading cause of sudden death in healthy young adults (13). When suspected, a non-contrast CT scan of the

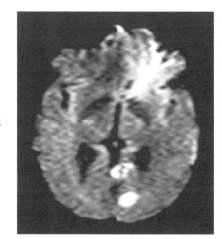

Figure 3-1   Occipital infarct on MRI study.

head should be performed. If no blood is seen, a lumbar puncture is necessary to exclude the possibility of a small leak that does not show up on imaging studies. Figure 3-2 shows a CT scan in which a subarachnoid hemorrhage is visible. SAH typically presents as a "thunderclap" headache of sudden onset, which reaches peak intensity in seconds to minutes. Headache is a very common symptom, occurring in 66% to 100% of cases (14). Characteristics of the headache vary tremendously, but in 70% of cases the pain causes incapacitation. Features of migraine, such as nausea, vomiting, and photophobia, may be present, although unilateral location is not common.

Brief or persistent non-localizing neurological signs, including loss of consciousness and lethargy, may occur, probably as a result of rapid rises in intracranial pressure, mass effect, or vasospasm (15). Meningeal irritation can cause stiff neck and even back pain. Fever, irritability, and confusion can occur. Retinal hemorrhages and papilledema are commonly seen by funduscopy.

The mean age of patients with SAH is 51 years. There is a female predominance, especially in the over-70 age group where the sex prevalence ratio is 10 females to 1 male. The incidence of aneurysmal SAH in the general population is 10 cases per 100,000 persons per year (16). Headache alone as a symptom of unruptured aneurysm is probably uncommon. Approximately one third of patients with an unruptured aneurysm get headaches, a prevalence similar to that observed in the general population. However, 11% of headache sufferers with aneurysm have other abnormal findings such as cranial nerve abnormalities, a fact which underscores the importance of careful evaluation in patients whose headaches are accompanied by abnormal neurological findings. An estimated 1% to 6% of the general population have asymptomatic intracranial aneurysms, and autopsy studies have found that 0.2% to 9.9% (average, 5%) of the general asymptomatic population have aneurysms. The prevalence of intracranial aneurysm may be as high as

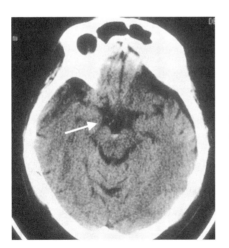

Figure 3-2   Subarachnoid hemorrhage *(arrow)* shown on CT scan.

20% in those with a family history of the disorder; those patients should be screened (17). The risk of aneurysmal rupture depends on location and size.

In addition to ruptured intracranial aneurysms, causes of SAH include arteriovenous malformations, hypertension, arteriosclerosis, cerebral emboli, bleeding diatheses, anticoagulants, tumor, and central nervous system (CNS) infection. Risk factors for SAH include hypertension, smoking, alcohol consumption, polycystic kidney disease, coarctation of the aorta, fibromuscular dysplasia, hereditary hemorrhagic telangiectasia, moya-moya disease, and Marfan's syndrome. Connective tissue disorders, including Ehlers-Danlos syndrome, impart a higher risk for aneurysm, subdural hematomas, and chronic recurrent headaches (50%) (18,19). The risk of rupture for cerebral aneurysms less than 10 mm in size with no prior SAH is 0.05% per year, whereas aneurysms larger than 10 mm have about a 1% risk of rupture per year (16).

The mortality from a ruptured aneurysm is 35%. Ruptured aneurysms and AVMs frequently rebleed, making prompt diagnosis important. Additionally, timely medical and surgical procedures markedly reduce death and morbidity. Over one half of patients with SAH recall an unusual warning, or "sentinel headache", in the weeks preceding their event. In the occasional patient who is evaluated more than 3 weeks after having typical SAH symptoms, findings on CAT and lumbar puncture (xanthochromia) may have resolved; here angiography is needed for definitive diagnosis.

Subdural Hematoma

Subdural hematoma may be acute, subacute, or chronic. Headaches occur in 11% to 55% of acute or subacute cases and in up to 81% of chronic cases. The headaches have no distinguishing characteristics, and a history of antecedent head trauma can be minor or completely lacking particularly within elderly patients (20). The diagnostic test of choice is a non-contrast CT scan.

Temporal Arteritis and Vasculitis

Temporal arteritis is usually seen in patients over age 50, especially Caucasian women. Headache is its most common manifestation and is often described as burning or throbbing. Findings on examination may include a tender superficial temporal artery, jaw claudication, elevated sedimentation rate, night sweats, low-grade fever, muscle aches, weight loss, and fatigue. Temporal artery biopsy is the definitive diagnostic test, and headache usually responds quickly upon treatment with glucocorticoids. Detection is important because untreated temporal arteritis will lead to permanent blindness in roughly one third of patients.

Other forms of vasculitis that cause headache may be more difficult to diagnose. Primary intracranial vasculitis, for example, requires brain biopsy for definitive diagnosis in many cases. It can be suspected based on symptoms that include seizures, stroke, transient ischemic attacks and confusion.

Carotid and Vertebral Dissection

Dissection of the carotid artery may cause pain and headache. The internal carotid artery in its extracranial location is the most common source of dissection (21). The headache and neck pain may persist for hours to days and culminate with the development of other signs of cerebral ischemia. The pain of carotid dissection is most likely due to dilation of the blood vessel. Headache onset is variable in duration and intensity but is unique compared with other headaches the patient may have experienced. It tends to be a localized pain condition and can last for days. The occurrence of neck pain, especially at the angle of jaw or near the midline in the posterior neck, associated with the development of a "new" headache should raise the suspicion for arterial dissection. Other neurological symptoms, including cranial nerve palsies and Horner's syndrome, are commonly associated with the headache (22). A history of trauma, cervical manipulation, and hypertension further raises the index of suspicion.

Vertebral dissection leads to headache in the occipital region and pain in the posterior neck. Generally there are signs of brainstem and cerebellar ischemia. Neurological symptoms may be delayed for up to a month after the onset of headache (23). Diagnosis is established with ultrasonography, MRI, MRA, and angiography. Once diagnosis is established it is imperative to reduce the risk of ischemic stroke. The use of appropriate anticoagulant therapy, including heparin followed by warfarin, is the treatment of choice. Bedrest is useful and should be maintained until evidence of circulation restoration is present on ultrasonography. The anticoagulant therapy should be maintained for up to about 6 months or until the internal diameter of the vessel approximates normal.

Meningitis, Encephalitis, and Brain Abscess

Intracranial infections such as meningitis, encephalitis, and brain abscess may cause headaches. There are no specific features of the headaches that distinguish those related to intracranial infections from other primary or secondary headache disorders. Meningitis (viral, bacterial, fungal) may be associated with headaches, fever, and nuchal rigidity. A recent prospective study, however, found that nuchal rigidity, Kernig's sign, and Brudzinski's sign were neither sensitive nor specific for a diagnosis of meningitis (24).

Headache is present in 81% of patients with herpes encephalitis. The primary features that differentiate encephalitis from other headache disorders are the presence of fever (92% of patients), altered mental status, and other neurological signs including alterations of consciousness (97%), changes in personality (71%), seizures (67%), hemiparesis (33%), cranial nerve defects (32%), and papilledema (14%) (25).

Headache is the most common symptom associated with brain abscess. The headache is often described as dull and aching, and its location may depend on the region of the brain involved with the abscess. Fever may be present in <50% of cases, and neurological signs occur in one third to one half of cases. Papilledema may be demonstrated in <25% of cases. The disease most often results from infections of the sinuses, middle ear, or teeth but can result from metastatic seeding from extracranial infections (sepsis, endocarditis, etc.). This diagnosis might be suspected in a patient with new headache or change in an existing headache *and* any of the following: 1) unexplained fever, 2) neurological signs, or 3) a recent history of intracranial or extracranial infections as mentioned above (26).

Key Points

- In most patients who seek medical care for headache, a benign, primary headache syndrome will be diagnosed.

- Headache history that does not suggest a primary headache requires that further evaluation for a dangerous or secondary cause of headache be undertaken.

- All new, changing, or progressive headaches, headaches occurring in the elderly, and headaches associated with systemic signs and symptoms are potentially serious and require prompt evaluation.

- Physical examination can identify conditions that may mimic or coexist with primary headache.

REFERENCES

1. **Silberstein SD, Lipton RB, Goadsby PJ.** Headache in Clinical Practice. Oxford: Isis Medical Media; 1998:17.
2. **Bates BA.** Guide to Physical Examination. Philadelphia: JB Lippincott; 1983:338.
3. **Silberstein SD.** Practice parameter: evidence-based guidelines for migraine headache (an evidence-based review): report of the Quality Standards Subcommittee of the American Academy of Neurology. Neurology. 2000;26;754-62.
4. **Campbell JK, Sakai F.** Diagnosis and differential diagnosis. In: Olesen J, Tfelt-Hansen P, Welch KMA, eds. The Headaches, 2nd ed. Philadelphia: Lippincott Williams and Wilkins; 2000:359-63.
5. **Vasquez-Barquero A, Ibanez FJ, Herrera S, et al.** Isolated headache as the presenting clinical manifestation of intracranial tumors: a prospective study. Cephalalgia. 1994;14:270-2.
6. **Forsyth PA, Posner JB.** Headaches in patients with brain tumors: a study of 111 patients. Neurology. 1993;43:1678-83.
7. **Hosokawa M, Asano A, Itioka O, et al.** Pituitary adenoma and headache. Jpn J Headache. 1987;14:59-63.

8. **Yokoyama S, Mamitsuka K, Tokimura H, Asakura T.** Headache in pituitary adenoma cases. J Jpn Soc Study Chron Pain. 1994;13:79-82.

9. **Abe T, Matsumoto K, Kuwazawa J, et al.** Headache associated with pituitary adenomas. Headache. 1998;38:782-6.

10. **Weinstein J, Isaacs S, Shore D, Blevins LS.** Diagnosis and management of pituitary tumors. Comp Ther. 1997;23:594-604.

11. **Jensen T, Gorelick P.** Headache associated with ischemic stroke and intracranial hematoma. In: Olesen J, Tfelt-Hansen P, Welch KMA, eds. The Headaches, 2nd ed. Philadelphia: Lippincott Williams and Wilkins; 2000:781-7.

12. **Kruit MC, van Buchem MA, Hofman PAM, et al.** Migraine as a risk factor for subclinical brain lesions. JAMA. 2004;291:427-34.

13. **Day JW, Raskin NH.** Thunderclap headache: symptom of unruptured cerebral aneurysm. Lancet. 1986;2:1247-8.

14. **Edlow JA, Caplan LR.** Avoiding pitfalls in the diagnosis of subarachnoid hemorrhage. N Engl J Med. 2000;342:29.

15. **Waga S, Ohtsubo K, Handa H.** Warning signs in intracranial aneurysms. Surg Neurol. 1975;3:15-20.

16. Unruptured intracranial aneurysms: risk of rupture and risks of surgical intervention. International Study of Unruptured Intracranial Aneurysms Investigators. N Engl J Med. 1998;339:1725-33.

17. **Obuchowski NA, Modic MT, Magdinec M.** Current implications for the efficacy of noninvasive screening for occult intracranial aneurysms in patients with a family history of aneurysms. J Neurosurg. 1995;83:42-9.

18. **Sacheti A, Szemere J, Bernstein B, et al.** Chronic pain is a manifestation of the Ehlers-Danlos syndrome. J Pain Symptom Manage. 1997;14:88-93.

19. **Jacome DE.** Headache in Ehlers-Danlos syndrome. Cephalalgia. 1999;19:791-6.

20. **Jensen T, Gorlick D.** Headache associated with ischemic stroke and intracranial hematoma. In: Olesen J, Tfelt-Hansen P, Welch KMA, eds. The Headaches, 2nd ed. Philadelphia: Lippincott Williams and Wilkins; 2000:781-7.

21 **Guillon B, Levy C, Bousser MG.** Internal carotid artery dissection: an update. J Neurol Sci. 1998;153:146-58.

22. **Mokri B, Sundt T, Houser O, Piepgras D.** Spontaneous dissection of the cervical internal carotid artery. Ann Neurol. 1986;19:126-34.

23. **Biousse V, Mitsias P**. Carotid or vertebral artery pain. In: Olesen J, Tfelt-Hansen P, Welch KMA, eds. The Headaches, 2nd ed. Philadelphia: Lippincott Williams and Wilkins; 2000:807-13.

24. **Thomas K, Hasbun R, Jekel J, Quagliarello V.** The diagnostic accuracy of Kernig's sign, Brudzinski's sign, and nuchal rigidity in adults with suspected meningitis. Clin Infect Dis. 2002;35:46-52.

25. **Whiteley R, Seng-Jaw S, Linneman C, et al.** Herpes simplex encephalitis: clinical assessment. JAMA.1982;247:317-20.

26. **Mathisen G, Johnson J.** Brain abscess. Clin Infect Dis. 1997;25:763-8.

4

Migraine Headache

Frederick R. Taylor, MD
Vincent T. Martin, MD

igraine headache is one of the most common disorders encountered by primary care physicians. It is more prevalent than diabetes, hypertension, and asthma. A day with migraine is considered by the World Health Organization to be as disabling as a day with quadriplegia, schizophrenia, or dementia (1). Migraine may also be associated with or lead to several serious and even life-threatening conditions, such as stroke, analgesic nephropathy, and medication dependence. Yet despite its high prevalence and the seriousness of its health consequences, migraine is under-recognized and frequently misdiagnosed.

Epidemiology

Prevalence in the General Population

The overall prevalence of migraine meeting International Headache Society (IHS) criteria in the US population is nearly 13%, with approximately 18% of women and 6% of men meeting strict diagnostic criteria for disease (2). One in every four households harbors at least one migraineur. It is most prevalent in young and middle-aged adults, with men most affected between 30 and 39 years of age and women between 40 and 49 years of age (3). The two most common patterns of migraine are migraine without aura, formerly called *common migraine,* and migraine with aura, or *classic migraine;* between 15% and 30% of sufferers experience aura with at least some attacks. Migraine can begin at any age but incidence peaks during the teens and early twenties.

Prevalence in the Primary Care Setting

The prevalence of migraine headache is much higher in patients that seek medical care from primary care physicians when compared with the general population. A study of primary care waiting rooms throughout the United States found a prevalence of migraine headache of 29% in patients presenting with any complaint to their primary care physician (4). The likelihood of migraine, however, increases in those that present with a chief complaint of headache. A study from a Seattle-based health maintenance organization found a prevalence of migraine headache of 57% in those that consult with their primary care physicians for a complaint of headache (5). Another study discovered a prevalence of migraine or migrainous headache (lacking one diagnostic criteria for migraine) of 94% in those visiting their primary care physicians for a complaint of episodic headache (<15 days per month) and no suspicion for secondary headache disorders (6).

Failure to Recognize Migraine and to Seek Medical Consultation

Those who suffer from migraine are often unaware of their diagnosis. In a population sample, 54% of individuals with IHS migraine did not know that they experienced the disorder (7). Stress headaches and sinus headaches are the most common labels patients erroneously give their migraine symptoms (7). Poor recognition of migraine may lead to delays in seeking appropriate care as well as inappropriate and ineffective utilization of treatments. It may also produce health care under-consultation and under-diagnosis.

In the 1999 American Migraine II study (AMSII), slightly less than 50% of migraine sufferers had consulted their physician during the past year for care (8). These lapsed or never consulters may miss opportunities for appropriate education and treatment of their headaches. Only 40% of migraine patients in a managed care organization (MCO) actually sought care for their headaches despite encouragement by the MCO to participate in a program including educational materials and/or consultation (9).

Misdiagnosis

Physicians correctly diagnose migraine in only 50% of all migraine patients. They are particularly likely to miss the diagnosis in patients who have concomitant tension-type headache (TTH), high levels of emotional distress, and a high number of headache days, and in patients who are male or over 65 years of age (10). The presence of depression and/or anxiety, for example, increases the tendency to diagnose TTH (11). Additional clinical practice barriers include insufficient office visit time, multiple complaints in one office visit, comorbid depression, and lack of familiarity with diagnostic criteria among primary care physicians. In particular, migraine is frequently misdiagnosed as TTH by primary care physicians. A recent study found that 82% of patients given a diagnosis of TTH by their primary care physicians actually had migraine headache when headache experts evaluated prospective diary results.

Primary care physicians may not apply a formal diagnostic label to headaches. A study of primary care physicians from a midwestern family practice group revealed that nearly 70% of all headache diagnoses were coded with the ICD-9 code of headache NOS (Not Otherwise Specified) (12). Nearly 30% of these charts contained sufficient data to reclassify patients as likely migraine or migrainous headache using a 20-item template based on IHS criteria. Lack of a specific migraine diagnosis had treatment implications: those not receiving an original ICD-9 diagnosis of migraine were less likely to receive migraine-specific therapy and more likely to receive nonspecific treatments such as barbiturates and opioids.

As the above study demonstrates, physicians are more likely to treat with nonspecific and often ineffective abortive therapies when migraine is not diagnosed. Effective abortive treatment is important from an ethical as well as from a public health perspective (13). Ineffective treatment leads to unnecessary suffering and may affect personal and professional relationships. It may also facilitate the progression of episodic migraine to chronic daily headache (14). Unfortunately, recent studies suggest the situation has not changed over the past decade (1989-1999), with migraine remaining underrecognized, under-diagnosed, and under-treated in clinical practice (15).

Impact

The severity of migraine symptoms can vary from one attack to another, but generally some degree of disability exists with migraine headaches (16). Patterns that emerge from population-based studies reveal on average that migraine headaches are more disabling and painful and longer in duration than other types of headache. Females report more pain and disability than do males. Dramatic differences exist between headache sufferers regarding their level of functioning at work, at home, or socially when experiencing headache (17).

Migraine headache can also have a profound impact on society. The American Productivity Audit, an ongoing week-to-week telephone survey of the workforce, was used to estimate the indirect costs from headache. Lost productive time in hours/week was estimated to cost $23.7 billion per year, with the most severe impact among those without a college degree, African-Americans, and those in high-demand, low-control occupations (18).

Etiology

The exact cause of the common forms of migraine headache is unknown. Migraine frequently runs in families, and genetic vulnerabilities play an important role in its development (19). Study of a very rare form of migraine known as familial hemiplegic migraine reveals a missense mutation in the alpha-1A subunit of a neuronal specific P/Q calcium channel in 50% of affected cases (20,21). Another study reported a missense mutation in the Na+, K+-ATPase pump gene in a separate kindred with familial hemiplegic migraine and benign infantile convulsions (22). These mutations create changes in channel expression and kinetics that result in a gain or loss of function (23). This and additional work suggests that genetic factors influence the clinical expression of migraine and may be responsible for altering the threshold for development of a migraine headache after exposure to a trigger factor.

Genes involved in the more common varieties of migraine with and without aura have not yet been identified. A study of migraine sibling pairs indicates an excess allele-sharing of markers in the CACNA1A region, occurring almost exclusively in those with migraine aura (23). While this study suggests that the CACNA1A gene may be involved in the more common forms of migraine, its precise role in influencing susceptibility to typical migraine remains speculative (24). Other genetic association studies have reported positive results, but their clinical significance remains unclear (25).

Twin and family studies indicate clearly that both genetic and environmental factors affect vulnerability to migraine. A large population-based study has shown that first-degree relatives of an individual with migraine aura have a relative risk of 3.8 of developing migraine aura (20). Migraine appears in nearly three of four offspring if both parents have migraine, in two of four if one parent has migraine, and in less than one of four if neither parent expresses the migraine phenotype (20).

It is important to distinguish between the underlying central nervous system (CNS) abnormalities that render a person susceptible to attacks of migraine (the cause) and environmental or other triggering or aggravating factors that bring out this vulnerability (triggers or aggravating factors). A number of triggers are characteristic of migraine, although individual patients vary widely in their sensitivity to them. Attempts to avoid all possible triggers are generally not feasible and are of questionable value in many cases, since individual triggers may be only weak or intermittent causes of migraine. A trigger load factor (i.e., the simultaneous presence of more than one trigger) may be necessary to trigger headaches in many patients. So, for example, a woman with migraine may be able to have a glass of wine or stay up late on occasion without incurring a subsequent headache, but if these two triggers are combined she may be more prone to headache.

Commonly mentioned triggers for migraine include alcohol, caffeine withdrawal, falling estrogen levels (such as occur during the week off the birth control pill or with naturally occurring menstrual periods), lack of sleep, and emotional or physical stress. Physicians may be likely to diagnose TTH if the patient reports that headaches are triggered by emotional stress. However, migraine is also commonly associated with stress. In a study of 69 consecutive patients with migraine, 72% of patients indicated that stress was at least sometimes responsible for triggering their migraines.

Pathophysiology

Migraine is a neurovascular disorder. Neurophysiological studies show differences between the central nervous systems of those with and without migraine. Studies have demonstrated hyperexcitability of neurons within the occipital cortex and elsewhere, whereas other studies support hypoexcitability (26,27). Brainstem auditory-evoked potentials may be abnormal in migraine patients. Auditory-evoked potentials dampen with a repetitive auditory stimulus in normal individuals (referred to as *habituation*), while this fails to happen in migraine patients (27,28). This suggests that migraineurs may not be not able to filter out repeated sensory stimuli. Subtle hypermetria (a sign of cerebellar dysfunction) may also exist in migraine patients, perhaps suggesting a possible CACNA1A-associated dysfunction (29). Other explanations for migraine have suggested serotonergic abnormalities in the central nervous system, mitochondrial dysfunction, or alterations in levels or activity of nitric oxide. These explanations are not mutually exclusive, but their significance remains to be clarified.

Aura Phase

The vascular theory of migraine postulated that the aura was secondary to vasospasm of cerebral arteries leading to the neurologic symptoms of the migraine aura. Recent studies have demonstrated that the aura is a primarily a neurological event, as evidenced by 1) a mismatch of hypoperfusion and hyperperfusion of cerebral blood flow to that of the pattern of head pain in migraine clinically (30), and 2) discovery of cortical spreading depression (CSD), which is a depolarization wave that moves across the brain cortex at 2 to 3 mm/min followed by decreased neuronal activity. CSD is associated with the failure of brain cell homeostasis with influx of calcium ions and efflux of excitatory amino acids, potassium, and hydrogen ions from cortical nerve cells (31). Oligemia often accompanies the wave of cortical depression, because cortical blood flow decreases in response to decreased neuronal activity. However, this oligemia is rarely in the ischemia range and is not thought to account for the neurological symptoms of migraine aura. The location of the spreading wave will influence the neurological symptoms. If the wave of cortical depression involves the visual cortex, a visual aura will result, and if it involves the motor cortex, motor symptoms will ensue. Experimental CSD can activate the trigeminovascular system, providing a possible link between aura and the headache phase of migraine (32).

Headache Phase

The trigeminal nerve and its innervation of dural blood vessels are important in the pathogenesis of the headache phase of migraine (Fig. 4-1) (33). During the headache phase of migraine, trigeminal nerve terminals release neuropeptides such as calcitonin gene-related peptide (CGRP). CGRP release leads to dilation of dural arteries, in turn causing further activation of the trigeminal nerve, sending orthodromic impulses to second- and third-order neurons in the brainstem and thalamus, respectively, and finally to the parietal cortex where further pain processing occurs (34). Additional trigeminal nerve release of other neuropeptides (possibly substance P) creates a sterile neurogenic inflammation around dural arteries. The trigeminal pain pathways are modulated by serotonergic (5-HT) receptors that reside on the peripheral trigeminal nerve, as well as second-order brainstem neurons and the dural arteries. 5-HT1D and 5-HT1F receptors are located on the trigeminal nerve and second-order nerves (trigeminal nucleus caudalis) within the brainstem; 5-HT1B receptors reside on dural arteries. Agonists of the 5-HT1D receptor deactivate the trigeminal nerve, and agonists of the 5-HT1B receptor cause vasoconstriction of the dural arteries (35). Both the triptans and ergots work as agonists of these two serotonin receptors, which accounts for their ability to decrease pain transmission in first-,

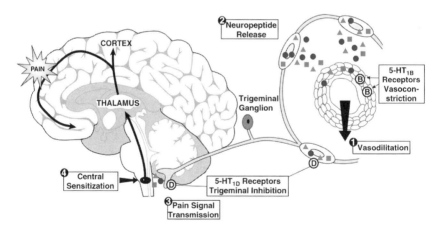

Figure 4-1   Pathophysiology of migraine headache. (1) Vasodilatation occurs and the trigeminal nerve becomes activated. (2) Neuropeptides such as calcitonin gene-related peptide are released from the trigeminal nerve, leading to further vasodilatation of the dural blood vessels. The vasodilatation is perceived as a painful stimulus by the trigeminal nerve. (3) The painful stimulus is transmitted from the peripheral trigeminal nerve to second-order neurons in the brainstem. (4) Second-order neurons in the brainstem are activated and sensitized, leading to a relay of the painful stimulus to third-order neurons in the thalamus and later to the cerebral cortex, where pain is perceived. (Adapted from Hargreaves RJ, Shepheard SL. Pathophysiology of migraine: new insights. Can J Neurol Sci. 1999;26(Suppl 3):S16.)

second-, and third-order neurons of the trigeminovascular pain pathways. Nitric oxide is another potent vasodilator whose precise role in migraine remains to be determined. A CGRP inhibitor has recently shown efficacy in the treatment of migraine, suggesting that a new class of migraine treatment may eventually be available (35a).

Diagnosis

International Headache Society Criteria

The diagnosis of migraine is made on the basis of patient history because no biochemical marker is available. According to the IHS's classification of headache disorders, first published in 1988, migraine headache may be classified as migraine with aura and migraine without aura (36). The classification was updated in 2004, although few substantive changes were made to the diagnostic criteria for migraine in adults.

A diagnosis of migraine cannot be made based on description or observation of a single attack. Rather, the diagnosis is based on a pattern of attacks. The IHS criteria outline a set of symptoms that constitute migraine, no one of which is necessary or sufficient to make a diagnosis of migraine.

Signs and Symptoms

Migraine is a recurrent headache disorder marked by combinations of characteristic signs and symptoms, including

- A severe, often unilateral headache most commonly located over the temple
- Pain that is described as throbbing, pounding, or pulsating
- Nausea, vomiting, and other gastrointestinal disturbances
- Aversion to strong sensory stimuli such as bright light, loud sounds, or strong smells
- Temporary intensification of pain with movement or physical activity

Although none of these characteristics is required for the diagnosis of migraine, the presence of a combination of these features should prompt consideration of the diagnosis. Very frequent migraine attacks (occurring 15 or more days per month) are termed *chronic migraine*. Since the majority of sufferers have intermittent attacks, separated by periods of headache-free time, chronic migraine is now considered a complication of migraine. The migraine attack can be arbitrarily divided into various phases, each of which may be missing, mild, or prominent in an individual patient, and which are characterized by certain recognizable features.

Prodrome, experienced by many patients, consists of a premonitory phase occurring hours or days before the onset of aura or headache. It is marked by vague symptoms such as changes in mood, food cravings, yawning, or changes in gastrointestinal activity. In some patients, prodrome occurs consistently enough that it can be considered a valuable warning sign of impending headache and prompt early action such as use of relaxation techniques, sleep, or medication intake that may forestall a headache. Aura is described below. Only 15% to 30% of patients with migraine experience aura. Patients may find it difficult to describe their aura symptoms, and asking them to record them may clarify diagnosis.

Headache generally begins at mild intensity and builds up slowly over several hours to reach peak intensity. If untreated, most headaches will progress to moderate or severe intensity that either makes normal activities difficult or prevents them entirely. Prompt treatment of the mild phase of headache (with medication or nonmedication strategies) may be more successful than later treatment in limiting both the severity and duration of the attack. Patients typically describe the pain as throbbing or pounding, especially if they are describing an untreated or unsuccessfully treated attack. Many patients, though, deny such characteristics of the pain, and it is important to remember that pounding or throbbing, while characteristic of migraine, is not required for diagnosis. While the location of the pain is often unilateral, over one temple or the other, generalized pain, pain felt in the neck or occiput, or even pain over the face or sinus area all can occur in migraine.

Postdrome is a phase that is commented upon by many patients and consists of symptoms very similar to those noted in the prodromal phase of an attack. Soreness of neck muscles, fatigue, and aversion to physical exertion are especially commonly mentioned aspects of this part of migraine.

Migraine with Typical Aura

According to IHS criteria, migraine with aura is defined by the characteristics of the aura and does not even require a headache to fulfill criteria for the diagnosis (Table 4-1). Migraine aura is a transient neurological disturbance that evolves gradually, lasts for 4 to 60 minutes and generally precedes the headache by 15 to 30 minutes. These transient neurological disturbances can take many forms:

1. Visual symptoms, which are the most common symptoms of aura, such as blind spots, flashing lights, geometric shapes, or zigzag lines
2. Sensory symptoms such as numbness or paresthesias of the trunk and/or extremities
3. Motor symptoms such as aphasia and hemiparesis

Aura may precede and disappear before the onset of headache. Less commonly, it can last into or even beyond the headache. Aura without

---

Table 4-1   International Headache Society Diagnostic Criteria for Migraine with Aura*

A. At least two attacks meeting criteria B-D
B. Aura must be fully reversible and consist of at least one of the following symptoms:
   1. Visual
   2. Sensory
   3. Dysphasic speech
C. At least two of the following:
   1. Homonymous visual symptoms and/or unilateral sensory symptoms
   2. Aura symptoms that develop gradually over more than 5 minutes and/or different aura symptoms occur in succession over 5 minutes
   3. Each aura symptom lasts longer than 5 minutes but less than 24 hours
D. Headache begins during the aura or follows the onset of aura within 60 minutes
E. Not attributed to another disorder

From International Headache Society. The International Classification of Headache Disorders, 2nd ed. Cephalalgia. 2004;24(Suppl 1):9-160; with permission.
*"Migraine with aura" headaches are termed "typical aura with migraine headache" under the new diagnostic criteria. If the patient has hemiplegia as the aura symptom, the headaches are termed "hemiplegic migraine".

---

headache can occur on occasion in patients who usually experience the two together. Migraine with aura is experienced by 15% to 30% of all migraineurs, although aura may not occur with every headache (36).

Migraine without Aura

Migraine without aura is diagnosed through identification of a constellation of symptoms. Current IHS criteria require seven questions to be answered to diagnose migraine headache: four related to the characteristic symptoms of the headaches, two related to associated symptoms, and one combining requirements for the minimum number of occurrences and typical duration (Table 4-2). Although no one symptom absolutely rules in or out the diagnosis, individual symptoms vary in their sensitivity and specificity (Table 4-3) (37). Characteristics with high sensitivity include nausea, moderate-to-severe intensity, and photophonia/phonophobia, and their absence makes migraine less likely. A connection of headaches with menstruation is very frequent in migraine (see Chapter 9). Migraine headache is more likely if symptoms with high specificity are present: nausea, worsening of pain with physical activity, pulsating/throbbing, and unilaterality. Migraine without aura comprises 70% to 85% of all migraine headache, and both varieties of migraine can coexist in the same patient.

    It is important to bear in mind that the strict IHS criteria for migraine were constructed to ensure a uniform population of migraineurs for clinical trials, not designed for use in clinical practice. While adopted worldwide

Table 4-2   International Headache Society Criteria for Migraine without Aura

A. At least 5 attacks fulfilling criteria B-D
B. Headache attacks lasting 4-72 hours (untreated or unsuccessfully treated)
C. Headache has at least two of the following characteristics:
   1. Unilateral location
   2. Pulsating quality
   3. Moderate or severe pain intensity
   4. Aggravation of or causing avoidance of routine physical activity (e.g., walking or climbing stairs)
D. During headache at least one of the following:
   1. Nausea and/or vomiting
   2. Photophobia and phonophobia
E. Not attributed to another disorder

From International Headache Society. The International Classification of Headache Disorders, 2nd ed. Cephalalgia. 2004;24(Suppl 1):9-160; with permission.

Table 4-3   Sensitivity and Specificity of Individual IHS Migraine Criteria

IHS Criteria	Sensitivity	Specificity
Nausea	0.81	0.83
Photophonia or phonophobia	0.88	0.63
Worse with physical activity	0.66	0.75
Unilateral	0.52	0.74
Moderate-to-severe pain	0.91	0.41
Throbbing or pulsating	0.62	0.76

Adapted from Martin V, Penzien D, Andrews M, Houle T. The predictive value of abbreviated diagnostic criteria for migraine headache [Abstract]. Headache. 2002;42:417.

by nearly all headache specialists, strict IHS criteria are used uncommonly. Only two thirds of the membership of the American Headache Society use IHS criteria, and they are often used alongside clinical judgment to make the diagnosis (38). The IHS criteria are even less commonly used within primary care practices and have been criticized as being too lengthy and cumbersome for use within this setting.

Coexisting Migraine and Tension-Type Headache and Resultant Misdiagnosis

Although TTH is known to be the most commonly experienced headache in the general population, pure episodic TTH is encountered infrequently in clinical practice because patients rarely consult for this condition alone (39,40). The Spectrum Study required patients to have disabling headache, and all patients were assigned an IHS diagnosis of migraine, migrainous (probable migraine or migraine minus one IHS criteria), or TTH. All 432 patients then recorded the characteristics of their headaches in a headache diary for up to 10 attacks. Headache experts compared the initial diagnosis of headache with a final diagnosis of headache after review of the headache diaries. Twenty-four of the 75 patients initially diagnosed with TTH met criteria for migraine or migrainous disorder. Among study participants, 90% of subjects with disabling headache ultimately met IHS criteria for a migraine-related disorder. Therefore, disabling headaches, even if initially diagnosed as migrainous or tension-type headaches, likely represent migraine headache (40).

The Landmark Study evaluated the diagnosis of headache in primary care patients. Patients were included if they reported episodic headache (<15 days per month with headache) and had no secondary cause of headache. Patients received an initial diagnosis of headache by their primary care physician and kept a diary describing the characteristics of six headache attacks. Headache experts later reviewed the headache diaries, and a final headache diagnosis was assigned. Upon review of the headache diaries, 94% of all patients had one or more attacks that met IHS criteria for migraine or migrainous headache. When the initial diagnosis of the primary care physician was migraine headache, it was correct 98% of the time (using the review of headache diaries as the gold standard for the diagnosis). When the clinician diagnosed non-migraine TTH, 87% of patients still met IHS criteria for migraine-related disorders.

The aforementioned studies as well as others demonstrate that symptoms of both migraine and TTH are often reported by the same patient. The combination of migraine and TTH was formerly termed *mixed headache syndrome* but is now identified as *coexisting migraine and TTH*. Migraine and TTH coexist in more than 50% of patients. Patients often do not describe the headache characteristics well and typically report symptoms of more than one type of headache or mix features of both in their description. These overlapping factors may lead to misdiagnosis.

Chronic Migraine

The revised IHS criteria include a new type of migraine. Chronic migraine is defined as migraine headache occurring on 15 or more days per month for more than 3 months in the absence of medication overuse. Most patients do not develop chronic migraine de novo; rather, it develops over time in patients who initially experience episodic migraine without aura. The new criteria require careful distinction of coexisting migraine and TTH from chronic migraine.

Abbreviated Migraine Diagnostic Criteria

There have been various attempts to develop abbreviated migraine diagnostic criteria or algorithms to facilitate diagnosis in primary care. These approaches can be categorized into symptom-based, disability/impact-based, or combined. Most attempts to simplify the diagnosis have focused on a symptom-based approach using current IHS criteria. Solomon found that a four-variable model requiring nausea/vomiting, throbbing, unilaterality, and phonophobia/photophobia had a sensitivity of 99% and a specificity of 62% in the diagnosis of migraine headache when two or more variables were present (41). Martin reported that a one-variable model of nausea had a sensitivity of 81% and a specificity of 83% in the diagnosis of migraine and migrainous headache (37).

Disability-based approaches have focused on the impact of disability of the patients from their headaches. It is postulated that headaches which impair the function of the patient in work, social, or household activities likely represent migraine headache (42). Maizels reported that episodic severe or disabling headaches had a sensitivity of 93% and specificity of 63% for episodic migraine headache (43). The Headache Impact Test-6 (HIT-6), a validated questionnaire assessing the impact of migraine on the function of patients, had a sensitivity and specificity of 83% and 85%, respectively, for the diagnosis of migraine headache when a cutoff score of 54 was used (44). HIT-6 and other disability assessment tools are discussed in more detail in the following section.

A third approach represents a combination of symptom- and disability-based approaches. A recent Canadian study first labeled patients with daily headaches as nonmigraineurs. Those remaining were sequentially asked the following questions:

1. Is your headache on one side of your head?
2. Does your headache stop you from doing things?

A positive response to either question yielded a sensitivity of 86% and specificity of 73% for the diagnosis of migraine headache (45). Lipton found that a three-variable model of nausea, disability, and photophobia (any two) had a sensitivity of 81% and a specificity of 75%. This three-question screener was administered as a written questionnaire and was tested in primary care patients with disabling headache or in those that wanted to discuss their headache with their physicians (46).

It is believed that these abbreviated diagnostic tools could simplify the diagnosis of migraine in primary care if confirmed in validation studies. An algorithm has been proposed for their use in primary care and involves just two steps (Fig. 4-2) (47). The first step consists of excluding any possible secondary headache disorders (47,48). If there is no suspicion for a secondary headache disorder, then the second step is to use one of the abbreviated tools to diagnose migraine headache. Although no tool has been shown to be superior to any other, the one-variable models of nausea and disabling headaches are appealing because of their simplicity. It should also be noted that only one of the abbreviated tools has been developed

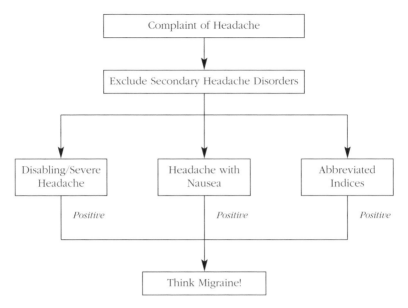

Figure 4-2   Algorithm for diagnosis of migraine headache.

exclusively in a primary care population and none has been validated in a second study to test their transportability (46). Until such validation by a second study, the abbreviated tools serve best as guides and not as absolute gold standards for the diagnosis of migraine headache.

Assessing Disability

Two questionnaires have been developed to assess the disability of migraine headache and can be useful in primary care. The Migraine Disability Assessment (MIDAS) Questionnaire was developed to determine the impact of migraine on the individual, the family, and society (see Appendix V). It is scientifically valid and measures disability by determining disability days (49). Disability days are defined as lost days or days with 50% or less function for work, housework, and social/family activities during the preceding 3 months. The number of disability days are totaled, and the total is graded on a scale of 1 to 4 based on the number of disability days per 3-month period. Severe disability is determined when there are 21 or more disability days during the past 3 months. In addition to its usefulness in diagnosing migraine, this questionnaire may be particularly helpful in guiding choice of therapy, as well as in determining a response to abortive and preventive therapies when measured serially (42).

HIT-6 (see Appendix IV) covers a broad range of headache impact and accurately estimates the severity of that impact. It is easy for patients and physicians to score and may be useful as a first-stage screener to identify migraine sufferers. Seventy-five percent of those with a score above 60 meet migraine diagnostic criteria (44,50).

Comorbidities and Consequences

Although comorbid and coexistent conditions may confound the diagnosis of migraine, they also provide an opportunity to streamline management of several conditions simultaneously. Comorbid conditions include respiratory, gastrointestinal, gynecological, cardiac, psychological, and neurological dysfunctions. A partial list includes allergy/asthma, irritable bowel syndrome, colitis, patent foramen ovale, and stroke. Because stroke and depression can be life-threatening, comorbid and coexistent conditions must be considered when planning a treatment strategy for a given patient. By doing so, therapies can be chosen that treat both migraine and the comorbid condition or a treatment that may be contraindicated for a comorbid disease can be avoided.

Psychological and Neurological Comorbidities

Important psychological and neurological comorbidity exists between migraine and the following disorders: depression, anxiety, panic, bipolar disorder, epilepsy, and essential tremor. Twenty-six percent of patients with bipolar disorder met IHS migraine criteria, indicating a greater risk for bipolar patients to develop migraine (51). Migraine prevalence was 77% in bipolar II disorder patients admitted consecutively to an open psychiatric ward, whereas prevalence was only 14% in bipolar I disorder (52). The risk of depression and migraine has been shown to be bi-directional, with each increasing the risk of first onset for the other. There was a three-fold increase in the expression of migraine following depression, while previous migraine predicted subsequent depression with a nearly six-fold increased risk (53). Anxiety and migraine reveal similar associations, with a relative risk of approximately four-fold. The converse has not been proven. Studies of epilepsy-migraine comorbidity revealed prevalence of migraine of 24% in probands with epilepsy, 26% in relatives with epilepsy, and 15% in relatives without epilepsy (54). In a small study of essential tremor, migraine was present in 36% of essential tremor patients and 18% of controls. Controlling for gender differences between groups yielded an odds ratio (OR) of 3.2, indicating significant comorbidity (55).

Stroke Comorbidity

Migraine increases the risk for stroke in any individual under age 45 and particularly for women under age 35. This association is independent of atherogenic risk factors in women and persists after controlling for vertigo, syncope, and epilepsy (56). The risk of stroke increases approximately two-to three-fold for migraine without aura and approximately six- to eight-fold for migraine with aura. The risk is complicated by use of combined oral contraceptives (OCs) (OR, 13.9) and in those who smoke one or more packs per day (OR, 10) (57). Combined or sequential pills containing 30 μg estrogen are associated with one third reduced risk compared with a higher dose, and no increased risk is associated with progestogen-only contraception (58). One study found that the risk for stroke was the same in female migraineurs with and without aura but that a multiplicative effect occurred in women using combined OCs or with a history of high blood pressure or smoking. Furthermore, a change in the frequency or type of migraine while using OCs did not predict stroke. This study found that between 20% and 40% of strokes in women with migraine seemed to develop directly from a migraine attack (59).

The risk of cerebral ischemia attributable to migraine is 20% in women below 35 years of age. Due to the very low incidence of cerebral ischemia in the young, the absolute risk for stoke remains low overall, at 8 per 100,000 non-migraine population, 17 per 100,000 any migraine individual, and 52 per 100,000 in individuals with migraine with aura (59).

Migraine with aura is approximately twice as common in individuals with patent foramen ovale and cryptogenic stroke as in those without patent foramen ovale, particularly when associated with atrial septum aneurysm (60,61). The influence of patent foramen ovale on the frequency of stroke and the effects of closure on migraine with aura continues to be investigated (62).

Neurological Consequences

Recent studies suggest that frequent migraine headache might be associated with neurological consequences. Kruit et al reported a higher incidence of asymptomatic cerebellar infarcts in migraine patients with more frequent migraine (>1 attack per month) when compared with controls (OR, 9.3 [95% CI, 1.1 to 76]) (63). Another study suggested increased iron deposition in the periaqueductal gray in those with more frequent migraine headaches (64). It is unknown if these potential neurological consequences are clinically significant or whether therapies might prevent their development.

Treatment

Identifying Migraine Triggers and Making Lifestyle Changes

Some patients find no appeal in nonpharmacological therapy, whereas others prefer non-drug therapy. For still others, modification of headache trigger factors is critical if disability is to be avoided. Overall patient satisfaction increases when attention is paid to these and other behavioral issues (65). Especially, accurate knowledge of potential migraine triggers increases a patient's sense of control over the disorder.

Understanding the complexity of migraine triggers is necessary for educating patients and interpreting their diary information. Not all triggers are equally potent. Patients consistently report stress, menstruation, changes in sleep, fasting or skipping meals, and weather changes (in that order) as their most common provokers. A small minority of patients reported exogenous dietary triggers, with alcohol the most frequent (66). The time from exposure to a trigger to the onset of migraine depends on the specific trigger but generally ranges from several hours to 72 hours (67). Exposure to multiple triggers at the same time may be more likely to lead to migraine headache. On the other hand, a trigger may not inevitably provoke a headache. The likelihood that trigger exposure will lead to a migraine probably depends on the potency of the trigger as well as the vulnerability of the central nervous system at the time of exposure (68).

It is not practicable for patients with migraine to avoid exposure to *all* known migraine triggers. A good general recommendation is to avoid the most common triggers (stress, change in sleep habits, and fasting or skipping meals) by making the following healthy lifestyle changes:

- Practice good sleep hygiene
- Avoid skipping meals
- Exercise regularly and keep well hydrated
- Maintain consistent work/school routines and minimize exposure to stress

Biofeedback, yoga, and meditation, along with reduction of work and social obligations that are unrealistic to maintain, all make sense as well.

No evidence supports the routine recommendation of a migraine diet because dietary triggers are reported by fewer than 30% of migraineurs, and diets have not shown efficacy in prospective trials. For patients who want to identify dietary triggers, use of a headache diary is recommended (see Appendix III). A potential dietary trigger can be suspected if a food or beverage leads to a new headache or worsening of an existing headache within 24 hours in more than 50% of exposures (68).

Abortive Migraine Therapy

The primary goal of acute episodic migraine therapy is to achieve freedom or relief from the pain, associated symptoms, and disability of migraine headache within 2 hours after treatment, while using abortives on two or fewer days per week. Most patients with infrequent migraine will not require preventive medications if provided with migraine-specific therapies to treat the specific attack. Even in patients who do receive preventive medication, abortive agents will still be required by essentially all patients because

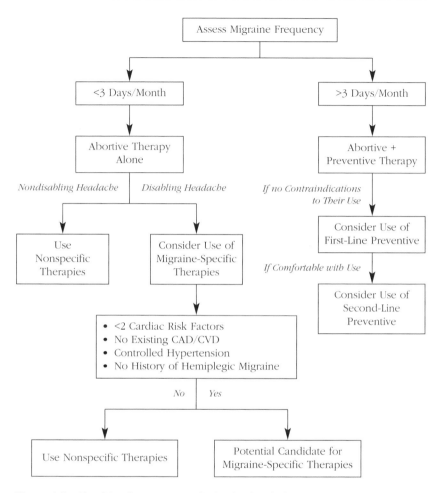

Figure 4-3 Algorithm for treatment of migraine headache. CAD = coronary artery disease; CVD = cerebrovascular disease.

preventive regimens tend to reduce migraine frequency by no more than 50%. Secondary goals of treatment include the minimization of rescue medications (i.e., back-up medications) and the prevention of a recurrence of migraine (a return of moderate-to-severe migraine 2 to 24 hours after administration of an abortive). However, no acute therapy is universally effective for every patient. Approximately 80% of attacks respond to first-line abortive medications. Many patients will therefore require a rescue medication (e.g., anti-inflammatories, triptans or dihydroergotamine, combination analgesics, narcotics, butalbital-containing medications*) for migraines that are inadequately treated (Fig. 4-3).

---

*Quantities of the last two should be limited to prevent medication overuse.

Medication Options and Their Efficacy

Abortive medications for migraine are categorized as either specific or non-specific. Migraine-specific medications are used to treat headache attacks in patients with a diagnosis of migraine headache (or cluster headaches), whereas migraine-nonspecific medications can be used to treat those with migraine as well as other headache disorders. In 2001, the United States Headache Consortium published efficacy-based guidelines for the choice of abortive medications for migraine. With these recommendations, the efficacy of a treatment was based on the strength of evidence demonstrated by randomized controlled trials. Medications were rated as A if more than one randomized controlled trial were positive, B if at least one randomized controlled trial were positive, and C if expert consensus suggested efficacy (but no randomized trial existed). The levels of evidence for the efficacy of the various specific and nonspecific migraine treatments are shown in Table 4-4.

Timing of Treatment

Older studies of the triptans (a group of medications including sumatriptan etc.) were conducted in migraine patients who were experiencing

Table 4-4   Options for Abortive Migraine Medication

Medication Class	Common Examples	Level of Evidence*
Migraine-nonspecific		
NSAIDS	Aspirin, ibuprofen, naproxen	B
Butalbital-containing medications	Butalbital/aspirin/caffeine	C
Combination analgesics	Aspirin/acetaminophen/caffeine[†]	A
	Isometheptene	B
Opioids	Butorphanol	A (nasal spray)
	Acetaminophen with codeine	A
	Meperidine	B
D2-receptor antagonists	Metoclopramide, prochlorperazine	A
Migraine-specific		
Triptans	Almotriptan, eletriptan, frovatriptan, naratriptan, rizatriptan, sumatriptan, zolmitriptan	A
Ergots	Dihydroergotamine	A (nasal spray), B (parenteral)
	Ergotamine/caffeine	B

* Level of evidence: A = multiple randomized controlled trials supporting efficacy; B = at least one randomized controlled trial supporting efficacy; C = expert panel consensus.
[†] Studies conducted in migraineurs with mild-to-moderate pain and no vomiting.

moderate-to-severe pain intensity. Triptans were very good at reducing the severity of pain at 2 hours, but migraineurs were pain free only 20% to 40% of the time. More recent studies have suggested that early treatment of migraine (when the pain is mild) may improve pain-free rates at 2 hours (69,70). Pooled results from two prospective studies of early treatment of migraine with sumatriptan found a 2-hour pain-free rate of 68% (71). There are also some data that early treatment of migraine with ergots and NSAIDS may improve its outcome (72).

Scalp Tingling or Pain When Touched During a Migraine

This is an example of allodynia, which is defined as pain resulting from stimuli that would not normally be perceived as noxious (e.g., a light touch of the skin). The presence of allodynia during a migraine attack indicates that second- and third-order neurons of the trigeminal nerve (located within the brainstem and thalamus) have become sensitized to painful/nonpainful stimuli. This central sensitization may alter the effectiveness of the triptans. A recent study reported that a 6 mg subcutaneous dose of sumatriptan produced a 2-hour pain-free rate of 93% in nonallodynic patients and a 15% pain-free rate in allodynic patients (72a).

Allodynia occurs in 79% of migraine attacks and begins during the first hour of migraine, reaching maximal severity 2 to 4 hours after onset (72b). These data suggest that there is a critical time period in which to treat migraine. Patients should treat migraine as early as possible after the start of pain but before the development of allodynia. However, this approach may not be practicable in those with daily or frequent migraine because it could lead to medication overuse.

Stratified and Stepped-Care Approaches to Treatment

Primary care physicians commonly use a step-care approach to the treatment of diseases such as hypertension and asthma. Step-care uses less expensive and sometimes less effective therapies before proceeding to more expensive and possibly more effective therapies, whereas a stratified approach matches the therapy to the treatment needs of the patient. A recent study compared step-care with the stratified approach in the abortive treatment of migraine headache (73). The stratified approach used a triptan for patients with more disabling migraine and a combination of aspirin/metoclopramide for patients with less disabling migraine. The stratified approach was found to be superior to the step-care approach, with improved pain relief at 1 and 2 hours post-dose. This has led to the recommendation that migraineurs with moderate-to-severe disability should use migraine-specific therapy as initial treatment but may start with non-specific therapy when disability is believed likely to be mild (74).

With the stratified approach, if a patient can reliably predict a low-impact attack, high-dose aspirin or NSAIDs, combination analgesics, anti-emetics, and isometheptene are recommended (47,48,73,74). Acetaminophen monotherapy is not recommended due to lack of efficacy and high recurrence rate (73). These treatments need to be taken at the first sign of the headache process, which may be at the warning pre-headache stage or at prodrome when identifiable (75). For patients in whom a higher-impact headache can be predicted, migraine-specific medications such as the triptans or dihydroergotamine are recommended (47,70).

Migraine-Specific Medications

Triptans
Seven triptans are commercially available in the United States:

- Almotriptan
- Eletriptan
- Frovatriptan
- Naratriptan
- Rizatriptan
- Sumatriptan
- Zolmitriptan

Available evidence indicates that all seven triptans are effective and tolerable. Table 4-5 lists their formulations and recommended doses. All work by mimicking the actions of serotonin at 5HT1-B and -D receptors on the trigeminovascular pain pathways. Triptans can be divided into those that are faster or slower acting, based on pooled research data. Almotriptan, eletriptan, rizatriptan, sumatritpan, and zolmitriptan are faster acting (achieving pain relief within 2 hours), whereas frovatriptan and naratriptan are slower acting (achieving pain relief within 4 hours). Frovatriptan and naratriptan

Table 4-5   Dosages of the Triptans

Generic	Tablet Strength	Optimum Dose*	Maximum Daily Dose	Additional Formulations
Almotriptan	6.25 & 12.5 mg	12.5 mg	25 mg	—
Eletriptan	20 & 40 mg	40 mg	80 mg	—
Frovatriptan	2.5 mg	2.5 mg	7.5 mg	—
Naratriptan	2.5 mg	2.5 mg	5 mg	—
Rizatriptan	5 & 10 mg	10 mg	30 mg	MLT
Sumatriptan	25, 50, & 100 mg	50 mg	200 mg	SC, NS, PR (Europe)
Zolmitriptan	2.5 & 5 mg	2.5 mg	10 mg	ZMT, NS

Data from Spierings ELH. Optimum-dose determination of the triptans [Abstract]. Headache. 2000;40:433-4.
*Two criteria have been applied to the optimum-dose determination for the triptans: 1) the highest effective dose that is associated with side effects numerically similar to placebo, and 2) the lowest dose that provides maximum therapeutic benefit where the therapeutic effect levels off at a certain point.

have significantly longer half-lives (6 hours for naratriptan and 26 hours for frovatriptan) than the other triptans, and it appears that they have a longer duration of action, perhaps with lower headache recurrence (76). These medications may be helpful for headaches with high recurrence rates, for long-duration headaches, and for the prophylaxis of menstrual migraine (an off-label use for these drugs) (77). Almotriptan and naratriptan have better tolerability and may be useful in patients who experience side effects from other triptans (Table 4-6) (78).

Small differences in outcome measures were reported between the triptans in a recent meta-analysis (78). The clinical significance of these differences is controversial, especially because all the trials were derived from the treatment of migraine headache with moderate-to-severe pain. It is unknown if these differences would persist if trials were conducted with early treatment. No studies have been conducted comparing the triptans when treating mild pain.

SIDE EFFECTS

Triptans are well tolerated, with side effects occurring in fewer than 15% of patients. Before use, however, patients should be warned about side effects, which include paresthesia of the extremities, neck/jaw tightness, chest tightness, dizziness, and difficulty with concentration.

CONTRAINDICATIONS

Contraindications for triptan use include known coronary artery disease, having more than two risk factors for coronary artery disease, cerebrovascular disease, uncontrolled hypertension, and hemiplegic and basilar migraine. If triptans must be used in those with two or more cardiovascular risk factors, an appropriate cardiac evaluation should be performed beforehand.

Triptans are weak vasoconstrictors of cerebral and coronary arteries through their agonism of 5HT1-B receptors. Although rare, cardiac and cerebrovascular events have been reported within 24 hours after the

Table 4-6 Clinical Uses of the Triptans	
Faster-acting	Almotriptan, eletriptan, rizatriptan, sumatriptan, zolmitriptan
Lower recurrence rates*	Eletriptan, naratriptan, frovatriptan
Lower side effect rates	Almotriptan, naratriptan
Prophylaxis of menstrual migraine[†]	Naratriptan, frovatriptan

Data based on meta-analysis from Ferrari MD, Roon KI, Lipton RB, et al. Oral triptans (serotonin 5-HT 1B/1D agonists) in acute migraine treatment: a meta-analysis of 53 trials. Lancet. 2001;358:1668-75.
* Recurrence is defined as a headache that improves from moderate to severe at baseline to mild or no headache at 2 hours post-dose, then returns to moderate to severe at 2 to 24 hours post-dose. The significance of recurrence rates is controversial because recurrence is predicated on an initial response to therapy.
[†] Not FDA approved for this indication.

administration of the triptans. Because both migraine and cardiovascular events are common, it is uncertain whether the triptans directly caused the event or were associated by chance occurrence. Prospective clinical trials of the triptans have demonstrated a very low risk of cardiovascular events in patients with fewer than two cardiac risk factors (79). Post-marketing data of sumatriptan found an incidence of 1.9 cardiac events per million administrations of the drug. Such data should be interpreted cautiously, however, because some cardiac events may not have been reported. Therefore triptans should only be used in patients with a low risk of cardiovascular disease.

DRUG INTERACTIONS

Drug interactions have been reported with some of the triptans. Monoamine oxidase (MAO) inhibitors should be not administered in patients receiving triptans metabolized by MAO pathways, which include sumatriptan, rizatriptan, and zolmitriptan. Sumatriptan contains a sulfa moiety and should be avoided in patients with sulfa allergies. Eletriptan is a substrate for the CYP3A4 metabolic pathways, so its use should be avoided with administration of CYP3A4 inhibitors such as clarithromycin, ketoconazole, itraconazole, nelfinavir, ritonavir, nefazadone, and troleandromycin. Rizatriptan should be reduced to 5 mg in those receiving propranolol therapy because it can alter the metabolism of rizatriptan (80).

Ergots

From a cardiac perspective, ergots are less safe than triptans because of their greater and more prolonged agonism of 5HT2 receptors, which cause coronary vasoconstriction. Oral ergotamine is no longer a recommended acute treatment for migraine. An expert consensus panel compared ergotamine with triptans and offered six reasons for avoiding the use of ergots, including poor efficacy, poor tolerability, and cardiovascular concerns due to duration of vasoactive effects (81).

Dihydroergotamine, an ergot derivative, may be administered intranasally, intramuscularly, subcutaneously, or intravenously and represents a very good migraine-specific abortive agent, but it may cause more nausea than the triptans. Because it is an ergot derivative, coronary vasoconstriction remains a concern.

Nonspecific Analgesics

Analgesics that are not specific for migraine include

- NSAIDs
- Butalbital-containing medications
- Opioids
- D2-receptor antagonists
- Tramadol

Nonspecific analgesics (especially barbiturates and opioids, including butorphanol nasal spray) generally do not terminate the migraine attack but can reduce the pain severity and discomfort of the headache. However, although nonspecific analgesics address the discomfort of the pain, they do so only if absorbed. Oral opioids are poorly absorbed in migraine and are associated with nausea and subsequent sedation, which may be problematic. Addiction is rare, but psychological and physical dependence are practical realities, as is the progression of the headache syndrome if overuse ensues. Opioids may be necessary in some patients as rescue medication, but they must be strictly regulated to, ideally, not more than 10 to 15 tablets or capsules per month. Barbiturates were recommended as rescue therapy by one guideline but are rarely effective if not used early in the course of migraine (82). Tramadol is sometimes effective and has a lower abuse potential than opioids or barbiturates, and it may be considered in patients who are unable to use specific therapy or NSAIDs.

Combined Migraine-Specific and Nonspecific Therapy

Combined therapy is the co-administration of a triptan with an NSAID or other analgesic. Package insert labeling does not contraindicate such combined therapy nor does it provide data on proven tolerability, safety, or efficacy. It is believed, based on clinical and anecdotal experience, that such an approach increases efficacy without significant side effects. The Disabilities in Strategies of Care trial showed a benefit of co-therapy: those who started with aspirin therapy and added a triptan 4 hours later were slightly more likely to have benefited from treatment than those who received the triptan or aspirin alone (73). One should not, however, use a triptan and ergot (or two different triptans) within 24 hours of one another, because their combined use could theoretically increase the risk of vasospastic events.

Medication-Overuse Headaches

Most headache experts believe that any acute medication can cause medication overuse or rebound headaches, although good-quality clinical evidence of this is lacking. The use of analgesic medications 3 or more days per week is considered analgesic overuse and may lead to the progression of episodic migraine to chronic migraine. Therefore acute medication use should be monitored to prevent development of analgesic overuse and headache (82). This can be done by the prescription of reasonable but appropriate amounts of acute drugs with written instructions not to exceed 2 days per week on average. Refills should be monitored because frequent refill requests are a red flag for medication overuse. Generally, it is recommended that not more than 2 days per week of triptan or simple analgesic medication use be allowed as abortive therapy for migraine headache. Medication-overuse headache and its treatment are discussed in Chapter 7.

Preventive Therapy

The traditional goals of migraine prevention therapy are to

1. Reduce attack frequency, severity, and duration
2. Improve responsiveness and reduce use of abortive medications
3. Improve ability to function
4. Reduce the disability of migraine while minimizing side effects

Prevention may also improve outcomes for comorbid or coexistent disorders (e.g., depression, hypertension, seizure disorders) because many preventives treat both disorders.

Preventive therapies should be considered in patients with frequent migraines (more than 3 to 5 days per month with migraine), a poor response or intolerance to migraine abortive medications, or significant disability with migraine headache. Acute medication use (more than 2 days per week on average) should also prompt consideration of prophylaxis. Preventive therapy is also indicated for patients who simply prefer it over abortive therapy. It should be kept in mind that recommendations for initiation of preventive therapy are by consensus and are not evidence-based.

Setting Realistic Expectations

It is important for the patient to have realistic expectations. *No prophylactic treatment eliminates all headaches.* Prophylactic medications for migraine are only 50% effective, at best, in reducing the frequency of migraine attacks (83). Also, it may take 1 to 2 months of preventive therapy to experience a reduction in migraine headache. Therefore patients need to be told that a complete cure for headache is not possible with current migraine preventives and that it may take some time to see an improvement.

General Principles

Low doses of preventive medication are used initially, then gradually increased. The dose may need to be increased until there is

1. A 50% or better reduction in frequency, severity, or duration of existing migraines, or
2. Intolerable side effects are experienced, or
3. Maximal beneficial dose is reached

The effective dose of the preventive is then maintained for 4 to 6 months. After 6 to 12 months, the patient should be weaned off the medication. A headache calendar (diary) may be used to monitor the success of a preventive therapy. Patients can record the average severity of their migraines on a calendar and bring it in for review at the time of the office visit. Periodic office visits will be necessary to attain the goals of preventive therapy.

No clinical trial data exist to guide the decision about how long a patient should be maintained on preventive medication. Many physicians attempt to taper and discontinue medication once the patient has had 4 to 6 months of a stable, acceptable level of headache activity. If headaches worsen, the effective medication can be restarted.

Side Effects

Side effects are the main determinant of compliance. Discussing the most frequent and serious adverse effects of preventives with the patient will enhance patient ownership of the process. Some of the most common side effects include weight gain, teratogenicity, GI problems, fatigue and lethargy, and cognitive disturbances (Table 4-7).

A nearly universal adverse effect of migraine drug prevention is weight gain, particularly with antidepressants such as the tricyclic antidepressants and the anticonvulsants such as divalproex sodium and gabapentin. Topiramate, with recent trials demonstrating good efficacy in migraine prevention, is associated with weight loss, making it a good choice for obese or overweight patients. Other preventive medications should be used cautiously in those with obesity.

Another major concern is teratogenicity in women of child-bearing age. Most of the migraine preventives have a C or D classification (a C category designation indicates that risk to the fetus cannot be excluded; a D designation indicates possible evidence of risk) by the Food and Drug Administration's Use in Pregnancy Rating System. For example, two commonly used preventive medications, divalproex sodium and amitryptyline, have a D rating in the FDA classification. For these reasons, adequate contraception and plans for pregnancy should be discussed with women of child-bearing age who require the use of migraine preventives. Some of the anticonvulsants can alter the effectiveness of OCs, so patients may need to use other forms of contraception. Other anticonvulsants do not require dose adjustment. For example, a recent study of topiramate (84) showed that doses of 50 to 200 mg did not alter the pharmacokinetics of OCs containing norethindrone and ethinyl estradiol. Caution, however, should still be exercised when using topiramate at doses over 200 mg/day with OCs.

Medication Options and Their Efficacy

The choice of preventive medications depends on efficacy, side effects, potential teratogenicity, and cost, as well as physician familiarity and comfort with their use. Based on these criteria, preventive drugs have been categorized as first-, second-, and third-line agents. First-line agents include the beta-blockers, tricyclic antidepressants, calcium channel blockers, NSAIDs,

Table 4-7   Dosages and Side Effects of Common Migraine Preventives

Preventives	Dosages	Common Side Effects
Propranolol	*Short-acting* • Starting dose: 10-20 mg tid • Titration: increase daily dose by 30-60 mg every 4 wks • Maintenance dose: 40-240 mg/day *Long-acting* • Starting dose: 80 mg PO qd • Titration: increase by 80 mg every 4 wks • Maintenance dose: 80-240 mg PO qd	Fatigue, atrioventricular block, nightmares, bradycardia, decreased exercise tolerance, sexual dysfunction
Verapamil	*Long-acting* • Starting dose: 180-240 mg PO qd • Titration: Increase by 180-240 mg every month • Maintenance dose: 180-240 mg PO qd or bid	Constipation, dizziness, peripheral edema, bradycardia, hypo-tension, tremors
Amitriptyline	• Starting dose: 10 mg PO qhs • Titration: Increase by 10 mg incre-ments as tolerated at 2-4 wk intervals • Maintenance dose: 10-75 mg PO qhs	Sedation, dry mouth, weight gain
Ibuprofen	• Starting dose: 400-800 mg tid • Titration: Uncertain if necessary • Maintenance dose: Same	GI side effects; avoid in renal failure
Naproxen sodium	• Starting dose: 550 mg PO bid • Titration: None • Maintenance dose: Same	GI side effects; avoid in renal failure
Rofecoxib	• Starting dose: 12.5 -25 mg qd • Titration: None • Maintenance dose: 12.5 -25 mg qd	Diarrhea; avoid in renal failure
Celecoxib	• Starting dose: 100 mg qd • Titration: Uncertain if necessary • Maintenance dose: 100-200 mg bid	Rash in sulfa allergic patients; avoid in renal failure
Fluoxetine	• Starting dose: 20 mg PO qd • Titration: Uncertain if necessary • Maintenance dose: 20-40 mg PO qd	Insomnia, induction of mania in those with bipolar disorder
Divalproex sodium	*Short-acting* • Starting dose: 125 mg tid • Titration: Increase to 250 mg PO tid at 2-4 wks, then 500 mg PO tid 2-4 wks later if tolerated • Maintenance dose: 250-500 mg PO tid	Weight gain, tremulous-ness, teratogenic side effects, hepatotoxicity, pancreatitis

(cont'd)

Table 4-7   Dosages and Side Effects of Common Migraine Preventives
(cont'd)

Preventives	Dosages	Common Side Effects
Divalproex sodium (cont'd)	*Extended-release* • Starting dose: 500 mg PO qhs • Titration: Increase from 500 to 1000 mg at 1 wk to 1 month • Maintenance dose: 500-1500 mg PO qhs	
Gabapentin	• Starting dose: 100 mg PO tid • Titration: If tolerated, increase to 300 mg PO tid for 2-4 wks, then 400 mg PO tid for 2-4 wks, then 600 mg PO tid for 2-4 wks, then 800 mg PO tid • Maintenance dose: 100-800 mg PO tid	Lethargy, dizziness, teratogenic side effects
Topiramate	• Starting dose: 25 mg PO qhs • Titration: Increase by 25 mg increments at 2-4 wk intervals • Maintenance dose: 25-200 mg PO qhs or 25-100 mg PO bid	Weight loss, kidney stones in 1-2%, metabolic acidosis, paresthesia, short-term memory loss (not permanent), glaucoma, teratogenic side effects

and fluoxetine. Cost-effectiveness analysis supports the use of tricyclic antidepressants and beta-blockers as starting treatments in primary care (83). Second-line therapies include anticonvulsants such as divalproex sodium, gabapentin, and topiramate. Although effective for treating migraine, anticonvulsants are listed as second-line agents because of their relative unfamiliarity among primary care physicians and their potential teratogenicity in women. The use of gabapentin in primary care, however, appears to be rapidly increasing. Third-line agents such as MAO inhibitors, botulinum toxin injections, and methysergide are uncommonly used in primary care settings and require special oversight for optimal efficacy and safety. At the time of this writing, methysergide is unavailable in the United States. Table 4-7 lists dosages of the common migraine preventives.

As was done for abortive medications, in 2001 the US Headache Consortium published recommendations regarding the strength of evidence for preventive therapies in treatment of migraine headache (85). At that time, there were no published preventive studies of topiramate, but the Consortium rated topiramate as having level A evidence (i.e., more than one randomized control was positive) based on preliminary trial results (86,87). As more experience with and evidence about the drug are gained, it is likely to become a first-line preventive agent. The ratings of other preventive medications are shown in Table 4-8.

Table 4-8   Strength of Evidence for Preventive Medications

Medication Class	Common Examples	Level of Evidence*
Category 1	**Proven high efficacy and mild-to-moderate side effects**	
Amitriptyline	TCA	A
Divalproex sodium	AED	A
Propranolol	Beta-blocker	A
Timolol	Beta-blocker	A
Methysergide	Serotonin antagonists	A
Topiramate[†]	Anticonvulsant	A
Category 2	**Lower efficacy and mild-to-moderate side effects**	
Aspirin, fenoprofen, flurbiprofen, ketoprofen, mefenamic acid, naproxen, naproxen sodium	NSAIDs	B
Atenolol	Beta-blocker	B
Gabapentin	AED	
Nimodipine, verapamil	Calcium channel blocker	B
Fluoxetine	SSRI	B
Botulinum toxin type A[††]	Neuromuscular blocker	B
Category 3	**Based on opinion, not controlled trials**	
Bupropion, venlafaxine, fluvox-amine, sertraline, mirtazapine, paroxetine, protriptyline, imipramine, doxepin, nortrip-tyline, trazodone, diltiazem	SSRI, subsets; TCAs and single tetra-ploid	C

*Level of evidence: A = multiple randomized controlled trials supporting efficacy; B = at least one randomized controlled trial supporting efficacy; C = expert panel consensus.
[†] Topiramate was not included in the US Consortium statement because studies were not complete at that time. The present authors, however, believe that there are sufficient data to place topiramate in the A category.)
[††] Botulinum toxin was not included in the US Consortium statement because studies were not complete at that time. The present authors, however, believe that there are sufficient data to place botulinum toxin in the B category.)

Beta-Blockers

Beta-blocker trials consistently show efficacy in migraine, with more than 40 controlled trials for propranolol alone (88). Others with proof of benefit, albeit much less studied, include metoprolol, timolol, atenolol, and nadolol. The FDA has approved propranolol and timolol for migraine prophylaxis. Their mechanism of action is theorized to be via inhibition of adrenergic pathways and modulating effects on the serotonergic system (89). Common side effects include fatigue, positional dizziness, nausea, depression, insomnia (often with associated nightmares), bradycardia, decreased exercise tolerance, and sexual dysfunction.

Calcium Channel Blockers

Trials of calcium channel blockers (CCB) trials have consistently provided evidence of efficacy for flunarizine, which is not available in the United States (88). Verapamil is the best studied and most widely used CCB in the United States, yet two of three studies suffered problems from high drop-out rates, while the third did not show significant benefit. Other CCBs are not adequately studied because of limited open-label trials (diltiazem and amlodipine), a likely poor cost-effectiveness ratio (nimodipine), or failed placebo-controlled trials (nifedipine). The mechanism of action of CCBs is not known, although they may decrease contraction of vascular smooth muscle, neuronal hypoxia, and prostaglandin synthesis. Side effects include constipation, dizziness, peripheral edema, bradycardia, hypotension, and tremors. Overall, calcium channel blockers are considered migraine preventive agents with mild-to-moderate efficacy, although anecdotal experience suggests that, for unknown reasons, they may be more effective in those with migraine with aura.

NSAIDs

NSAIDs have grade B evidence of efficacy as reported in the US Headache Consortium Guidelines and include fenoprofen, flurbiprofen, ketoprofen, mefenamic acid, naproxen, and naproxen sodium. Of these, naproxen sodium has the best supporting evidence (90,91). One as-yet unpublished trial showed modest efficacy for the Cox II antagonist rofecoxib 25 mg daily compared with placebo. Typical side effects include gastrointestinal and renal toxicities with low-intensity anti-platelet effects.

Tricyclic Antidepressants

Trials of tricyclic antidepressants support the use of amitriptyline as a preventive for migraine headache (92). The use of other tricyclic antidepressants such as doxepin, imipramine, nortriptyline, desipramine, and protriptyline has been based on uncontrolled studies, anecdotal reports, and clinical habit. They are most commonly used in those with comorbid depression. The choice of a tricyclic antidepressant is based on its side-effect profile, with some causing more sedation and weight gain than others. The drugs listed below are ranked from most-to-least sedative and appetite stimulating:

- Amitryptyline
- Doxepin
- Imipramine

- Nortriptyline
- Desipramine
- Protriptyline

It would thus be appropriate to choose amitryptyline or doxepin if a patient has insomnia, and nortriptyline, desipramine, imipramine, or protryptyline if there is no insomnia. If weight gain is undesirable, then protriptyline or desipramine would be preferable. All tricyclic antidepressants are nonspecific reuptake inhibitors of multiple monoamines such as serotonin, dopamine, and noradrenaline, and they affect the regulation of these synaptic receptors and second messenger systems as well. In addition, side effects typically include dry mouth, blurred vision up close, constipation, palpitations, urinary retention, tremors, and confusion. Inducement of mania in bipolar patients with depression and seizures due to lowering of the seizure threshold in susceptible individuals may occur.

Divalproex Sodium

Five prospective trials have yielded definitive proof of the efficacy of divalproex sodium, and it has obtained FDA approval for migraine prophylaxis (93-96). It exists in short-acting and long-acting formulations; both have proven efficacy in migraine prevention (97). There have been no head-to-head comparisons of the short- and long-acting formulations, but cross-study comparisons suggest that the short-acting formulation may have higher efficacy. Efficacy appears to be to due to the ability of divalproex sodium to increase GABA activity in the brainstem and to block Na- and T-type Ca channels. Glutamate receptor antagonism is uncertain. A one-year open-label safety and tolerability trial revealed side effects of sedation, tremors, hair loss, confusion, and a low incidence of weight gain (98). Rare hepatotoxic reactions, teratogenicity, platelet dysfunction, pancreatitis, and idiosyncratic reactions including elevation of barbiturate levels have been reported.

Gabapentin

Gabapentin is perhaps the most widely used anticonvulsant of the class but has limited data supporting its use for migraine prophylaxis. Two randomized placebo-controlled trials exist, and one undersized comparator trial is available for analysis (99,100). Mechanistic activity on GABA potentiation is thought important with L-type calcium channel activity with uncertain sodium and glutamate antagonism. Side effects are primarily sedation and dizziness with little drug-drug interaction or organ dysfunction.

Topiramate

Topiramate trials have demonstrated efficacy for migraine prophylaxis, with an anticipated FDA migraine indication in 2004 (86,92,101,101a). A recent randomized placebo-controlled trial evaluated the efficacy of topiramate in the prevention of migraine headache. Participants receiving daily doses of 100 and 200 mg of topiramate experienced a 50% or greater reduction in migraine frequency in 47% and 49%, respectively (102). This anticonvulsant is structurally unique in that it is the only monosaccharide-derivative neuronal stabilizing agent (NSA). Besides having a mechanism of action similar to divalproex sodium, topiramate has additional calcium channel effects, definite glutamate receptor antagonism, and carbonic anhydrase inhibition. These additional actions produce the broadest spectrum of CNS effects of currently available NSAs. Side effects of topiramate include weight loss, paresthesia, cognitive dysfunction such as language disorders, blurred vision due to secondary angle closure glaucoma, and predisposition to kidney stone formation. Metabolic acidosis may occur, and periodic measurements of serum biocarbonate are recommended for patients on topiramate. It is worth noting that the clinical trial size and methodological rigor of the topiramate migraine prevention trials are impressive and set a new standard for the field (102).

Botulinum Toxin

Subcutaneous injections of botulinum toxin type A have been demonstrated in one randomized controled trial to be effective in the prevention of migraine headache; in addition, there are numerous open-label trials supporting its use (103,104). The most effective dosage remains to be clarified, but most studies have injected 25 to 150 U into 12 to 20 sites in the supraorbital, frontal, temporal, occipital, and cervical regions. Its mechanism of action is uncertain, but botulinum toxin is believed to work by muscle paralysis as well as by sensory modulation through decreased release of neuropeptides (104). Side effects are few but include pain at the injection site and possible eyebrow or eyelid ptosis.

Monoamine Oxidase Inhibitors

Monoamine oxidase inhibitors are specialty headache center drugs for refractory headache patients. Benefit is based primarily on anecdotal experience; the US Headache Consortium rated phenelzine as a Group 3 drug whose use was based on consensus and clinical experience with no scientific evidence of efficacy (85). Drug-drug interactions contraindicate their use with meperidine, sympathomimetics, and MAO inhibitor metabolized triptans. Dietary restrictions abound and require special dietary education with a nutritionist for optimal safety. The mechanism of action is the blockade of monoamine deamination of norepinephrine and serotonin. Side effects are significant and include, but are not limited to, insomnia or excess sedation, orthostatic hypotension, weight gain, sexual dysfunction, hyperhidrosis, edema, depression, and irritability.

Common Migraine Myths

Myth: Migraine is always one-sided.

Fact: Up to 40% of attacks may be described as generalized or bilateral.

Myth: To avoid medication overuse, patients should be instructed to treat only when the headache is intense.

Fact: Treatment is more effective and headache recurrence less likely if treatment occurs early, while the headache is still mild.

Myth: Children do not get migraine.

Fact: Migraine is quite common in children. Diagnostic criteria in children allow for headache duration of 1 to 72 hours because attacks are generally shorter than those occurring in adults.

Myth: If a migraine occurs with menstruation, it is a menstrual migraine and requires special treatment.

Fact: Although falling estrogen levels associated with menstruation do increase the chance that a migraine will occur (in at least 70% of women with migraine), usual treatments for migraine (e.g., the triptans) are generally effective for these attacks. In addition, some headaches occur with the menstrual period by chance alone.

Myth: People who have migraine are often under a lot of stress. Telling them to relax is helpful.

Fact: Stress is a well-recognized trigger or aggravating factor for migraine, but it is not the underlying cause. Patients resent being told "just relax" but respond well to suggestions that learning to cope more effectively with stress is one way they can gain control over headaches.

■   ■   ▓

Key Points

- Migraine is the most common primary headache disorder encountered in primary care but is frequently misdiagnosed or missed.
- Headache associated with nausea or disability is likely migraine.
- Migraine-specific therapies (e.g., the triptans) are preferred for patients who have migraine that is disabling. They work best when used early in the headache.
- Preventive therapy is necessary when patients have frequent or disabling headaches or a poor response to abortive therapies.

■   ▓   ▓

REFERENCES

1. **Menken M, Munsat TL, Toole JF.** The global burden of disease study: implications for neurology. Arch Neurol. 2000;57:418-20.
2. **Lipton RB, Stewart WF.** Migraine headaches: epidemiology and comorbidity. Clin Neurosci. 1998;5:2-9.

3. **Lipton RB, Stewart WF, Diamond S, et al.** Prevalence and burden of migraine in the United States: data from the American Migraine Study II. Headache. 2002;41: 646-57.

4. US Waiting Room Study: Headache World 2000 symposia. Pfizer; unpublished data on file.

5. **Osterhaus JT, Towsend RJ, Gandek B, et al.** Measuring the functional status and well-being of patients with migraine headache. Headache. 1994;34:337-43.

6. **Dowson AJ, Dahlof C, Tepper S, et al.** The spectrum of headaches experienced by migraineurs in a primary care setting [Abstract]. Cephalalgia. 2002;22:591.

7. **Lipton RB, Stewart WF, Liberman JN.** Self-awareness of migraine: interpreting the labels that headache sufferers apply to their headaches. Neurology. 2002; 58(Suppl 6):S21-S26.

8. **Lipton RB, Diamond S, Reed M, et al.** Migraine diagnosis and treatment: results from the American Migraine Study II. Headache. 2001;41:638-45.

9. **Solomon GD, Hu H, Conboy K, et al.** Impact of migraine disease management. The Medica Migraine Disease Management Study: Humanistic Outcomes [Abstract]. Cephalalgia. 2002;22:596.

10. **Stang PE, VonKorff M.** The diagnosis of headache in primary care: factors in the agreement of clinical and standardized diagnoses. Headache. 1994;34:138-42.

11. **Diamond ML.** The role of concomitant headache types and non-headache comorbidities in the underdiagnosis of migraine. Neurology. 2002;58(Suppl 6):S3-9.

12. **Smith R, Hasse LS, Ritchey PN.** Migraine and unspecified headaches and their treatment in family practice. Is there a headache treatment problem in family practice [Abstract]? Cephalalgia. 2002;22:604.

13. **Spierings ELH.** Abortive treatment. In: Migraine: Questions and Answers, 2nd ed. West Palm Beach, FL: Merit; 2002:80-1.

14. **Osterhaus JT, Towsend RJ, Gandek B, et al.** Measuring the functional status and well-being of patients with migraine headache. Headache. 1994;34:337-43.

15. **Lipton RB, Diamond S, Reed M, et al.** Migraine diagnosis and treatment: results from the American Migraine Study II. Headache. 2001;41:638-45.

16. **Stewart WF, Shechter A, Lipton RB.** Migraine heterogeneity: disability, pain intensity, and attack frequency and duration. Neurology. 1994;44:S24-39.

17. **Holroyd KA, Malinoski P, Davis MK, et al.** The three dimensions of headache impact: pain, disability and affective distress. Pain. 1999;83:571-8.

18. **Stewart WF, Ricci JA, Chee E, Lipton R.** Employer burden of headache in the United States: results from the American Productivity Audit [Abstract]. Cephalalgia. 2002;22:600.

19. **Russel MB, Olesen J.** Increased familial risk and evidence of genetic factor in migraine. BMJ. 1995;311:541-4.

20. **Ophoff R, Terwindt GM, Vergouwe MN, et al.** Familial hemiplegic migraine and episodic ataxia type-2 are caused by mutations in the Ca2+ channel gene CACNL1A4. Cell. 1996;887:543-96.

21. **Hans M, Luvisetto S, Williams ME, et al.** Functional consequences of mutations in the human alpha-1A calcium channel subunit linked to familial hemiplegic migraine. J Neurosci. 1999;19:1610-9.

22. **Vanmolkot K, Kors E, Hottenga J, et al.** Navel mutations in the Na+, K+ATP1A2 associated with familial hemiplegic migraine and benign familial infantile convulsions. Ann Neurol. 2003;54:360-6.

23. **Twerwindt GM, Ophoff RA, van Eijk R, et al.** Involvement of the CACNA1A gene containing region on 19p13 in migraine with and without aura. Neurology. 2001;56:1028-32.

24. **Lea RA, Curtain RP, Hutchins RP, et al.** Investigation of the CACNA1A gene as a candidate for typical migraine susceptibility. Am J Med Genet. 2001;105:707-12.

25. **Kors E, Haan J, Ferrari M.** Migraine genetics. Curr Pain Headache Reports. 2003; 7:212-7.

26. **Aurora SK, Cao Y, Bowyer SM, Welch KMA.** The occipital cortex is hyperexcitable in migraine: experimental evidence. Headache. 1999;39:469-76.

27. **Ambrosini A, de Noordhout AM Sandor PS, Schoenen J.** Cephalalgia. 2003; 23(Suppl 1):13-31.

28. **Wang W, Timsit-Berthier M, Schoenen J.** Intensity dependence of auditory evoked potentials is pronounced in migraine: an indication of cortical potentiation and low serotonergic neurotransmission? Neurology. 1996;46:1404-9.

29. **Sandor P, Seidel L, de Pasqua V, Schoenen J.** Subclinical cerebellar impairment in the common types of migraine: a three-dimensional analysis of reaching movements. Neurology. 2001;49:668-72.

30. **Lauritzen M, Olesen J.** Regional cerebral blood flow during migraine attacks by Xenon-133 inhalation and emission tomography. Brain. 1984;107:447-61.

31. **Lauritzen M.** Pathophysiology of the migraine aura: the spreading depression theory. Brain. 1994;117:199-210.

32. **Bolay H, Reuter U, Dunn AK, et al.** Intrinsic brain activity triggers trigeminal meningeal afferents in a migraine model. Nat Med. 2002;8:136-42.

33. **Hargreaves RJ, Shepheard SL.** Pathophysiology of migraine: new insights. Can J Neurol Sci. 1999;26:S12-S19.

34. **May A, Goadsby PJ.** The trigeminovascular system in humans: pathophysiologic implication for primary headache syncromes of the neural influences on the cerebral circulation. J Cereb Blood Flow Metab. 1999;19:115-27.

35. **Ferrari MD.** Migraine. Lancet. 1998;351:1043-51.

35a. **Olesen J, Diener HC, Husstedt IW, et al.** Calcitonin gene-related peptide receptor antagonist BIBN 4096 BS for the acute treatment of migraine. N Engl J Med. 2004;350:1104-10.

36. **Headache Classification Committee of the International Headache Society.** Classification and Diagnostic Criteria for Headache Disorder, Cranial Neuralgias and Facial Pain. Cephalalgia. 1988;8(Suppl 7):1-96.

37. **Martin V, Penzien D, Andrews M, Houle T.** The predictive value of abbreviated diagnostic criteria for migraine headache [Abstract]. Headache. 2002;42:417.

38. **Nash JM, Lipchik GL, Holroyd KA, et al.** American Headache Society members assessment of headache diagnostic criteria. Headache. 2003;43:2-13.

39. **Rasmussen BK, Jensen R, Schroll M, Olesen J.** Epidemiology of headache in a general population: a prevalence study. J Clin Epidemiol. 1991;44:1147-57.

40. **Lipton RB, Cady RK, Stewart WF, et al.** Diagnostic lessons from the Spectrum Study. Neurology. 2002;58:S27-S31.

41. **Solomon S.** Diagnosis of primary headache disorder: validity of the International Headache Society criteria in clinical practice. Neurol Clin. 1997;15:15-26.

42. **Lipton RB, Goadsby PJ, Sawyer JPC, et al.** Migraine: diagnosis and assessment of disability. Rev Contemp Pharmacother. 2000;1:63-73.

43. **Maizels M, Burchette R.** Rapid and sensitive paradigm for screening patients with headache in primary care settings. Headache. 2003;43:441-50.

44. **Ware J, Bayliss M, Kosinski M, et al.** Accuracy of the headache impact test (HIT) for migraine case finding [Abstract]. Cephalagia. 2000;20:305.

45. **Pryse-Phillips W, Aube M, Gawel, et al.** A headache diagnosis project. Headache. 2002;42:728-37.

46. **Lipton R, Kolodner K, Dodick D, et al.** A self-administered screener for migraine in primary care: the ID migraine validation study [Abstract]. Headache. 2003; 43:511.

47. **Dowson AJ, Lipscombe S, Sender J, et al.** New guidelines for the management of migraine in primary care. Curr Med Res Opin. 2002;18:414-39.

48. **Dowson AJ, Sender J, Lipscombe S, et al.** Establishing principles for migraine management in primary care. Int J Clin Prac. 2003;57:493-507.

49. **Stewart WF. Lipton RB, Kolodner K, et al.** Reliability of the migraine disability assessment score in a population-based sample of headache sufferers. Cephalalgia. 1999;19:107-14.

50. **Ware JE, Bjorner JB, Dahlof C, et al.** Development for the headache impact test (HIT) using item response theory (IRT) [Abstract]. Cephalalgia. 2000;20:309.

51. **Mahmood T, Romans S, Silverstone T.** Prevalence of migraine in bipolar disorder. J Affect Disord. 1999;52:238-41.

52. **Fasmer OB.** The prevalence of migraine in patients with bipolar and unipolar affective disorders. Cephalalgia. 2001;21:894-9.

53. **Breslau N, Lipton RB, Stewart WF, et al.** Comorbidity of migraine and depression: investigating potential etiology and prognosis. Neuorology. 2003;60:1308-12.

54. **Ottman R. Lipton RB.** Comorbidity of migraine and epilepsy. Neurology. 1994; 44:2105-10.

55. **Biary N, Koller W, Langenberg P.** Correlation between essential tremor and migraine headache. J Neurol Neurosurg Psychiatry. 1990;53:1060-2.

56. **Carolei A, Marinir C, De Matteis G.** Italian National Research Council Study on Stroke in the Young. Lancet. 1996;347:1503-6.

57. **Tzourio C, Tehindrazanarivelo A, Iglesias S, et al.** Case-control study of migraine and risk of ischaemic stroke in young women. BMJ. 1995;310:830-3.

58. **Lidegaard O.** Oral contraception and risk of a cerebral thromboembolic attack: results of a case-control study. BMJ. 1993;306:956-63.

59. **Chang CL, Donaghy M, Poulter N.** World Health Organization Collaborative Study of Cardiovascular Disease and Steroid Hormone Contraception. BMJ. 1999; 318:13-8.

60. **Lamy C, Giannesini C, Zuber M, et al.** Clinical and imaging findings in cryptogenic stroke patients with and without patent foramen ovale: the PFO-ASA Study. Atrial Septal Aneurysm. Stroke. 2002;33:706-11.

61. **Anzola GP, Magnoni M, Guindani M, et al.** Potential source of cerebral embolism in migraine with aura: a transcranial Doppler study. Neurology. 1999;52: 1622-5.

62. **Sztazel R, Genoud D, Roth S, et al.** Patent foramen ovale, a possible cause of symptomatic migraine: a study of 74 patients with acute ischemic stroke. Cerebrovasc Dis. 2002;13:102-6.

63. **Kruit MC, van Buchem MA, Hofman PAM, et al.** Migraine as a risk factor for subclinical brain lesions. JAMA. 2004;29:427-34.

64. **Welch K, Nagesh V, Aurora S, et al.** Periaqueductal gray matter dysfunction in migraine: the cause or the burden of illness? Headache. 2001;41:629-37.

65. **Lake AE.** Behavioral and nonpharmacological therapy of headache. Med Clin North Am. 2001;85:1055-75.

66. **Peatfield RC, Glover V, Littlewood JT, et al.** The prevalence of diet-induced migraine. Cephalalgia. 1984;4:179-83.

67. **Gettis A.** Viewpoint: food induced "delayed reaction" headaches in relation to tyramine studies. Headache. 1987;27:444-5.

68. **Martin VT, Behbehani MM.** Toward a rational understanding of migraine trigger factors. Med Clin North Am. 2001;85:911-41.

69. **Cady RK, Lipton RB, Hall C, et al.** Treatment of mild headache in disabled migraine sufferers: results of the Spectrum Study. Headache. 2000;40:792-7.

70. **Klapper JA, Charlesworth B, Rosjo O, et al.** Treatment of mild migraine with oral zolmitriptan 2.5 mg prevents progression to more severe migraine and reduces the impact on normal activities in patients with significant migraine-related disability. Neurology. 2002;58:A291.

71. **Winner P, et al.** Platform presentation at American Headache Society Meeting, 21-23 June 2002, Seattle. GlaxoSmithKline; data on file.

72. **Cady RK, Sheftell F, Lipton RB, et al.** Effect of early intervention with sumatriptan on migraine pain: retrospective analyses of data from three clinical trials. Clin Ther. 2000;22:1035-48.

72a. **Burstein R, Collins B, Jakubowski M.** Defeating migraine pain with triptans: a race against the development of cutaneous allodynia. Ann Neurol. 2004;55: 19-26.

72b. **Burstein R, Yarnitsky D, Boor-Aryeh I, et al.** An association between migraine and cutaneous allodynia. Ann Neurol. 2000;47:614-24.

73. **Lipton RB, Stewart WF, Stone AM, et al.** Stratified care vs. step care strategies for migraine: the Disability in Strategies of Care (DISC) Study: a randomized trial. JAMA. 2000;284:2599-605.

74. **Bedell AW, Cady RK, Diamond ML, et al.** Patient-centered strategies for effective management of migraine. Primary Care Network; 2000.

75. **Luciani R, Carter D, Mannix L, et al.** Prevention of migraine during prodrome with naratriptan. Cephalalgia. 2000;20:122-6.

76. **Geraud G, Keywood C, Senard JM.** Migrane headache recurrence: relationship to clinical, pharmacological, and pharmacokinetic properties of triptans. Headache. 2003;43:376-88.

77. **Silberstein SD, Elkind AH, Schreiber C.** Frovatriptan, a 5-HT1B/1D agonist, is effective for prophylaxis of menstrually-associated migraine [Abstract]. Neurology. 2003;60(Suppl 1):A94.

78. **Ferrari MD, Roon KI, Lipton RB, et al.** Oral triptans (serotonin 5-HT 1B/1D agonists) in acute migraine treatment: a meta-analysis of 53 trials. Lancet. 2001;358: 1668-75.

79. **Welch KM, Mathew NT, Stone P, et al.** Tolerability of sumatriptan: clinical trials and post-marketing experience. Cephalalgia. 2000;20:687-95.

80. **Tepper SJ, Millson D.** Safety profile of the triptans. Expert Opin Drug Safety. 2003;2:123-32.

81. **Tfelt-Hansen P, Saxena PR, Dahlof C, et al.** Ergotamine in the acute treatment of migraine: a review and European consensus. Brain. 2000;123:9-18.

82. **Snow V, Weiss K, Wall EM, Mottur-Pilson C.** Pharmacologic management of acute attacks of migraine and prevention of migraine headache. Ann Intern Med. 2002;137:840-9.

83. **Adelman JU, Adelman LC, VonSeggern R.** Cost-effectiveness of antiepileptic drugs in migraine prophylaxis. Headache. 2002;42:978-83.

84. **Doose D, Wang S, Padmanabhan M, et al.** Effect of topiramate or carbamazepine on the pharmacokinetics of an oral contraceptive containing norethindrone and ethinyl estradiol in healthy obese and nonobese female subjects. Epilepsia. 2003; 44:540-9.

85. **Silberstein SB for the US Headache Consortium. Practice Parameter:** Evidence-based guidelines for migraine headache (an evidence-based review): Report of the Quality Standards Subcommittee of the American Academy of Neurology. Neurology. 2000;55:754-62; and at www.aan.com/professionals/practice/pdfs/gl0085.pdf.

86. **Silberstein SD, Karim R Jordan D, et al.** Treatment effect for topiramate in migraine prophylaxis: utllity of repeated measures and weighted regression analyses. Cephalalgia. 2002;22:610.

87. **Dodick D, Neto W, Schmitt J, Jacobs D.** Topiramate in migraine prevention (MIGR-001): secondary efficacy measures from a randomized, double-blind, placebo-controlled trial [Abstract]. Neurology. 2003;60(Suppl 1):A237.

88. **Silberstein S, Saper J, Freitag F.** Migraine: diagnosis and treatment. In: Silberstein S, Lipton R, Dalessio D, eds. Wolff's Headache and Other Head Pain, 7th ed. New York: Oxford University Press; 2001:78.

89. **Silbertstein S, Silberstein M.** New concepts in the pathogenesis of headache. Part II. Pain Management. 1990;3:334-42.

90. **Bellavance AJ, Meloche JP.** Comparative study of naproxen sodium, pizotifen and placebo in migraine prophylaxis. Headache. 1990;30:710-5.

91. **Sargent J, Solbach P, Damasio H, et al.** A comparison of naproxen sodium to propranolol hydrochloride and a placebo control for the prophylaxis of migraine headache. Headache. 1985;25:320-4.

92. **Ziegler D.** The treatment of migraine. In: Silberstein S, Lipton R, Dalessio D, eds. Wolff's Headache and Other Head Pain, 7th ed. New York; Oxford University Press; 2001:87-111.

93. **Jensen R, Kurzitzky A.** Sodium valproate has a prophylactic effect in migraine without aura: a triple-blind, placebo-controlled crossover study. Neurology. 1994; 44:647-51.

94. **Klapper J, for the Divalproex Sodium in Migraine Prophylaxis Study Group.** Divalproex sodium in migraine prophylaxis: a dose-controlled study. Cephalalgia. 1997;17:103-8.

95. **Mathew NT, Saper Jr, Silberstein SD, et al.** Migraine prophylaxis with divalproex. Arch Neurol. 1995;52:281-6.

96. **Silberstein SD.** Divalproex sodium in headache: literature review and clinical guidelines. Headache. 1996;36:547-55.

97. **Freitag F, Collins SD, Carlson H, et al, for the Depakote ER Migraine Study Group.** A randomized trial of divalproex sodium extended release tablets in migraine prophylaxis. Neurology. 2001;58:1652-9.

98. **Siberstein SD, Collins SD, for the Long-Term Safety of Depakote in Headache Prophylaxis Study Group.** Safety of divalproex sodium in migraine prophylaxis: an open-label, long-term study. Headache. 1999;39:633-43.

99. **Mathew NT, Rapoport A, Saper J, et al.** Efficacy of gabapentin in migraine pro-phylaxis. Headache. 2001;41:119-28.

100. **Hernandez J, Narvaez T, Acebal F.** Effectiveness and safety of gabapentin in the preventive treatment of migraine. Rev Neurol. 2002;35:603-6.

101. **Brandes J, Jacobs D, Neto W, Bhattacharya S, for the MIGR-002 Study Group.** Topiramate in the prevention of migraine headache: a randomized, double-blind, placebo-controlled, parellel study (MIGR-002) [Abstract]. Neurology. 2003;60(Suppl 1):A238.

101a. **Silberstein S, Neto W, Schmitt J, Jacobs D.** Topiramate in migraine preven-tion: results of a large controlled trial. Arch Neurol. 2004;61:490-5.

102. **Brandes JL, Saper JR, Diamond M, et al.** Topiramate for migraine prevention: a randomized controlled trial. JAMA. 2004;291:965-73.

103. **Silberstein SD, Mathew N, Sapter J, Jenkins S.** Botulinum toxin type A as a mi-graine preventative treatment. Headache. 2000;40:445-50.

104. **Evers S.** Is there a role for botulinum toxin in the treatment of migraine? Current Pain Headache Reports. 2003;7:229-34.

5

Tension-Type Headache

Roger K. Cady, MD

Curtis P. Schreiber, MD

Kathleen Farmer, PsyD

ension-type headache (TTH) is the most common and most commonly misdiagnosed headache condition. The experience of episodic TTH is almost universal, yet most of these headaches are mild and respond well to self-treatment; sufferers of episodic TTH rarely seek medical attention (1). In contrast, migraine, although less common than TTH, is on average more disabling and less amenable to over-the-counter (OTC) treatment. For this reason, most patients presenting in a primary care setting with a chief complaint of headache are ultimately found to have some form of migraine, not TTH. The diagnosis of TTH should be made cautiously in a medical setting: 88% of TTH diagnoses are incorrect (2), usually because the possibility of migraine has been overlooked. However, TTH is far from being an unimportant disorder. Chronic forms of TTH are disabling and often do prompt medical consultation.

The confusion about TTH is understandable. TTH has no unique diagnostic features; in fact, it is a diagnosis made by default when the characteristic features of other primary headaches are absent. The pathophysiology of TTH is also poorly understood, with explanations ranging from muscle tension to psychological stress, none of which are supported by scientific evidence.

Epidemiology

Epidemiological studies of TTH are plagued by problems with diagnostic imprecision, population definitions, and other methodological issues. Estimates of the lifetime prevalence of TTH thus vary, but all show that non-migraine headache is very common. In a Danish study the lifetime prevalence of TTH was 69% in men and 88% in women (3). A recent United States study showed a 1-year prevalence of 38.3% for episodic TTH and 2.2% for chronic TTH. Episodic TTH prevalence was highest in the fourth decade of life and increased with level of education. Chronic TTH prevalence, in contrast, was inversely related to educational level. Episodic TTH most often occurred once or twice a month, and pain intensity was generally mild or moderate. TTH was noted to be slightly more common in women than in men, but the female predominance was not as marked as for migraine. This study concluded that although the individual burden imposed by episodic TTH is modest, the condition has a significant social impact because of its prevalence. In contrast, the individual burden of chronic TTH is high, but its impact on society is lower than that of episodic TTH because it occurs less commonly (4).

A family history of TTH is obtained in approximately 6% of the population; age at onset is generally in early adulthood. As noted earlier, many patients with migraine also have headaches that meet criteria for TTH. In the American Migraine II Study, most of a cohort of 1607 subjects defined as having migraine (according to International Headache Society [IHS] guidelines) by telephone interview reported on a follow-up questionnaire that in addition to migraine they experienced TTH (5). The clinical and epidemiological overlap between migraine and TTH has led to speculation that there are two different TTH phenotypes: those with TTH accompanied by migraine headache and TTH in the absence of migraine (6,7). However, this assertion is difficult to validate in population-based epidemiological studies, especially given the lack of formal prospective studies of the natural history of migraine and TTH.

Pathophysiology

One theory about the pathogenesis of TTH is that such headaches result from transient, reversible alterations of pain-perception mechanisms in the trigeminal system (8). When the nervous system cannot adequately adjust to the level of demands placed on it, second-order neurons in the trigeminal nucleus caudalis of the brainstem become disinhibited. This allows amplification of sensory input from the trigeminal and upper cervical (skin, vascular, and myofascial stimuli among them). As with migraine, there is little scientific evidence that psychological tension or muscle contraction is the underlying cause of TTH, although emotional stress, chronobiological changes, and caffeine withdrawal are triggers or aggravating factors for the disorder (8). No trigger is unique to TTH; in fact, almost all are shared with migraine (9,10).

Similar pathophysiological mechanisms may be shared by migraine and TTH. A study of more than 1900 patients who met IHS criteria for migraine with or without aura revealed that attacks of headache in patients who did not meet criteria for migraine responded just as well to treatment with subcutaneous sumatriptan as did attacks that clearly met criteria for migraine (11). Although drug response is not reliable as a method of diagnosis, such results call into question the presumed specificity of the 5-HT-1 agonists for migraine and suggest that, at least in subjects recognized as having migraine, similar pathophysiological mechanisms are shared by migraine and TTH attacks.

These observations were confirmed by a prospective, double-blind, placebo-controlled study that assigned subjects with disabling headache* to one of three groups based on a structured clinical interview using IHS criteria (12). The first group had IHS-defined migraine as well as other attacks of headache that met criteria for both TTH and migrainous headache. The second group had IHS-defined migrainous headache (i.e., probable migraine or migraine minus one IHS criteria) as well as some attacks that met criteria for TTH. The third group had only IHS-defined TTH. All groups were asked to treat up to 10 headaches of any type with 50 mg of oral sumatriptan and keep diaries of headache-associated symptoms and response to treatment. In the group with migraine, all attacks, whether migraine, migrainous, or TTH, responded equally well to sumatriptan 50 mg. In the small population of subjects with a diagnosis of disabling episodic TTH, though, response to sumatriptan was no better than response to placebo. These results suggest that the entire spectrum of headache attacks in patients who have IHS-defined migraine are triptan-responsive and that all headaches in these patients share similar underlying pathophysiological mechanisms. Results further suggest that patients who experience only disabling episodic TTH may have a different pathophysiology underlying their headaches.

A subset of patients violated the treatment protocol and treated their headaches when their pain was mild. Two-thirds of the subjects treating mild headache with placebo experienced worsening of headache to moderate-to-severe intensity within 1 hour (13). This prompted the suggestion that both migraine and TTH evolve from the same pathophysiological process and that clinical diagnosis of headache in migraine sufferers may vary depending upon how far the migraine process has evolved at the time of diagnosis (Fig. 5-1) (14). In other words, many headaches if left untreated or observed longer would develop signs and symptoms suggesting a diagnosis of migraine.

In clinical practice, patients with headaches significant enough to cause disability rarely have the sole diagnosis of episodic TTH; almost all patients seeking medical care who have some attacks characteristic of TTH will also have attacks that meet criteria for migraine or probable migraine (15). Patients with episodic tension-type attacks with disability are rare in clinical practice. It has been suggested by many observers that migraine and TTH are not distinct entities but represent the two ends of a continuum of benign headache (16,17); this view remains controversial.

---

*As measured on the Headache Impact Test (HIT-6), a validated disability instrument; see Appendix IV.

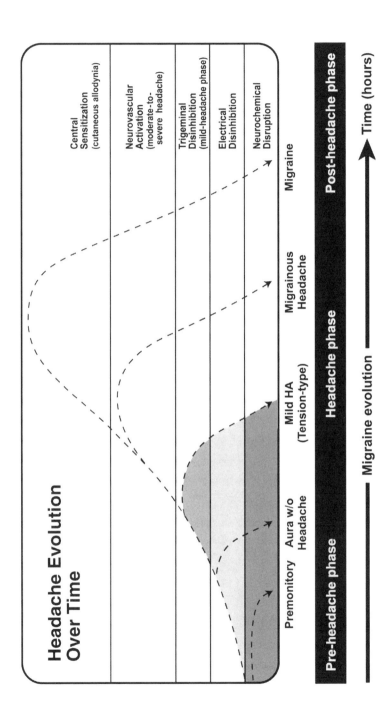

Figure 5-1 Convergence hypothesis. Tension-type and migraine headache may represent the opposite ends of a spectrum of headache. Early in the course of a headache, tension-type headache may be diagnosed, but if the headache evolves and other features such as nausea develop, a diagnosis of migraine may result.

Diagnostic Construct of Tension-Type Headache

Tension-type headache is a remarkably recent diagnostic construct. Although ancient references to migraine can be found, historical references to TTH do not occur until the mid-20th century. The first edition of the classic text *Headache and Other Head Pain,* for example, published in 1948, contains no chapter on TTH. It was not until the early 1950s that the idea of TTH became commonplace, with causation often ascribed to muscle tension or psychological stresses (18). These were attempts to describe and explain headaches that were not clearly migraine. Terms such as "muscle contraction", "stress", and "ordinary" headache were used for what is today classified as TTH.

By 1980, the authoritative textbook *Headache* included a TTH chapter. Its authors commented that "a daily, constantly recurring headache without associated focal neurological symptoms or prominent vomiting represents the clinical features that usually lead to the conclusion that a patient suffers from tension headache. The lack of boundaries between migrainous and tension headache unfortunately has led many physicians to assume that headache disorders that occur without organic explanation, and lack the stereotypic features of migraine, are tension-type headache" (19).

International Headache Society Diagnostic Criteria

In 1988 the IHS developed diagnostic criteria for the primary headache disorders and was faced with a host of descriptive terms that had traditionally been used for non-migraine primary headache. In general, these terms were diagnostically imprecise and implied causation that was not scientifically demonstrated. The IHS thus combined many of these terms (such as "tension headache", "muscle contraction headache", "idiopathic headache", and "psychogenic headache", as well as many other nonspecific headache labels) into the single category of TTH (20).

The IHS diagnostic criteria for TTH are listed in Table 5-1. The IHS recognizes infrequent and frequent episodic and chronic forms of TTH, and also distinguishes between TTH with and without associated muscle involvement. Critical features of diagnosis include a history of at least 10 attacks of primary headache that do not achieve symptoms of other primary headache disorders such as migraine, cluster, and chronic paroxysmal hemicrania.

TTH is thus defined as much by the signs and symptoms that are not present as it is by the symptoms that are present, leading some to describe TTH as the "photographic negative" of migraine. Episodic TTH is often bilateral in location, non-pulsating in quality, mild to moderate in intensity, not aggravated by activity, not associated with nausea or vomiting, and not associated with both photophobia and phonophobia (although one of these symptoms may be present). When TTH occurs more frequently than

---

**Table 5-1   International Headache Society Diagnostic Criteria for
Tension-Type Headache**

A. At least 10 previous headache episodes fulfilling criteria B-D listed below.
B. Headache lasting from 30 minutes to 7 days (except in chronic forms of the
   disorder, where headache may be longer or continuous).
C. At least two of the following pain characteristics:
   1. Pressing/tightening (non-pulsating) quality
   2. Mild or moderate intensity (may inhibit but does not prohibit activities)
   3. Bilateral location
   4. No aggravation by walking stairs or similar routine physical activity
D. Both of the following:
   1. No nausea or vomiting (anorexia may occur)*
   2. Photophobia and phonophobia are absent, or one but not the other is present
E. Not attributed to another disorder.
   Subdivision Diagnosis
   1. Infrequent episodic TTH (1 day/month on average (<12 days/year)
   2. Frequent episodic TTH (>1 day/month but <15 days/month for at least
      3 months)
   3. Chronic TTH (>15 days/month on average for >3 months)

From International Headache Society. The International Classification of Headache Disorders, 2nd ed.
Cephalagia. 2004;24(Suppl 1):9-160; with permission.
*Chronic tension-type headache may include one of these symptoms: nausea, photophobia, phonophobia.

15 days per month for at least 3 months it is classified as chronic TTH. For
unclear reasons, the diagnostic criteria for chronic TTH are more liberal
than those for episodic TTH in that they allow the presence of mild nausea
and either photophobia or phonophobia.

Episodic Tension-Type Headache

Episodic TTH is typically nondescript, usually bilateral and often described
as a "band-like" or pressure sensation. TTH is commonly devoid of associated symptoms: photophobia or phonophobia are only occasionally described; technically, only one of these associated symptoms can be present
during a single attack of TTH. Other symptoms, such as neck muscle pain,
fatigue, irritability, nasal congestion, rhinorrhea, and poor concentration
are also described by many sufferers but do not occur with enough regularity to be diagnostically useful (21). The duration of episodic headache
varies greatly but does not exceed 7 days.

Chronic Tension-Type Headache

Chronic TTH commonly presents as a daily or near-daily headache pattern.
TTH is defined as chronic when it occurs more than 15 days a month for
more than 6 months. Unlike episodic TTH, chronic TTH frequently leads to

missed work and social opportunities due to the chronicity rather than severity of the pain, and it can be difficult to treat. Clinically, chronic TTH is similar to the bilateral, pressure-like pain of episodic TTH, but it occurs on a daily or near-daily basis, presumably as a result of a nervous system that does not revert to a normal baseline state, with the result that symptoms of headache, autonomic disruption, and muscle pain persist. Chronic TTH characteristics are the same as those of episodic TTHs except that the duration can exceed 7 days. These patients frequently have other headaches with migrainous features superimposed on their background level of pain and may occasionally experience migraine-like symptoms (nausea or sensitivity to light or noise). Symptoms of neck muscle pain, fatigue, irritability, nasal congestion, rhinorrhea, and poor concentration are often more pronounced and troublesome in patients with chronic TTH than in those with episodic TTH. Chronic TTH affects 2% to 3% of the adult population (1)

In most cases, chronic TTH evolves over many years, suggesting that central sensitization of pain pathways over time may lower the threshold to future attacks of headache. Other factors that underly this transformational process may include medication overuse. Evaluation of a population of patients with daily or nearly daily headache in a tertiary headache center showed that most had transformed from migraine; only 20% began with episodic TTH, but there was significant overlap in the two populations with regard to headache-associated symptoms and response to treatment (22). Overuse of analgesics has been implicated in the transformational process, and discontinuation of these drugs often produces reversion to the episodic form of the disorder (23,24). Some patients with chronic TTH use substantial quantities of acute treatment medications, which can maintain the daily or near-daily headache pattern (a condition known as "medication overuse" or "rebound" headache). Psychological factors such as the development of entrenched medication use patterns, a sense of hopelessness, and poor coping techniques also play a role in the evolution of chronic TTH.

Why the Term "Tension-Type" Headache?

The term "tension-type" headache has replaced older terms such as "tension", "muscle contraction", and "stress" headache because there is no good evidence that patients with this variety of headache have elevated levels of either muscle or psychological tension. However, to foster research into the disorder, the IHS does allow for subdivision of TTH into those "with muscle involvement" and those "without muscle involvement". Similarly, if psychological or psychiatric factors are felt to be causative in the headache, a third-digit modifier can be added to the IHS diagnostic number. These distinctions have limited usefulness in clinical practice. Many experts consider the category of TTH to be an unsatisfactory one. Some view TTH as the mild end of a continuum of benign headaches, rather than as a separate diagnostic category.

Treatment

Episodic Tension-Type Headache

Episodic TTH is generally self-treated and rarely comes to medical attention. When TTH becomes chronic or co-exists with migraine or other conditions, it is more likely to lead to medical consultation. Particularly when a patient with episodic TTH presents for medical care, it is important to search for associated primary headache disorders or co-morbidities, especially affective disorders such as depression or anxiety, that might have influenced the decision to seek treatment. If episodic TTH is not well controlled, it can evolve into a chronic condition. Scrupulous management of individual attacks of headache, along with preventive mediations, may decrease the likelihood of progression, although this remains to be definitively demonstrated. Table 5-2 summarizes evidence-based treatments for episodic TTH (25).

Optimal treatment of episodic TTH often depends upon its association with migraine. These two primary headache disorders may occur independently of one another or, more commonly, mild TTH may evolve into a migraine headache. In the latter case, attacks may respond to migraine-specific

Table 5-2   Treatments for Episodic Tension-Type Headache

Class	Drug	Typical Individual Dosage	Comments
NSAIDs	Ibuprofen	200-800 mg	Short-term adverse effects include renal and hepatic toxicity; risk for analgesic-induced rebound headache is low; Pregnancy Category B
	Naproxen	250-500 mg	
	Ketoprofen	25-75 mg	
	Indomethacin	25-75 mg	
	Aspirin	500-100 mg	
Analgesics	Acetaminophen	650-1000 mg	
Combination analgesics	Acetaminophen/ aspirin/caffeine	1 or 2 tablets	
	Ibuprofen/caffeine	1 or 2 tablets	
	Acetaminophen/codeine	1 or 2 tablets	
	Aspirin or acetamino- phen/caffeine/ butalbital	1 or 2 tablets	
Muscle relaxants	Methocarbamol	500-750 mg	Minimal evidence exists for the efficacy of muscle relaxants with the exception of tizanidine
	Cyclobenzaprine	10 mg	
	Chloroxazone	250-500 mg	
	Tizanidine (27)	4 mg	

Adapted from Millea PJ, Brodie JJ. Tension-type headache. Am Fam Physician. 2002;66:797-804.

therapies such as triptans or ergots. In other words, in patients with a history of migraine, early symptoms of an episodic TTH attack should be treated as migraine, before migraine symptoms evolve over the course of the headache. The value of this approach has been demonstrated by a study in which stratifying patients to abortive headache treatment based on their historic pattern of headache disability yielded outcomes superior to treatment based on initial headache symptoms (26). However, although this approach is reasonable for patients with episodic headaches, it would not be practicable for those with chronic daily headaches because medication overuse could result.

When attacks of migraine and TTH occur separately, the TTH should be viewed as part of the total headache burden facing the patient. Poorly controlled TTH can lead to analgesic overuse and decrease the effectiveness of migraine therapy. As more headaches occur, TTH and migraine become symptomatically indistinct and eventually evolve into a chronic daily or near-daily headache pattern.

It is important to set therapeutic goals and limit the use of abortive medication for the treatment of episodic TTH. In most instances, a reasonable goal is improvement or elimination of the headache within 2 hours of treatment. Restricting use of acute treatment to no more than 2 days per week is also recommended to avoid medication side effects and inadvertent worsening of the headache due to analgesic rebound. If medication use routinely exceeds this limit, preventive therapy should be considered.

Reasonable lifestyle modifications include elimination or restriction of caffeine intake, regular sleep and wake patterns, regular meal schedules, and enjoyable physical activity. It is often useful to have a patient maintain a diary of headaches and treatment strategies for several months to improve compliance (see Appendix III).

Preventive treatment is rarely used for episodic TTH. Most episodes of TTH respond well to OTC medications, especially nonsteroidal anti-inflammatory drugs. If headaches are associated with significant disability, and particularly if there are symptoms characteristic of migraine, the diagnosis of TTH should be re-examined and consideration given to a migraine-specific medication such as a triptan for treatment.

Chronic Tension-Type Headache

In general, the same acute medications used for episodic TTH are employed for chronic TTH, but more care must be taken in supervising their appropriate use (Fig. 5-2). Lists of commonly used prophylactic therapies for chronic TTH are given in Tables 5-3 and 5-4. Low-dose tricyclic antidepressants are preferred by many clinicians.

Individual headache attacks in chronic TTH are often associated with more symptoms than in episodic TTH, and this form of the disorder is more frequently complicated by overuse of OTC or prescription medications.

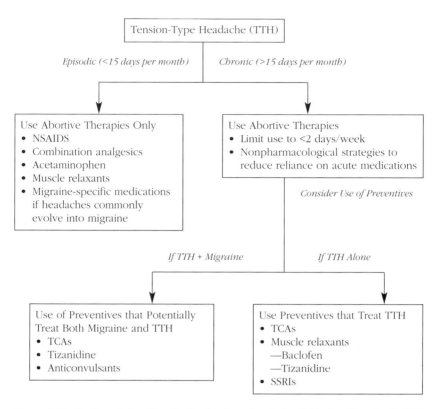

Figure 5-2   Treatment algorithm for tension-type headache. Patients with episodic TTH may only require treatment with abortive medications, whereas those with chronic TTH may require treatment with both abortive and preventive therapies. To prevent medication overuse, abortive therapies should not be administered >2 days per week in patients with chronic TTH. Patients with chronic TTH may require preventive therapies if the headaches are extremely bothersome or if abortive medications are routinely used >2 days per week. If patients have co-existing TTH and migraine, therapies should be selected that can prevent both disorders.

Medication use should be carefully assessed in all patients with this headache pattern. Non-pharmacological strategies should be emphasized as a means of reducing reliance on acute medications. Patients benefit from being taught pain-coping and cognitive-restructuring techniques, biofeedback-assisted relaxation, and other strategies for pain relief and prevention. These interventions are valuable in themselves, but they also augment the effectiveness of any medications that are used. The benefit from many of these non-pharmacological techniques is long lasting, as is the reduced reliance on pharmacological interventions (32).

Abortive treatment alone frequently elicits a poor response and can lead to medication overuse and lost school, work, or social time. Therefore, regardless of optimal abortive therapy, preventive treatment is indicated.

Table 5-3   Pharmacological Prophylaxis of Chronic Tension-Type Headache

Class	Drug	Typical Dosage	Comments
Tricyclic anti-depressants	Amitriptyline Nortriptyline Doxepin	10-150 mg/day 10-150 mg/day 10-150 mg/day	Begin at low dose and titrate slowly; efficacy may not be obvious for 2-6 months; sedation, constipation, fatigue, and weight gain are common side effects
Muscle relaxants	Tizanidine	4-8 mg tid	Trial results were in patients with chronic daily headache; some had chronic TTH, others had chronic migraine (27)
SSRIs	Fluoxetine	10-40 mg/day	Generally better tolerated than TCAs; other SSRIs may also be helpful but less data are available
Beta-blockers	Inderal Atenolol Nadolol	20-160 mg/day 10-40 mg/day 20-80 mg/day	Indicated when migraine and TTH co-exist; use with caution in asthma, diabetes, and depression; avoid in advanced heart block; fatigue and exercise intolerance are common side effects
Anti-epileptic drugs	Divalproate sodium	250-1000 mg/day	Indicated when migraine and TTH co-exist; weight gain, gastric upset, and occasional temporary hair loss are common side effects; rare hepatic toxicity; *known cause of birth defects*

Table 5-4   Nonpharmacological Prophylaxis of Chronic Tension-Type Headache

Treatment	Comments
Biofeedback, relaxation training, cognitive therapy (28)	Useful as primary treatment and as adjunctive therapy with pharmacological interventions; both thermal and EMG biofeedback effective; improvements maintained long-term
Physical therapy (29)	Massage, ice or heat, ergonomic corrections, and daily exercise likely beneficial
Acupuncture (30)	Trials of poor quality; recent review concludes that acupuncture "may" have a place in treatment
Spinal manipulation (31)	One trial comparing spinal manipulation to amitriptyline found them equally effective but benefits of spinal manipulation were not maintained

Unfortunately, preventive treatment for TTH has been less well-studied than that for migraine. Many treatments used for migraine prevention have some efficacy in TTH, although there is a clinical impression that tricyclic antidepressants, such as amitriptyline, are the most helpful. This class of medications is of benefit in many different pain disorders, which may explain its usefulness in treating several kinds of headache problems. Elevated levels of mood and anxiety disorders are seen in patients with chronic TTH, which may be another explanation for the effectiveness of tricyclic antidepressants. Other commonly used migraine preventives are anecdotally noted to be more useful when TTH and migraine co-exist. They include beta-blockers, calcium blockers, and antiepileptic drugs such as divalproex. Regarding duration of use for preventive treatment, however, there is no evidence from clinical trials on which to base recommendations. Most clinicians taper and discontinue preventive treatments after 4 to 6 months of a stable headache pattern and reinstitute the medication as headaches recur.

Nonpharmacological treatment strategies, particularly biofeedback-assisted relaxation training and use of ice, heat, or other physical therapies, are also beneficial. Given the lack of good-quality evidence for many of the drugs recommended for TTH, nonpharmacological treatments should be considered early in the course of treatment because a beneficial effect may eliminate or reduce the need to use medication on a daily basis. A systematic review of the literature has determined the efficacy of behavioral preventive therapies. The Technical Report of the Agency for Healthcare Research and Quality has identified 335 articles on behavioral treatments for migraine prevention (33). Because most patients with TTH requiring prophylaxis also have migraine, this therapy is appropriate. A review of these articles identified 70 controlled trials, of which 39 prospective randomized controlled studies that were aimed at migraine prevention met all data extraction requirements (33).

It is important to educate patients about appropriate expectations of treatment benefit. Preventive treatments are not likely to eliminate headaches entirely; most provide reductions in frequency and intensity of about 50% from the baseline headache problem. Most also take anywhere from 4 to 8 weeks to show maximal effect, so patience in assessing benefit is also important. Inadequate treatment trial length is a common reason for treatment failure. Patients who are using preventive treatment can still use abortive medications for more severe episodes of pain, particularly for the superimposed episodes of migraine that many of them experience. Those headaches, like migraine occurring in isolation from TTH, should be treated aggressively, with triptans or other disease-specific medications, unless contraindications to use exist. Special care to avoid medication overuse must be taken, though, because the frequency with which headaches occur, along with the fact that not all patients are able to judge accurately when to take medication, make medication overuse a particularly likely pitfall. Abortive treatment should still be limited to 2 to 3 days per week. It is helpful to allow patients to be in charge of deciding "when and where" they will use their allotted medication but necessary to be firm about limiting the overall quantities they are permitted.

Selection of a particular prophylactic medication strategy is often based on the side-effect profile of the medication. If patients have difficulty sleeping, a sedating tricyclic antidepressant may be most useful. If they have arthritis, scheduled use of an anti-inflammatory drug can be considered. (For more information on prophylactic medications, see Chapter 7.)

In patients with chronic and complex headache disorders, therapy must often be multifaceted. Over time, multiple mechanisms have become involved in perpetuating and maintaining headache. These include myofascial mechanisms, psychological factors, and the effects of co-morbid problems such as depression, family dysfunction, and workplace disability. A comprehensive treatment program that addresses as many of these factors as possible has the best chance of success in these cases. Sequential attention to each aspect of the problem is not as effective as intense, comprehensive treatment.

Summary

Episodic tension-type headache is extremely common. However, because it is generally mild in severity and occurs infrequently, TTH does not usually cause people to seek medical evaluation. As headaches become more frequent, however, medical consultation is increasingly likely. In patients known to have migraine, headaches with symptoms similar to those of TTH are most likely migraine and should be treated accordingly. The key goal in managing TTH is to carefully diagnose the headache and any co-morbid disorders. Management is directed towards preventing evolution to a chronic headache pattern and controlling overuse of acute treatment medications.

Key Points

- Episodic tension-type headache is common but rarely prompts medical consultation.
- Chronic tension-type headache (prevalence 2% to 3%) is disabling and likely to lead to medical consultation.
- There is considerable diagnostic and treatment overlap between migraine and tension-type headache.

REFERENCES

1. **Stewart WF, Liberman J, Lipton RB.** Prevalence of frequent headache in a population sample. Headache. 1998;38:497-506.

2. **Dowson A, Tepper SJ, Newman L, Dahlof C.** The Landmark Study. Cephalalgia. 2002;22:590-1.

3. **Rasmussen BK.** Migraine and tension-type headache in the general population: psychosocial factors. Int J Epidemiol. 1992;2:1138-43.

4. **Schwartz BS, Stewart WF, Simon D, Lipton RB.** Epidemiology of tension-type headache. JAMA. 1998;279:381-3.

5. **Lipton RB, Diamond S, Reed ML, et al.** Migraine diagnosis and treatment: results of the American Migraine Study II. Headache. 2001;41:538-45.

6. **Graham JR.** The natural history of migraine: some observations and a hypothesis. Trans Am Clin Climatol Assoc. 1952;4:1.

7. **Waters WE.** The epidemiological enigma of migraine. Int J Epidemiol. 1973;2:189-94.

8. **Silberstein SD, Lipton RB, Goadsby PJ.** Headache in Clinical Practice. Oxford: ISIS Medical Media; 1998:92-3.

9. **Spierings EL, Ranke AH, Honkoop PC.** Precipitating and aggravating factors of migraine versus tension-type headache. Headache. 2001;41:554-8.

10. **Schade AJ.** Quantitative assessment of the tension-type headache and migraine severity continuum. Headache. 1997;37:646-53.

11. **Cady RK, Gutterman, D, Saiers JA, Beach ME.** Responsiveness of non-IHS migraine and tension-type headache to sumatriptan. Cephalalgia. 1997;17:588-90.

12. **Lipton RB, Stewart WK, Cady RK, et al.** Sumatriptan for the range of headaches in migraine sufferers: results of the spectrum study. Headache. 2000;40:783-91.

13. **Cady RK, Lipton RB, Hall C, et al.** Treatment of mild headache in disabled migraine sufferers: results of the spectrum study. Headache. 2000;40:792-7.

14. **Cady RK, Schreiber CP, Farmer KU, Sheftell F.** Primary headaches: a convergence hypothesis. Headache. 2002;42:204-16.

15. **Lipton RB, Cady RK, Stewart WF.** Diagnostic lessons from the spectrum study. Neurology. 2002;58(Suppl 6):S27-S31.

16. **Featherstone HJ.** Migraine and muscle contraction headaches: a continuum. Headache. 1985;24:194-8.

17. **Raskin NH.** Headache, 2nd ed. New York: Churchill Livingstone; 1988.

18. **Friedman AP, von Storch TJ, Merritt HH.** Migraine and tension headaches: a clinical study of 2000 cases. Neurology. 1954;4:773-88.

19. **Raskin N, Appenzeller O.** Headache. Philadelphia: WB Saunders; 1980.

20. Classification and diagnostic criteria for headache disorders, cranial neuralgias, and facial pain. Headache Classification Committee of the International Headache Society. Cephalalgia. 1988;8(Suppl 7):1-96.

21. **Barbanti P, Fabbrini G, Pesare M, et al.** Neurovascular symptoms during migraine attacks [Abstract]. Cephalalgia. 2001;212-95.

22. **Mathew NT, Reuveni U, Perez F.** Transformed or evolutive migraine. Headache. 1987;27:102-6.

23. **Kudrow L.** Paradoxical effects of frequent analgesic use. In: Critchley M, Fridman A, Gorina S, Sicuteri F, eds. Advances in Neurology, volume 33. New York: Raven Press; 1982:335-41.

24. **Rapoport AM, Weeks RE, Sheftell FD.** Analgesic rebound headache: theoretical and practical implications. Cephalalgia. 1985;(Suppl 3):448-9.

25. **Millea PJ, Brodie JJ.** Tension-type headache. Am Fam Physician. 2002;66:797-804.

26. **Lipton RB, Stewart WF, Stone AM, et al.** Stratified care versus step care strategies for migraine: the Disability in Strategies of Care (DISC) study. A randomized trial. JAMA. 2000;284:2599-605.

27. **Saper JR, Lake AE, Cantrell DT, et al.** Chronic daily headache prophylaxis with tizanidine: a double-blind, placebo-controlled, multicenter outcome study. Headache. 2002;42:470-82.

28. **Attanasio V, Andrasik F, Blanchard EB.** Cognitive therapy and relaxation training in muscle contraction headache: efficacy and cost-effectiveness. Headache. 1987;27:580-3.

29. **Hammill JM, Cook TM, Rosecrance JC.** Effectiveness of a physical therapy regimen in the treatment of tension-type headache. Headache. 1996;36:149-53.

30. **Melchart D, Linde K, Fischer P, et al.** Acupuncture for recurrent headaches: a systematic review of randomized controlled trials. Cephalalgia. 1999;19:779-86.

31. **Boline PD, Kassak K, Bronfort G, et al.** Spinal manipulation versus amitriptyline for the treatment of chronic tension-type headaches: a randomized clinical trial. J Manipulative Physiol Ther. 1994;18:148-54.

32. **Holroyd KA.** Tension-type headaches, cluster headache, and miscellaneous headaches: psychological and behavioral techniques. In: Olesen J, Tfelt-Hansen P, Welch KMA, eds. The Headaches. New York: Raven Press; 1993:515-20.

33. **Campbell JK, Penzien D, Wall EM.** Evidence-based guidelines for migraine headache: behavior and physical treatments. Neurology. (Serial online; available at http://www.neurology.org. Accessed 2/25/04.)

6

Cluster Headache and Other
Autonomic Cephalalgias

C. David Gordon, MD

The typical primary care practitioner is likely to encounter only a few patients with cluster headache (CH) in a career, because this syndrome is
actually quite rare – in fact, much less common than migraine. So severe
that it is sometimes referred to as "suicide headache", CH responds to
treatment that overlaps with, but is not identical to, that for migraine.
Early recognition of CH thus has important treatment implications because
it decreases the pain and disability associated with delayed or incorrect
diagnosis.

Cluster headache is classified by the International Headache Society
(IHS) as one of a group of disorders known as the trigeminal autonomic
cephalalgias (TACs). These include cluster headache, chronic and episodic
paroxysmal hemicrania (PH), hemicrania continua (HC), and short-lasting
unilateral neuralgiform pain with conjunctival injection and tearing, generally referred to as SUNCT syndrome. Table 6-1 provides a comparison of
the important features of these related disorders.

Cluster headache is the main focus of this chapter; there are briefer discussions of the other TACs. Patients in whom a TAC besides CH is suspected should generally be referred for specialty consultation.

Cluster Headache

Epidemiology

The rarity of CH makes epidemiologic studies difficult to conduct. Perhaps
the most reliable estimates come from a study that examined the entire
population of the small Italian republic of San Marino, which produced a

Table 6-1   Differential Diagnosis of Trigeminal Autonomic Cephalalgias*

	Cluster Headache	EPH	CPH	SUNCT	HC	TN
Sex (M:F)	5:1	1:1	1:3	4:1	1:2	1:2
Age at onset (years)	20-40	6-81	6-81	30-68	11-58	50-60
Number of attacks	0-8/day	3-30/day	1-40/day	1/day – 30/hr	Varies	Up to hundreds
Duration of attacks	15-180 min	1-30 min	2-45 min	5-250 sec	Continuous	Seconds
Localization of pain	Orbital/temporal	Orbital/temporal	Orbital/temporal	Periorbital	Orbital/temporal	V1-V2
Autonomic features	++	++	++	++	+	–
Character of pain	Stabbing, boring	Stabbing, throbbing	Stabbing, boring	Lancinating	Throbbing or stabbing, superimposed upon constant dull ache	Lancinating
Precipitation by alcohol	++	+	+	+	+	–
Indomethacin responsive	+/–	++	++	–	++	–

*EPH, episodic paroxysmal hemicrania; CPH, chronic paroxysmal hemicrania; SUNCT, short-lasting unilateral neuralgiform pain with conjunctival injection and tearing; HC, hemicrania continua; TN, trigeminal neuralgia.

point prevalence estimate of 56/100,000 and a one-year incidence estimate of 2.5/100,000 (1). All studies show a male predominance for the disorder, which fact alone distinguishes it from essentially every other primary headache syndrome. The male-to-female ratio varies from study to study, though, ranging from 4:1 to almost 12:1. It has been suggested that the incidence of CH in women is increasing (2), although this may be as much due to improved recognition of the disorder as to an actual change in its epidemiology (3).

The onset of episodic cluster headache (ECH) is most commonly in the mid-to-late 20s, later than is seen for migraine and tension-type headache (1). In almost all patients, onset occurs before age 50 (2). Chronic cluster headache (CCH), in contrast, generally begins in the early 30s in men but much later in women (4). Clinical observation has suggested that certain facial characteristics (hazel eyes and seasoned facies, or peau d'orange skin) are more common in CH patients than in controls. The prevalence of alcohol use and co-morbid cardiac and peptic ulcer disease is also said to be increased among patients with CH (5). CCH appears to be associated with smoking as well, with heavy smokers also experiencing more attacks on a daily basis. Along with cigarette smoking, other unfavorable prognostic indicators associated with a high likelihood of conversion from ECH to CCH include onset at an older age (in women only), frequent cluster periods and sporadic attacks outside well-defined cluster periods, cluster periods longer than 8 weeks, and remissions of less than 6 months (6).

Cluster headache cycles seem most likely to begin following the summer or winter solstices; they are least likely to occur within several weeks of the initiation and termination of Daylight Saving Time. Once an active cycle of CH begins, individual headache attacks are characteristically provoked by the ingestion of alcohol, especially beer, although other vasodilators (such as nitroglycerin) will also trigger an attack (7).

Genetics

The contribution of genetic factors to CH is poorly understood. CH occurs with greater-than-expected frequency in relatives of patients, and various investigators have suggested a model of autosomal dominant transmission with a low co-occurrence of a separate susceptibility allele (8). CH is not associated with any of the known genetic abnormalities that have been identified in migraine (9).

Pathophysiology

The characteristic clinical presentation of CH suggests underlying pathophysiological mechanisms. The clockwork regularity of attacks strongly implicates involvement of a central brain pacemaker, almost certainly the hypothalamus. Positron emission tomography studies show increased cerebral blood flow in the region of the hypothalamus in CH patients during an attack, but not in normal controls experiencing capsaicin-induced pain in the same region (10). Structural abnormalities in the hypothalamus have also been demonstrated using voxel-based morphometric analysis of T1-weighted magnetic resonance imaging scans (11). Indirect evidence of hypothalamic dysfunction has been demonstrated in CH patients. Males with the disorder have low levels of melatonin, and there are differences in the levels of other substances secreted by the hypothalamus as well, including cortisol, endorphins, and prolactin (12). Overall, the suggestion is of hyperactivity of the hypothalamic-pituitary-adrenal system with disturbances in circadian rhythm, perhaps mediated by decreased responsiveness to melatonin.

The invariably unilateral location of CH behind one eye clearly implies involvement of the ophthalmic branch of the trigeminal nerve. The pain of CH is thought to be arise from activation of neurogenic inflammation within the trigeminovascular system, which is dependent on the participation of neuropeptides such as calcitonin gene-related peptide (CGRP), substance P, and neurokinin A, as well as vasoactive intestinal polypeptide (VIP) and nitric oxide. Finally, the characteristic autonomic features of the headache could only be produced through activation of the ipsilateral cranial parasympathetic system.

Differential Diagnosis

Some secondary causes of headache can be confused with CH. These include

- Temporal arteritis
- Cavernous sinus disease (e.g., thrombotic or vascular)
- Acute sphenoid sinus infection or other sinus disease (infection or malignancy)
- Vascular dissection
- Glaucoma
- Neoplasm within the brainstem
- Cervicogenic causes

In general, though, the cyclic presentation of stereotypic headaches conforming to a predictable circannual and circadian pattern of occurrence supports a diagnosis of recurrent CH; only a deviation from this well-established pattern suggests a need for further investigation (13). As already mentioned, other causes of headache to be considered in the differential are the other TACs. Although similarities exist between CH and other autonomic and indomethacin-responsive cephalalgias, they are usually comfortably distinguished from one another on the basis of frequency, duration, sex, age at onset, and autonomic specificity (see Table 6-1).

Diagnosis

Signs and Symptoms

Cluster headache is the most distinctive of the primary headache disorders. The individual headache attack is unmistakable and stereotyped. Sufferers report attacks of severe, strictly unilateral pain characteristically situated behind or around the eye. The attacks are much shorter than those of migraine, lasting 15-180 minutes and beginning abruptly, generally without warning. Maximal pain intensity is reached quickly, generally within 5 to 10 minutes. The headaches are accompanied by autonomic signs or symptoms such as ipsilateral ptosis, miosis, lacrimation, conjunctival injection, and nasal congestion or rhinorrhea (14).

Patients can have up to eight attacks per day and frequently note a clock-like regularity to the attacks that is uncommonly seen in any other headache disorder. In particular, the first rapid-eye-movement period during the night almost invariably provokes an attack, making many patients frightened of going to sleep. In contrast to migraine patients, who typically prefer quiet, dark rooms and avoid motion, CH sufferers commonly moan, pace, and thrash about in agony, often pounding their head or fist against the floor, even smashing furniture. Despite the headache's nickname, suicide is rarely attempted, due to the relative brevity of symptoms and suffering (15).

Cluster headache may be either episodic or chronic. *Episodic* is the most common form; sufferers experience attacks from once every other day up to eight times daily in distinct cluster cycles or periods lasting 7 days to 1 year in duration, after which they are completely free of headache for periods of at least one month, often up to years. Roughly 85% of CH patients suffer from the episodic form; of these, around 5% will eventually convert to the chronic form (7). *Chronic* cluster headache is defined by a pattern of headache activity occurring for not less than 1 year in duration, with less than 14 days of remission or no remission at all (14).

International Headache Society Diagnostic Criteria

The 2004 IHS diagnostic criteria for cluster headache are shown in Table 6-2. According to these criteria, besides being characterized by severe ulilateral pain in the orbit or surrounding area, the headache must be accompanied by *no fewer than one* of the autonomic signs or symptoms (e.g., ptosis or eyelid edema) mentioned earlier. If patients whose headache description suggests cluster headache do not report such signs, ask them to observe the next attack closely, perhaps with the aid of a mirror; this will often demonstrate the presence of additional features.

As with all headache syndromes, the diagnosis of CH relies heavily on an accurate history. Though typically benign, the physical examination is important to assess possible secondary causes of headache. Laboratory and neuroimaging studies (MRI) are normal; as with other primary headache

---

Table 6-2   International Headache Society Diagnostic Criteria for Cluster Headache

A. At least 5 attacks fulfilling criteria B-D
B. Severe or very severe unilateral orbital, supraorbital, and/or temporal pain lasting 15-180 minutes if untreated
C. Headache is accompanied by at least one of the following:
   1. Ipsilateral conjunctival injection and/or lacrimation
   2. Ipsilateral nasal congestion and/or rhinorrhoea
   3. Ipsilateral eyelid oedema
   4. Ipsilateral forehead and facial sweating
   5. Ipsilateral miosis and/or ptosis
   6. Sense of restlessness or agitation
D. Attacks have a frequency from one every other day to 8 per day
E. Not attributed to another disorder

From International Headache Society. The International Classification of Headache Disorders, 2nd ed. Cephalalgia. 2004;24(Suppl 1):9-160; with permission.

---

disorders, testing is principally useful to investigate suspected secondary causes of headache, not to "rule in" a diagnosis of CH. Diagnostic pitfalls exist, because there can be significant variability in cluster presentation from one patient to another, and occasionally from one cluster period to the next within a single individual. For example, though the pain of CH is strictly unilateral, it can change sides within or between cluster episodes. CH occasionally occurs with minimal autonomic symptoms, and some patients have a mixture of CH and migraine symptomatology. For the majority of patients, however, CH features, including duration of each headache, the associated autonomic features, distribution of pain, and duration of cluster period (periodicity), are remarkably consistent.

Treatment

Treatment of CH almost invariably involves medication. Unlike most other primary headache disorders, most forms of CH respond dramatically to pharmacologic treatment; in many cases, complete elimination of attacks is possible. Tracking headache frequency and treatment response with a diary is useful in many cases (Appendix III).Traditional management includes aggressive early intervention with corticosteroids (*transitional*) coupled with appropriate rescue (*abortive*) and maintenance (*prophylactic*) therapies (Figure 6-1 and Tables 6-3 and 6-4).

Transitional Treatment
The pain and autonomic symptoms of CH improve dramatically with the use of corticosteroids. Prednisone is typically given at a starting dosage of up to 60 mg per day (1 mg/kg/day taken in 3 divided doses) and tapered

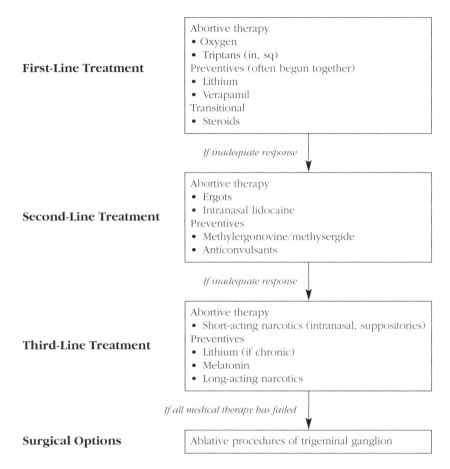

First-Line Treatment

Abortive therapy
- Oxygen
- Triptans (in, sq)
Preventives (often begun together)
- Lithium
- Verapamil
Transitional
- Steroids

If inadequate response

Second-Line Treatment

Abortive therapy
- Ergots
- Intranasal lidocaine
Preventives
- Methylergonovine/methysergide
- Anticonvulsants

If inadequate response

Third-Line Treatment

Abortive therapy
- Short-acting narcotics (intranasal, suppositories)
Preventives
- Lithium (if chronic)
- Melatonin
- Long-acting narcotics

If all medical therapy has failed

Surgical Options

Ablative procedures of trigeminal ganglion

Figure 6-1   Algorithm for treatment of cluster headache. Medical management involves the progression from first to second to third line treatments. Second and third line therapies are generally added to first-line therapies to achieve a therapeutic response (e.g., verapamil + anticonvulsant + methergine). Surgery is reserved for the most refractory cases because its side effects are irreversible. **First-line** abortive therapies include home oxygen and triptans (sq. or in.). Prednisone is often prescribed as a first-line preventive if there are no contraindications. **Second-line** abortive medications such as the oral ergots and intranasal lidocaine are administered if there is failure of first-line agents. Second-line preventives include the anticonvulsants and methylergonovine/methysergide; they are usually added to first-line preventives. Short-acting narcotics may be administered as a **third-line** abortive medication but cautiously because of the risk of overuse. Lithium may be helpful for chronic cluster headaches. Long-acting narcotics may be used as salvage therapy in patients that are refractory to all other treatment regimens.

gradually over a period of 2 to 4 weeks. Alternatively, dexamethasone 4 mg bid may be tapered over three weeks (13).

Although transitional treatment is highly effective in relieving symptoms, patients should be aware that unless it is begun in combination with a

Table 6-3 Selected Drugs Used in Cluster Headache Abortive Therapy

Agent	Dose	Comments
Oxygen	100% @7-10 L/min prn	Use high-flow regulator and face mask for up to 15 min
Dihydroergotamine (DHE)		Must not be used within 24 hr of a triptan, ergot, or methysergide; avoid in uncontrolled HTN, CAD, or basilar migraine; IV most potent, SQ least potent
Nasal spray	1 spray (0.5 mg) to each nostril; may repeat in 15 min	
Subcutaneous	1 mg/mL q1h prn	
Intramuscular	1 mg/mL q1h prn	
Intravenous	1 mg/mL q1h prn	
Sumatriptan		Avoid in HTN, CAD, or basilar migraine
Oral	25-100 mg initially; may repeat after 2 hr	Max: 200 mg/24 hr
Nasal spray	5, 10, or 20 mg single dose; may repeat after 2 hr	Max: 40 mg/24 hr
Subcutaneous	6 mg initially; may repeat after 1 hr	Max: 12 mg/24 hr
Zolmitriptan (oral)	1-2.5 mg initially; may repeat after 2 hr	Avoid in HTN, CAD, or basilar migraine; max: 10 mg/24 hr
4% Lidocaine (nasal spray)*	10-15 drops to ipsilateral nostril qid prn	Instill to the ipsilateral nostril with the head tilted backwards and to the affected side
Indomethacin (rectal suppository)*	50 mg tid-qid prn	—

*Not commercially available; must be formulated at compounding pharmacy.

suitable prophylactic regimen, the headaches will inevitably return as the steroid dose is tapered. The risks of steroid use should also be discussed with patients, particularly those who have frequent cluster periods. Over a lifetime of steroid use, complications may emerge, including avascular hip necrosis. The disability and suffering of uncontrolled CH are so great, though, that these risks are acceptable to patients in most cases.

Abortive Treatment

Abortive treatment is given at CH onset. Effective acute therapies include oxygen, dihydroergotamine, triptans (sumatriptan and others), lidocaine, indomethacin, and opioids (see Table 6-3), as well as sphenopalatine ganglion blockade. Which abortive agent is chosen depends upon factors such as convenience, ease of use, rapidity of onset, and safety. Many patients benefit from a combination of abortive agents, or they alternate treatments from attack to attack to minimize the overuse and side effects of any one

Table 6-4 Selected Drugs Used in Cluster Headache Prophylactic Therapy

Agent	Dose	Headache Response	Comments
Prednisone	1 mg/kg/day (up to 60 mg/day in 3 divided doses) tapered over 7-18 days	Within 24 hr	Avoid in cases of peptic ulcer, possible tuberculosis, pregnancy; beware possible ischemic hip necrosis; consider including as a "bridge" therapy (i.e., to be used until another drug kicks in)
Verapamil (short-acting)	80-160 mg tid	Within 7-10 days	Monitor blood pressure, pulse; beware edema, constipation
Verapamil (long-acting)	120-360 mg bid	Within 7-10 days	Monitor blood pressure, pulse; beware edema, constipation
Lithium carbonate	150-300 mg bid-tid	Within 7 days	Monitor renal and thyroid functions; beware tremor, diarrhea
Methysergide	2 mg tid-qid	Within 7 days	Monitor for evidence of vasoconstrictive symptoms; beware fibrotic complications
Methylergo-novine	0.2-0.4 mg tid-qid	Within 7 days	As for methysergide but less vasoconstrictive
Valproic acid	125-500 mg tid	Within 7 days	Monitor hepatic and platelet functions; beware pancreatitis and thrombocytopenia
Melatonin	Up to 10 mg qhs	Within 7 days	Further studies needed to demonstrate efficacy
Topiramate	25-50 mg bid	From 1 to 3 weeks	Further studies needed to demonstrate efficacy

treatment. With few exceptions, abortive treatment of CH should be non-oral; the rapid escalation to severe pain levels over a period of minutes means that oral therapy is inappropriate for the majority of patients.

OXYGEN

One hundred percent oxygen inhalation is a safe, rapid, and reliable method of aborting CH, bringing relief to 90% of cluster patients in over 90% of all attacks (16). It is used at the onset of the headache; a flow rate of 7 to10 L/min is administered through a non-rebreathing face mask with a high-flow regulator. Improvement occurs within 15 to 20 minutes. The mask should be applied firmly to the face, and the patient should remain seated in a forward position, with elbows situated on the knees, throughout the treatment. If ineffective, this procedure may be repeated after 5 minutes. Oxygen treatment is particularly helpful for nocturnal attacks; its major disadvantage is the cumbersome nature of the procedure and the equipment necessary to administer oxygen.

TRIPTANS

Almost all of the commercially available triptans are probably more effective than placebo for the abortive treatment of CH, although efficacy in clinical trials has been demonstrated only for subcutaneous sumatriptan and oral zolmitriptan; only the former has Food and Drug Administration approval for the CH indication. With few exceptions, oral therapy of individual attacks is inappropriate, given the rapid onset of severe pain and the generally short duration of the headaches; by the time an oral drug has become effective, many attacks will have ceased naturally. Triptans must be used cautiously, if at all, in patients with risk factors for coronary artery disease (CAD) and are thus contraindicated in those with known CAD (13).

LIDOCAINE

Lidocaine is effective abortive treatment for CH in about one third of patients. Since its efficacy does not compare favorably with other treatment alternatives, lidocaine is useful mainly as adjunctive therapy or in those patients who cannot use more effective treatments. Lidocaine may be applied as a 4% nasal spray solution to the nasal mucosa or be given as 10 to 15 drops to the ipsilateral nostril with the head tilted backwards to the affected side. This may be repeated once after 15 minutes, but total use should not exceed four times per day. Side effects include nervousness, dizziness, sore throat, and occasional allergic reactions (17).

OTHER NON-ORAL TREATMENTS

Anecdotal and clinical experience suggest that rectal suppositories offer a rapid-acting alternative to parenteral administration of abortive drugs for CH. Those that have been used include indomethacin (50 mg), chlorpromazine (50 to 100 mg), and certain opioids such as morphine sulphate (10 to 20 mg) and hydromorphone (3 mg). Butorphanol nasal spray is another nonoral option, but overuse is a serious risk in patients with frequent headache. Butorphanol should be reserved for situations in which alternative treatments are ineffective or contraindicated, and its use must be carefully monitored (13).

NEURAL BLOCKADE

Anesthetizing the sphenopalatine ganglion (SPG) through the local application of cocaine or other anesthetics may help abort cluster headache (18).

This technique is not widely used, however, because it offers little advantage over other more acceptable abortive agents and is inconvenient and unpleasant.

ERGOTAMINE

Several ergotamine-based drugs have been used for decades for both migraine and cluster abortive therapy. These include ergotamine tartrate (oral, sublingual, rectal) and dihydroergotamine (DHE-45, provided in intravenous, intramuscular, subcutaneous, or nasal spray forms). Their limited therapeutic benefits are often outweighed by their side effects, including nausea and emesis, as well as their potential vasoconstrictive activity, making them generally obsolete choices for treatment (13). Ergotamine must be avoided in patients with uncontrolled hypertension or ischemic vascular conditions.

Prophylactic Treatment

Because corticosteroids induce only a brief remission of cluster symptoms, therapy must also include prevention, which generally requires several weeks to take effect. Prophylaxis is usually initiated at the start of the cluster period, often in tandem with an initial corticosteroid burst, and continued for the duration of the cluster cycle, then tapered and discontinued. In patients with CCH, prevention may continue indefinitely. Medication is selected on the basis of intended duration of treatment, tolerability, and previous effectiveness in the individual patient. Table 6-4 lists commonly used prophylactic treatments for CH.

VERAPAMIL

Verapamil is used for both migraine and CH but is much more effective in the latter; in fact, most headache experts regard it as the preventive agent of choice for the majority of patients. Dosages range from 80 mg tid to 160 mg qid for the short-acting form, and from 120 to 360 mg bid for the long-acting form. The short-acting drug is widely believed to be more reliable, but the sustained-release form is also used, with typical total daily dosage ranging from 240 to 720 mg, given in divided doses (19). Constipation and ankle edema are the most common side effects, but dizziness, hypotension, bradycardia, and fatigue may also occur. Heart block is rare but, at high dosages, an electrocardiogram to identify conduction delay is probably wise. Verapamil may be combined with other preventive agents, including lithium carbonate, valproic acid, and methysergide (or its metabolite, methylergonovine), but doses may have to be reduced to avert side effects.

LITHIUM

Lithium carbonate is highly effective for CH and is used by itself and in combination with verapamil. It is both safe and well-tolerated at the doses used for CH, which range from 150 mg bid to 300 mg tid (20). The principal side effect is tremor, chiefly affecting the hands, although some patients may also complain of diarrhea. When used for extended periods, serum trough levels should not exceed 1.0 mEq/L, and electrolytes as well as thyroid functions should be monitored.

SODIUM VALPROATE

Open-label evidence suggests some effect for sodium valproate in CH prophylaxis (21). Sodium valproate is often started at 125 to 250 mg bid and gradually increased to as much as 2 g daily, given in divided doses. Patients may tolerate the encapsulated sprinkles better than the tablet form. Side effects include nausea, weight gain, fatigue or somnolence, hair loss, and tremor. These disturbances may remit over time or with dosage reduction. Prolonged valproate use may cause pancreatitis and thrombocytopenia. It is a known teratogen and thus relatively contraindicated in women of childbearing age.

METHYSERGIDE/METHYLERGONOVINE

These ergotamine-based drugs have been used for cluster and migraine prophylaxis for many years, but popularity waned after discovery of the rare but serious side effects of retroperitoneal, pleural, and pericardial fibrosis. Thought to occur idiosyncratically and only after prolonged use, this complication nonetheless is frightening to many clinicians unfamiliar with these drugs, who often fear using them, even for relatively short duration. This is unfortunate, because methysergide and methylergonovine are effective and ordinarily tolerated well by most patients. A one-month drug holiday is recommended for those using the drugs for more than 6 consecutive months to prevent retroperitoneal fibrosis. Also, periodic abdominal CT scans may be indicated at yearly intervals to screen for this disorder in those with chronic use. Valvular abnormalities such as mitral and tricuspid regurgitation have also been reported with prolonged use, and some physicians recommend periodic echocardiograms to identify these abnormalities.

Methysergide is dosed at 2 mg tid to qid; methylergonovine, a metabolite of methysergide, is usually prescribed at 0.2 mg tid to 0.4 mg qid. Short-term adverse effects include arthralgias, peripheral edema and abdominal pain, but these improve with prolonged therapy or dosage reduction. Neither drug should be used in conjunction with other vasoconstrictive agents (e.g., sumatriptan), and both are contraindicated in ischemic vascular and active peptic ulcer disease (13).

OTHER AGENTS

Some newer agents that show promise in CH prophylaxis are topiramate, gabapentin, and melatonin. Topiramate has been used in doses ranging from 50 to 125 mg/day (22). Gabapentin, sometimes in very high doses, also appears useful in some cases (23). Melatonin may act to stabilize impaired circadian rhythms; a dose of 10 mg at bedtime appears most effective (24). In addition, at least two recent reports have documented the successful use of daily naratriptan in refractory CH (25,26). Some evidence also exists for the use of baclofen in cluster headache (27). Although evidence is inadequate to recommend these agents as initial treatment, they are alternatives for those refractory to traditional therapy.

Inpatient Hospitalization for Intractable Cluster Headache

Intractable CH occurs in 10% of sufferers and requires aggressive treatment that may include polypharmacy and parenteral therapy. These treatments frequently require hospitalization. Hospitalization is also necessary for patients with co-morbidities that require careful supervision of therapy and for desperate or suicidal patients. Hospitalization allows initiation of parenteral (IV) DHE over a 3-day period or longer, with simultaneous and aggressive institution and dose escalations of CH preventive therapy. Other parenteral agents such as IV valproate, droperidol, or even hydrocortisone may also be used. In refractory cases, it is not uncommon to use three or four preventive agents; close monitoring is essential. Such patients should ideally be treated in well-established headache treatment facilities with broad experience in this type of intensive care (13).

Surgical Treatment for Refractory Cluster Headache

Surgical treatment of CH is appropriate only after medical options for therapy have proved ineffective. Only patients with strictly unilateral, side-locked headaches are likely to benefit; if attacks have ever switched sides there is an unacceptably high risk of recurrence after surgery. Surgical procedures invariably involve some degree of unwanted injury to the trigeminal nerve, leaving patients with facial analgesia in all cases and occasionally serious side effects such as deafferentation pain known as anesthesia dolorosa (28).

   Surgical treatment is generally aimed at the sensory trigeminal nerve or the cranial parasympathetic system. Techniques that involve surgery on the sensory trigeminal nerve include radiofrequency (RF) thermocoagulation of the trigeminal ganglion or glycerol or alcohol gangliorhizolysis. The former is more popular, given its track record of safety, efficacy, and durability. RF may provide up to 75% of patients with satisfactory or excellent results, with remission lasting in some patients up to 20 years, but recurrence is seen in 20% of patients.

   Post-surgical complications depend on the site and extent of the surgical lesion (V1, V2, or V3) and can include visual and auditory changes, sharp or stabbing pain, deviation of the jaw, and corneal anesthesia. Satisfactory results may also be obtained with sensory trigeminal rhizotomy procedures through various approaches that transect the nerve at the root exit zone. In all of these procedures, however, unless the presenting CH is strictly unilateral, contralateral pain may recur following initial success (28). Microvascular decompression (MVD) of the trigeminal nerve (and nervus intermedius) is another surgical approach to recalcitrant CH pain but involves craniectomy; its role in treatment is currently poorly defined. A recent small study suggests that gamma knife radiosurgery provided relative or absolute pain relief in six refractory CH patients. Pain resolved, partially or totally, within one week, and in some lasted up to eight months or more. This procedure is noninvasive, and side effects are minimal compared with ablative procedures. Nevertheless, further studies will be necessary to confirm its safety and efficacy (29).

Surgical treatments aimed at the cranial parasympathetic system include trigeminal RF or sphenopalatine ganglion and nervus intermedius resection. These techniques provide inconsistent pain relief, although they seem more effective in eliminating autonomic symptoms associated with CH (28).

Stimulation of the ipsilateral hypothalamic area in a patient with chronic cluster headache through use of stereotactically implanted electrodes is a novel treatment that requires more evaluation (30).

Other Trigeminal Autonomic Cephalalgias

Chronic Paroxysmal Hemicrania

A headache disorder potentially related to cluster headache, and one that occurs more commonly in women, is chronic paroxysmal hemicrania. This disorder can also have an episodic version as may occur in cluster headache. The headaches are brief, lasting from 2 to 25 minutes. Like cluster headache, they are strictly unilateral and generally located in the periorbital and temporal regions. The attacks typically occur five times per day or more and have ipsilateral autonomic symptoms such as lacrimation, rhinorrhea, conjunctival injection, nasal congestion, ptosis, and eyelid edema. Table 6-5 gives the IHS criteria for chronic paroxysmal hemicrania.

Chronic paroxysmal hemicrania is twice as common in women than men and often begins in the adult years. A family history of similar headaches is uncommon. The cervical spine may play a role in this disorder. About one fifth of patients may elicit the headache by bending or turning the neck. Others find that pressure on the nerve roots of C2 or the transverse processes of the upper cervical vertebrae may bring on the attacks (13).

The treatment of choice is indomethacin 25 to 300 mg/day. An initial dose of 25 mg three times a day may be increased to 50 mg three times a day if the response is incomplete. The failure of the patient to respond to indomethacin should be cause to rethink the diagnosis. Patients failing to achieve satisfactory results with indomethacin may be tried with other anti-inflammatory agents, verapamil, and even acetazolamide (13).

Table 6-5   International Headache Society Diagnostic Criteria for Chronic and Episodic Paroxysmal Hemicrania*

A. At least 20 attacks fulfilling criteria B-D
B. Attacks of severe unilateral orbital, supraorbital, or temporal pain lasting 2 to 30 minutes
C. Headache is accompanied by at least one of the following:
   1. Ipsilateral conjunctival injection and/or lacrimation
   2. Ipsilateral nasal congestion and/or rhinorrhoea
   3. Ipsilateral eyelid oedema
   4. Ipsilateral forehead and facial sweating
   5. Ipsilateral miosis and/or ptosis
D. Attacks have a frequency above 5 per day for more than one half of the time, although periods with lower frequency may occur
E. Attacks are prevented completely by therapeutic doses of indomethacin
F. Not attributed to another disorder

From International Headache Society. The International Classification of Headache Disorders, 2nd ed. Cephalalgia. 2004;24(Suppl 1):9-160; with permission.
*Episodic paroxysmal hemicrania must fulfill above criteria and have at least 2 attack periods lasting 7 to 365 days and separated by pain-free remission periods of >1 month. Chronic paroxysmal hemicrania must fulfill above criteria and have attacks recur over >1 year without remission periods or with remission periods lasting <1 month.

Episodic Paroxysmal Hemicrania

The characteristics of episodic paroxysmal hemicrania are virtually indistinguishable from those of chronic paroxysmal hemicrania; the IHS criteria are also very similar (see Table 6-5). The main difference is that attack periods of episodic paroxysmal hemicrania last 7 to 365 days as opposed to the more than one year for chronic paroxysmal hemicrania.

Hemicrania Continua

Hemicrania continua is another rare headache disorder that is exquisitely indomethacin responsive. It is more common in women and presents with side-locked (i.e., always on the same side) unilateral headaches. The headaches are generally daily and continuous, but the pain severity tends to wax and wane from moderate to severe. For definitive diagnosis, the headaches must be associated with ipsilateral autonomic symptoms and there must be a complete response to therapeutic doses of indomethacin (Table 6-6). (Hemicrania continua is discussed in detail in Chapter 8.)

SUNCT Syndrome

SUNCT syndrome is characterized by brief unilateral headaches that are associated with ipsilateral autonomic symptoms. Its main distinguishing factor from the other autonomic cephalalgias is short duration (5 to 240 seconds).

**Table 6-6   International Headache Society Diagnostic Criteria for
Hemicrania Continua**

A. Headache for >3 months fulfilling criteria B-D
B. All of the following characteristics
   1. Unilateral pain without side-shift
   2. Daily and continuous, without pain-free periods
   3. Moderate intensity, but with exacerbations of severe pain
C. At least one of the following autonomic features occurs during exacerbations
   and ipsilateral to the side of pain:
   1. Conjunctival injection and/or lacrimation
   2. Nasal congestion and/or rhinorrhoea
   3. Ptosis and/or miosis
D. Complete response to therapeutic doses of indomethacin
E. Not attributed to another disorder

From International Headache Society. The International Classification of Headache Disorders, 2nd ed.
Cephalalgia. 2004;24(Suppl 1):9-160; with permission.

**Table 6-7   International Headache Society Diagnostic Criteria for
SUNCT Syndrome**

A. At least 20 attacks fulfilling criteria B-D
B. Attacks of unilateral orbital, supraorbital or temporal stabbing or pulsating pain
   lasting 5 to 240 seconds
C. Pain is accompanied by ipsilateral conjunctival injection and lacrimation
D. Attacks occur with a frequency of 3 to 200 per day
E. Not attributed to another disorder

From International Headache Society. The International Classification of Headache Disorders, 2nd ed.
Cephalalgia. 2004;24(Suppl 1):9-160; with permission.

SUNCT syndrome is more common in men, and attacks may occur 3 to 200
times per day. Rare potential secondary causes of SUNCT syndrome are
lesion of the posterior fossa and pituitary gland. These headaches tend to
be resistant to most therapies, but there have been reports of improvement
with carbamazepine, gabapentin (31), lamotrigine (32), and topiramate.
Indomethacin has not been shown to be helpful in this syndrome. Table 6-7
gives the IHS diagnostic criteria for SUNCT syndrome.

Key Points

Cluster headache is rare but distinctive and highly disabling.
'cognition is important to avoid unnecessary patient suffering
   to delayed or incorrect diagnosis.

- Effective abortive treatments for cluster headache include oxygen inhalation and parenteral sumatriptan.

- Transitional and preventive therapies for cluster headache, including verapamil, lithium, and methysergide, are necessary for almost all patients.

- Interventional treatment is reserved for refractory headaches.

- The trigeminal autonomic cephalalgias should be considered in those patients with strictly unilateral headaches associated with ipsilateral autonomic symptoms.

REFERENCES

1. **Tonon C, Guttmann S, Volpinin M, et al.** Prevalence and incidence of cluster headache in the Republic of San Marino. Neurology. 2002;58:1407-9.

2. **Manzoni G.** Male preponderance of cluster headache is progressively decreasing over the years. Headache. 1997;37:588-9.

3. **Finkel AG.** Epidemiology of cluster headache. Current Pain and Headache Reports. 2003;7:144-9.

4. **Ekbom K, Svensson D, Traff H, Waldenlind E.** Age at onset and sex ratio in cluster headache: observations over three decades. Cephalalgia. 2002;22:94-100.

5. **Horton BT.** Histaminic cephalgias: differential diagnosis and treatment—1176 patients, 1937-1955. Mayo Clin Proc. 1956;31:325-33.

6. **Torelli P, Cologna D, Cademartiri C, Manzoni G.** Possible predictive factors in the evolution of episodic to chronic cluster headache. Headache. 2000;40:798-808.

7. **Kudrow L.** Cluster headache: diagnosis, management, and treatment. In: Dalessio DJ, Silberstein SD, eds. Wolff's Headache and Other Head Pain, 6th ed. New York: Oxford University Press; 1993:171-97.

8. **Russell M, Andersson P, Thomsen L.** Familial occurrence of cluster headache. J Neurol Neurosurg Psychiatry. 1995;58:341-3.

9. **Haan J, van Vliet J, Kors E, et al.** No involvement of the calcium channel gene in a family with cluster headache. Cephalalgia. 2001;21:959-62.

10. **May A, Bahra A, Buchel C, et al.** Hypothalamic activation in cluster headache attacks. Lancet. 1998;351:275-8.

11. **May A, Ashburner J, Buchel C, et al.** Correlation between structural and functional changes in brain in an idiopathic headache syndrome. Nat Med. 1999;5: 836-8.

12. **Aurora SK.** Etiology and pathogenesis of cluster headache. Current Pain and Headache Reports. 2002;6:71-5.

13. **Saper JR, Silberstein SD, Gordon CD, et al.** Handbook of Headache Management: A Practical Guide to Diagnosis and Treatment of Head, Neck, and Facial Pain, 2nd ed. Baltimore: Lippincott Williams & Wilkins; 1999.

14. **International Headache Society.** The International Classification of Headache Disorders, 2nd ed. Cephalalgia. 2004;24(Suppl 1):9-160.

15. **Dodick DW, Campbell JK.** Cluster headache: diagnosis, management, and treatment. In: Silberstein SD, Lipton RB, Dalessio DJ, eds. Wolff's Headache and Other Head Pain, 7th ed. New York: Oxford University Press; 2001:283-321.

16. **Fogan L.** Treatment of cluster headache: a double-blind comparison of oxygen versus air inhalation. Arch Neurol. 1985;42:362-3.

17. **Maizels M, Scott B, Cohen W, et al.** Intranasal lidocaine for the treatment of migraine: a randomized, double-blind, controlled study. JAMA.1996;276:319-21.

18. **Kitelle JP, Grouse DS, Seyboro ME.** Cluster headache: local anesthetic abortive agents. Arch Neurol. 1985;42:496-8.

19. **Leone M, D'Amico D, Attanasio A, et al.** Verapamil is an effective prophylactic for cluster headache: results of a double-blind multicenter study versus placebo. In: Olesen J, Goadsby PJ, eds. Cluster Headache and Related Conditions. Oxford: Oxford University Press; 1999:296-9.

20. **Steiner RJ, Hering R, Couturier ECM, et al.** Double-blind placebo-controlled trial of lithium in episodic cluster headache. Cephalalgia. 1997;17:673-5.

21. **Hering R, Kuritzky A.** Sodium valproate in the treatment of cluster headache: an open clinical trial. Cephalalgia. 1989;9:195-8.

22. **Lainez MJ, Pascual J, Santonja JM, et al.** Topiramate in the prophylactic treatment of cluster heaache. Cephalalgia. 2001;21:369.

23. **Leandri M, Luzzani M, Cruccu G, Gottlieb A.** Drug-resistant cluster headache responding to gabapentin: a pilot study. Cephalalgia. 2001;21:744-6.

24. **Leone M, Damico D, Moschiano F, et al.** Melatonin versus placebo in the prophylaxis of cluster headache: a double-blind pilot study with parallel groups. Cephalalgia. 1996;16:494-6.

25. **Loder E.** Naratriptan in the prophylaxis of cluster headache. Headache. 2002;42:56-7.

26. **Eekers PJ, Koehler PJ.** Naratriptan prophylactic treatment in cluster headache. Cephalgia. 2001;21:75-6.

27. **Hering-Hanit R, Gadoth N.** The use of baclofen in cluster headache. Curr Pain Headache Rep. 2001;5:79-82.

28. **Rozen TD.** Interventional treatment for cluster headache: a review of the options. Current Pain and Headache Reports. 2002;6:57-64.

29. **Ford RG, Ford KT, Swain S, et al.** Gamma knife treatment of refractory cluster headache. Headache. 1998:38:1-9.

30. **Leone M, Franzini A, D'Amico D, et al.** Intractable chronic cluster headache relieved by electrode implant to posterior inferior hypothalamus. Cephalalgia. 2001;21:503.

31. **Hunt C, Dodick D, Bosch E.** SUNCT responsive to gabapentin. Headache. 2002; 42:525-6.

32. **Piovesan E, Slow C, Kowacs P, et al.** Influence of lamotrigine over the SUNCT syndrome: one patient follow-up for 2 years. Arq Neuropsiquiatr. 2003;61:691-4.

7

Daily or Frequent Headaches

Glen D. Solomon, MD

Vincent T. Martin, MD

One of the most vexing issues in clinical medicine is the management of patients suffering with daily or very frequent headaches. Chronic daily headache encompasses a group of disorders characterized by a frequency of 15 or more days per month (averaged over the preceding 6 months) and a duration of more than 4 hours for each individual headache attack (1). These patients present both diagnostic and therapeutic challenges. The goal of this chapter is to simplify the diagnostic approach to these patients and provide a therapeutic framework for their management.

Diagnostic Classification and Clinical Characteristics

Chronic daily headache is not a diagnostic entity included in the International Headache Society (IHS) classification schema. Diagnostic criteria have been proposed, however, and these will be described below (2). Although not included in formal diagnostic systems, the term is so clinically useful that it remains in wide use to describe a frequently encountered clinical situation. See Tables 7-1 and 7-2 for clinical characteristics of the common and uncommon types of chronic daily headache.

"Chronic Daily Headache": Every Day?

"Chronic daily headache" is a misnomer. Daily headaches are not required to make the diagnosis! Headaches that occur more frequently than *every other day* are considered chronic daily headache.

Conversely, headaches of short duration (lasting less than 4 hours) can occur on a daily basis (i.e., cluster headache, chronic paroxysmal hemicrania, idiopathic stabbing headache, hypnic headache, cranial neuralgias), but they are *not* considered chronic daily headache.

Table 7-1   Common Types of Chronic Daily Headache

Type of Headache	Clinical Characteristics
Chronic migraine headache	Chronic daily headache in a patient with past history of migraine headache; some of the headaches resemble episodic migraine, others may resemble tension-type headaches
Chronic tension-type headache	Characteristics are the same as for episodic tension-type headaches except that duration can be longer than 7 days and more frequent than every 15 days
Medication overuse headache	Chronic daily headache that occurs in patients with analgesic overuse; suspect in those who use abortive headache medications more than 2 days/week; often exists concomitantly with diagnosis of migraine or tension-type headaches and may lead to their transformation into chronic daily headache

Table 7-2   Uncommon Types of Chronic Daily Headache

Type of Headache	Clinical Characteristics
Pseudotumor cerebri	May resemble chronic migraine or tension-type headache; results from increased intracranial pressure (opening pressures on lumbar puncture >250); suspect in obese women with chronic daily headache
Post-traumatic headache	Begin within 14 days of known head trauma, which may be minor or major; may resemble chronic migraine or tension-type headache
Cervicogenic headache	Commonly located in the unilateral cervical/occipital region and result from pathology of the cervical spine (e.g., radiculopathy of the C1 and C2 nerve root, cervical facet disease, greater occipital neuralgia); suspect in patients with headaches in cervical/occipital location who have history of neck injury or cervical spine disease; anesthetic blocks may aid in diagnosis
New daily persistent headache	Abrupt onset (developing over fewer than 3 days) in patients with no past history of migraine or tension-type headache
Hemicrania continua	Headaches strictly unilateral, continuous, and have ipsilateral automonic symptoms such as lacrimation, rhinorrhea, ptosis, and conjunctival injection; headache severity can wax and wane; complete resolution of headaches with indomethacin therapy

Epidemiology

Population-based studies in the United States, Europe, and Asia report that approximately 4% of the general population suffer from chronic daily headache (3-9). In addition, 0.5% of the population have severe headache on a daily basis (10).

Chronic daily headache is roughly twice as prevalent in women as in men (11). The average age at onset of chronic daily headache is in the thirties. The prevalence of chronic daily headache appears consistent across age groups from childhood and adolescence to adults and the elderly (11). This is in contrast to episodic migraine, which decreases in prevalence after the sixth decade.

In the most detailed epidemiological study of tension-type headache, the Danish Glostrup Population Studies (12), the 1-year prevalence of chronic tension-type headache was 3% (2% in men and 5% in women). The gender difference was statistically significant, with a male-to-female ratio of 4:5. The prevalence of tension-type headache decreased with increasing age.

Population-based studies report that the most common cause of chronic daily headache is chronic tension-type headache (1.4%-2.7%), followed by chronic migraine (1.0%-1.7%) (11). However, in tertiary headache centers and other medical settings, the most common cause of chronic daily headache is migraine that has evolved over time from an episodic to a chronic form. This is important to keep in mind when evaluating patients with frequent headache.

Pathophysiology

The pathophysiology of chronic headache is poorly understood. Chronic migraine and tension-type headache often evolve from their episodic forms. Factors associated with the development of chronic daily headache include head or back injury, stress, pregnancy, use of oral contraceptives/hormone replacement therapies, surgery, and viral illness (13). Analgesic overuse may also play a role in the transformation of episodic into chronic headache disorders. Psychological factors, myofascial mechanisms, and other medical conditions may also contribute.

Most current theories suggest that chronic migraine and possibly tension-type headaches may result from sensitization of second- and third-order neurons of the trigeminal pain pathways located within the brainstem and the thalamus/parietal cortex, respectively (14-16). Such sensitization leads to lower pain thresholds within the trigeminal nerve to a variety of painful stimuli (e.g., thermal, pressure) and has been termed "central sensitization". Sensitization of these neurons within the central nervous system could theoretically lead to chronic daily headache. Additionally, medication overuse, depression, and use of caffeine may contribute to perpetuation of the headache once it is well established.

Risk Factors

A recent cohort study followed 1134 patients with headache and 798 patients without headache (the headache status was defined at patient entry into study) for an average of 11 months (17). Factors associated with the new onset of chronic daily headache were higher baseline headache frequency ($P < 0.005$), obesity (OR 5.53 for BMI > 30), self-reported physician-diagnosed arthritis (OR 3.29), and self-reported physician-diagnosed diabetes (OR 3.43 with borderline statistical significance). Another recent study reported that habitual snoring was associated with chronic daily headache (18).

Psychiatric Comorbidity

Psychiatric comorbidity is more frequent in patients with migraine than in the general population. Anxiety, depression, panic disorder, and bipolar disease have all been found to be more common in migraine sufferers (19,20). Because migraine is a component of many daily or frequent headache syndromes, psychiatric comorbidity with these disorders can be expected. Generalized anxiety was reported in 70% of "chronic migraine" patients and somatoform disorders (including somatization, conversion disorder, factitious disorder, and hypochondriasis) were reported in 5.7% (21). Depression has been reported in 25% to 80% of chronic migraine patients (21,22). Coexisting depression does not influence the persistence, frequency, or disability of migraine headache in patients with a history of migraine (23). Conversely, migraine does not increase the probability of future episodes of depression. This suggests that the chronic headache is not the result of major depression in migraine patients, or vice versa. Rather, shared underlying abnormalities in the central nervous system may predispose patients to develop one or both of these disorders. Behavioral or personality factors, in contrast to affective illness, do appear to play a role in perpetuation or worsening of headache, perhaps by affecting treatment compliance or leading to medication overuse.

Patients with chronic tension-type headache, like patients with other chronic pain disorders, have about a 25% likelihood of developing secondary depression. Half of these patients develop depression simultaneously with the onset of headache, while in the other half the development of depression is more insidious (24). Tension-type headache may be present in almost all psychiatric disturbances (25).

Chronic Tension-Type Headache

The IHS defines tension-type headache as a bilateral headache having a pressing or tightening quality of mild-to-moderate severity (2). Unlike migraine, it is not aggravated by physical activity nor is it associated with vomiting. Phonophobia or photophobia may be present, but not both. In chronic tension-type headache, but not episodic tension-type headache, patients may experience nausea. By definition, chronic tension-type headache occurs at least 15 days per month for longer than 6 months, although in clinical practice it is usually a daily or almost daily headache (2).

Transformed Migraine

Transformed migraine is a syndrome of daily or very frequent headaches, occurring in patients with a history of episodic migraine, in which superimposed severe headache attacks have the characteristics of migraine (1). Typically, the patient describes a history of distinct attacks of migraine with or without aura, starting in the teens or early twenties, which eventually become more frequent. In addition, the patient develops tension-type headaches between the attacks of migraine, which also become more frequent, eventually leading to a daily or near-daily headache. Patients may suffer from migraine on one day and from tension-type headache the next. The evolution from paroxysmal headaches into a near-daily headache pattern is often associated with overuse of analgesic medication (26). The term "chronic migraine" is defined by the IHS as attacks meeting criteria for migraine occurring 15 or more days per month. Note that many patients with transformed migraine have frequent attacks but such attacks may not all be severe enough to qualify for a diagnosis of chronic migraine.

Headache Attributed to a Substance or Its Withdrawal

An important condition contributing to the development of headaches in a chronic daily pattern is overuse of abortive medication. Ironically, this is most likely to occur in patients with frequent headaches. Analgesic overuse was reported in 25% to 38% of the chronic daily headache population (11). In headache referral centers, among chronic daily headache sufferers, rates of analgesic overuse range from 46% to 87% (1). Because drug habituation is a common accompaniment of many chronic headache syndromes, this is often the first issue that must be considered in patient management.

Classifications

The revised IHS criteria include a category of "Headache Attributed to a Substance or Its Withdrawal". They have been classified as

1. Headache induced by acute substance use or exposure
2. Medication overuse headache (MOH)
3. Headache as an adverse event attributed to chronic medication
4. Headache attributed to withdrawal from chronic use of other substances

Headache induced by acute substance use or exposure includes such things as headache attributed to use of nitrates, carbon monoxide exposure, or cocaine or alcohol use. The headaches generally begin within 3 to 5 hours of exposure and resolve within 72 hours. The character of the headache varies depending on the substance to which one was exposed and on the baseline characteristics of the patient. For example, acute ingestion of nitrates may produce a delayed headache in migraineurs that meets IHS criteria for migraine without aura. The same exposure in a nonmigraineur may not produce such a headache.

Medication overuse headache is induced by overzealous use of abortive medication. The amount of medication and duration of its use thought necessary to produce the headache are frequently specified in the IHS criteria. MOH diagnosis can only be made in retrospect, after discontinuation of the suspect medication has produced resolution or improvement of the headache. The time required for this to occur varies depending on the medication involved.

Headache as an adverse event attributed to chronic medication is a diagnosis made when headache develops during chronic use of medication for any medical condition and resolves after that medication has been discontinued. Examples include headache occurring with the use of drugs such as tetracycline-class antibiotics, anabolic steroids, or lithium carbonate.

Finally, *headache attributed to substance withdrawal* is a category that describes headache syndromes that may occur when substances such as caffeine, exogenous estrogens, or opioids are withdrawn. Patients with preexisting headache disorders may be especially prone to developing these headache syndromes; careful evaluation may identify one of these disorders as a complicating factor in many chronic headache patients. Caffeine withdrawal, in particular, may occur over the course of a single day in patients whose caffeine intake, particularly in the morning, is high. Headache present upon awakening that is relieved or improved with the first morning cup of coffee should lead to suspicion that variations in caffeine intake may be an aggravating factor in headache.

Caffeine: Friend or Foe?

Many headache sufferers and even clinicians find the relationship between caffeine and headache to be confusing. Caffeine is an ingredient in many widely used headache medications whether over-the-counter (e.g., Excedrin) or prescription (e.g., Fiorinal, Cafergot). All can be effective when used to treat an individual headache. Furthermore, many patients recognize that caffeine in the form of a cup of coffee or a can of soda can occasionally be used to abort a headache, especially while the headache is still mild. Yet caffeine reduction or elimination is frequently advised for patients with troublesome headaches, a seemingly contra-dictory recommendation.

The fact is that caffeine itself, used occasionally, can be an effective treatment for mild tension-type or migraine headaches, especially if it is used early in their course. Caffeine is a vasoconstrictor, has modest analgesic properties of its own, and augments the absorption and effectiveness of other analgesics when it is used in combination medications. Used regularly, however, withdrawal headaches can occur when caffeine levels drop. For those who drink many cups of coffee throughout the day, this may be most noticeable in the early morning hours. The longest period without caffeine for these patients is likely to be while they are sleeping, accounting for the not-infrequent story that "I have headaches, but as soon as I have my morn-ing cup of coffee they go away." If the person recounting this is not trou-bled by the headaches, treatment may not be necessary. On the other hand, if the physician is being consulted for a headache problem, advising elimi-nation or reduction of caffeine makes sense.

No threshold intake has been clearly established below which headache will not occur and above which it definitely will, but most clinicians recom-mend no more than two regular-sized cups of coffee per day for patients who cannot or will not eliminate it altogether. Intake of caffeinated sodas or "energy drinks" should also be assessed, especially in children and adoles-cents. Finally, the patient should be questioned about caffeine intake in over-the-counter or prescription medications. Many patients are unaware that these medicines may contain caffeine.

Caffeine withdrawal headache may be more common than generally recognized. One study of headaches occurring after general anesthesia, for example, found that it was probably not the anesthetics that were to blame but rather the instruction "Nothing to eat or drink after midnight" before the surgery. The result: Missing the usual morning cup of coffee led to caffeine-withdrawal headache!

Medication Overuse Headache

Medication overuse headache is associated with chronic substance use or exposure. Patients with chronic headache disorders who are using large amounts of abortive headache medications should be evaluated for the presence of this disorder. In the preface to the diagnostic criteria for MOH, the IHS comments that "by far the most common cause of migraine-like headache occurring on 15 or more days per month and of a mixed picture of migraine-like and tension-type-like headaches on 15 or more days per month is overuse of symptomatic migraine drugs and/or analgesics." Clinically, MOH is likely to occur only with frequent, regular use of abortive medications. The frequency of dosing required to induce MOH is not well established, but nevertheless general guidelines have been proposed by the IHS.

IHS criteria define medication overuse as more than 15 days per month of intake of simple analgesics and narcotics for longer than 3 months, and more than 10 days per month of intake of triptans, ergots, and combination analgesics for longer than 3 months. Furthermore, not all abortive medications seem equally likely to cause MOH. There may be a threshold level of quantity or duration of use necessary to produce the condition, and this may vary from person to person and even within the same person at different times. Finally, MOH does not appear to occur at all in those who do not have a previous susceptibility to primary headache disorders, thus the comment by the IHS that "Medication overuse headache is an interaction between a therapeutic agent used excessively and a susceptible patient . . . ." Because the diagnosis of MOH depends on resolution or reversion of the headache to its previous pattern within 2 months after discontinuation of the suspected medication, it is a diagnosis that can be made only in retrospect.

Not all patients who are "overusing" abortive medication for headache have MOH. A substantial percentage (approximately 75%) of patients who meet criteria for overuse as defined in Table 7-3 will have improvement in their headaches after discontinuation of the medication, but the other 25% will not. Additionally, there seem to be at least some situations in which regular use of triptans or ergotamine preparations may actually have a prophylactic effect on headache (27). Thus, although MOH should be sought in patients with chronic headache, it is important to remember that medication

---

Table 7-3   International Headache Society Criteria for Medication Overuse Headache

A. Headache present more than 15 days per month
B. Intake of:
   1. Opioids and simple analgesics more than 15 days per month for longer than 3 months
   2. Ergots, triptans, and combination analgesics more than 10 days per month for 3 months
C. Headache has developed or markedly worsened during use of abortive medication
D. Headache resolves or reverts to its previous pattern within 2 months after discontinuation of abortive medication

Adapted from International Headache Society. The International Classification of Headache Disorders, 2nd ed. Cephalalgia. 2004;24(Suppl 1):9-160; with permission. Specific headache characteristics are required for classification of MOH for triptans, ergots, and simple and combination analgesics; these are not listed in the above criteria. In addition, a designation of "probable medication-overuse headache" has been given to those who fulfill all of the above criteria but whose headaches have not fully resolved or reverted to the original pattern after 2 months of medication withdrawal.

Table 7-4   Common Medications Associated with Medication Overuse Headache

Medication Class	Examples
Combination analgesics[†]	Butalbital-containing medications, ASA/caffeine/acetaminophen, narcotic-combination pills
Opioids	Codeine, hydrocodone, meperidine, oxycodone, hydromorphone
Ergots	Ergotamine, ergotamine/caffeine combinations
Triptans	Almotriptan, eletritpan, frovatriptan, naratriptan, sumatriptan, rizatriptan, zolmitriptan
Simple analgesics*	NSAIDs, aspirin, acetaminophen

[†] Combination analgesics (particularly those that contain caffeine and butalbital) and opioids are especially common causes of MOH.
* Whether NSAIDs and ASA lead to MOH is controversial.

overuse can be an associated, not causative, feature of the headache disorder in some patients. Table 7-4 lists common medications associated with MOH.

There remains considerable controversy, even among headache experts, about which substances can produce MOH. Many experts believe that plain NSAIDs, used without added caffeine, are unlikely to produce headache and may even be used to treat it. Other experts disagree. Thus, in an individual patient with refractory, frequent headache, it may be reasonable to try a course of scheduled NSAIDs as a replacement for other, overused medications, or to attempt discontinuation if they are already being used in order to assess whether they might, in a particular case, be aggravating the situation. There is consensus, however, that ergots, caffeine-containing medications, and opioids are frequently associated with MOH.

Use of abortive medications more than 2 or 3 days per week for longer than 3 months can lead to MOH. Primary care physicians should ask patients about the quantity of abortive medications consumed and the frequency of dosing. Because over-the-counter medications are frequently overused, patients should be specifically queried about them.

The characteristics of the headaches induced by medication overuse depend on the underlying headache disorder. Most commonly, they present as a constant, diffuse, dull headache without associated symptoms in migraine patients (28). Clinically, this syndrome cannot be differentiated from migraine with chronic tension-type headache or chronic migraine. Withdrawal headache in migraine patients resembles a severe and prolonged migraine attack. In patients with chronic tension-type or post-traumatic headache, MOH cannot be distinguished from primary headache (28).

Daily use of ergots may lead to a throbbing, pulsating headache in the early morning, sometimes with nausea. The headache disappears between 30 and 60 minutes after intake of ergotamine. It may be distinguished from migraine by the absence of an attack pattern or associated migraine symptoms (28). Anecdotal reports suggest that the daily use of triptans may provoke a similar syndrome (28).

Because of the problems with defining the disorder, the epidemiology of medication-induced headache remains poorly documented. Reliable prevalence and incidence rates are not available. A Spanish study estimates that 1% of the population has daily headache combined with MOH (4). Approximately 5% to 10% of all patients seen in headache centers are reported to have MOH (28).

Medication overuse is also common in headache patients within primary care practices. A study of primary care headache patients in Seattle found that 22% were chronic or frequent users of analgesics. The group of analgesics most commonly overused was over-the-counter medications (29).

In their meta-analysis of studies of chronic MOH in patients seeking care in specialty headache centers, Diener and Dahlof (28) reviewed 29 studies including 2612 patients. Sixty-five percent of patients had migraine as their principal underlying headache disorder, 27% had tension-type headache, and 8% had mixed headache. Women were 3.5 times as likely as men to suffer from chronic MOH. These results differ from those of population-based studies, in which tension-type headache predominates. Patients developing chronic MOH had an average duration of primary headache exceeding 20 years and frequent analgesic or ergot intake for more than 10 years. The mean duration of daily headache was almost 6 years. The average number of tablets or suppositories taken per day was 5. Patients used either combination drugs or several products, averaging 2.5 to 5.8 different pharmacological components taken simultaneously.

Treatment

The first step in the treatment of chronic daily headache syndrome is to identify specific contributing behaviors or problems that can be targeted. Although there is no single treatment for chronic daily headache, there are potentially effective approaches for MOH, chronic tension-type headache, and migraine, as well as for comorbid illnesses such as depression that may contribute to poor treatment compliance (Fig. 7-1). The first step is to identify, if possible, the underlying primary headache disorder(s). The management approach may include treatment of the analgesic overuse by analgesic withdrawal, abortive and prophylactic therapy for the chronic tension-type headaches, and abortive and prophylactic therapy for the migraine attacks. It is especially important to carefully limit use of abortive therapies to avoid aggravation of the headache problem.

In clinical practice, it is not uncommon to see improvements in some components of the headache syndrome and intractability in other components. After drug withdrawal and initiation of abortive and prophylactic

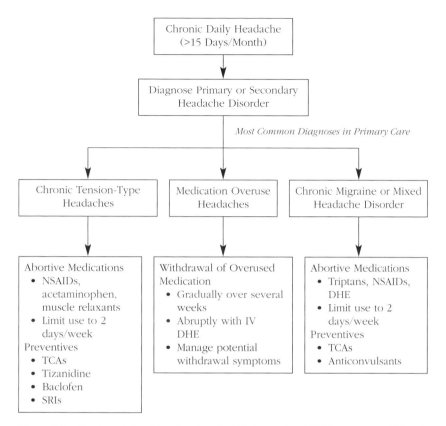

Figure 7-1   Treatment algorithm for chronic daily headache. NSAIDs = nonsteroidal anti-inflammatories; SSRIs = selective serotonin reuptake inhibitors; DHE = dihydroergotamine; TCAs = tricyclic antidepressants.

therapies, patients may improve in their ability to manage their acute migraine attacks but continue to be burdened by the frequency of their migraine or tension-type headache attacks. Their quality of life and functional ability are often significantly improved, yet they may still report having frequent headaches. In these cases, practitioners should rely on quality of life or functional (disability) measures, rather than number of headache days, to judge the outcome of therapy. Only by separating chronic daily headache into individual components that can be targeted for treatment can the overall situation be improved.

The use of biofeedback-assisted relaxation and other nonpharmacological treatments, as outlined in Chapter 5, are often extraordinarily helpful in chronic daily headache. Their use can decrease reliance on medication and thus assist in tapering or discontinuation protocols. Cognitive behavioral techniques are also useful because they challenge long-established and counterproductive behavior patterns (e.g., taking medication "just in case" of a headache, beliefs that absence from school is appropriate for mild headache, expectations of treatment failure). The practitioner can modify therapy to improve the poorly controlled component(s) of the headache syndrome without giving up the gains achieved in other components.

Withdrawal of Medications and Detoxification

Detoxification from habituating drugs is the initial step in the treatment of patients who are taking excessive pain medications. Prophylactic medication is generally ineffective for patients suffering from overuse or withdrawal headaches but becomes effective once medication overuse has resolved. Frequently patients will say that they "would stop taking pain medication if only the preventive medication prevented the headaches". Patients must be instructed that the "pain medication" is part of the cause of the headaches, and that headache therapy is futile until the rebound/habituation cycle is resolved.

Management of the habituated patient can be difficult, and the medical literature offers little insight into proper techniques of detoxification. Detoxification can be accomplished on an outpatient or inpatient basis, and the offending medications can be withdrawn abruptly or gradually.

Gradual withdrawal of the offending analgesic medications on an outpatient basis can often be accomplished and may represent the most reasonable approach for most primary care physicians. The quantity of abortive medication is gradually reduced every week until the offending medication is withdrawn or reduced to acceptable quantities. It may take 8 to 12 weeks to detoxify patients in this fashion depending on the quantity of abortive medication consumed by the patient. To accomplish such a withdrawal, patients should be seen in the office every 2 weeks, and decreasing quantities of the abortive medication should be dispensed at the time of each visit.

Abrupt outpatient withdrawal of abortive medications can also be undertaken. Several protocols have been proposed. Hering and Steiner reported successful outpatient management of patients with analgesic-overuse headache using a technique consisting of abrupt drug withdrawal, explanation of the disorder, regular follow-up, amitriptyline 10 mg at bedtime for prophylaxis, and naproxen 500 mg for acute relief (30). Smith reported an effective outpatient treatment plan for analgesic rebound headache that included abrupt drug withdrawal, tizanidine 2 mg at bedtime titrated every 3-5 days to 2-16 mg at bedtime, and a long-acting NSAID or coxib in the morning (31).

Abrupt withdrawal of medications carries with it the risk for withdrawal syndromes. Typical analgesic withdrawal symptoms last 2 to 10 days (average 3.5) and include headache, nausea, vomiting, hypotension, tachycardia, sleep disturbances, restlessness, and anxiety. Seizures and hallucinations are rare, even for patients using barbiturate-combination drugs. Patients who are habituated to opioids may benefit from clonidine therapy to prevent withdrawal, and those taking butalbital-containing medications may benefit from phenobarbital. In the absence of good scientific evidence, glucocorticoids and phenothiazines are sometimes prescribed for outpatient detoxification from butalbital, ergotamine, or low doses of opioids. Generally, a 6 to 14 day tapering course of glucocorticoid is given, with phenothiazine suppositories prescribed for severe withdrawal headaches associated with vomiting. See Table 7-5 for recommended strategies for the prevention of withdrawal symptoms.

Attempts of outpatient withdrawal sometimes are not successful, so inpatient therapy is occasionally required. Most primary care physicians would probably refer to a specialist at this time. During hospitalization, all offending analgesic medications are stopped abruptly and the patient may be administered intravenous dihydroergotamine to prevent withdrawal headaches. Generally, the intravenous dihydroergotamine provides a "bridge" to enable the patient to cease use of the offending medication.

Prevention of Relapse

Prevention of relapse after detoxification is critical to prevent recurrence. About one third of patients will relapse into drug overuse within the first 5 years after detoxification. Almost 90% of patients who relapse use the same drug that they initially overused (28).

To reduce the risk of relapse in patients treated for analgesic overuse, patients should be instructed to follow these recommendations:

- Use specific antimigraine drugs only for migraine attacks.
- Restrict the dose of ergots and triptans per attack and per week.
- Avoid mixed analgesics, butalbital, opioids, and tranquilizers.
- Start prophylactic drugs early (start prophylaxis for 2 or 3 attacks per month rather than for the 3 to 5 attacks per month in patients with headache not induced by analgesic overuse).

Table 7-5   Strategies for Preventing Withdrawal Symptoms

Medication Withdrawn	Prevention Strategies
Opioids	Clonidine tablets 0.1-0.3 mg bid or a clonidine patch TTS 1, 2, or 3 applied q wk
Butalbital-containing medications	For patients taking fewer than 5 butalbital-containing meds, can wean over 5 days; for those taking more than 5 tabs, can substitute phenobarbital at a dose of 30 mg for every 100 mg of butalbital, then wean by 10%/day or 30 mg/day

Pharmacological Treatment

Preventive Therapy

The goals of preventive therapy in chronic daily headache are similar to those in migraine: 1) reduction in headache frequency and severity, 2) improved responsiveness to abortive medications, and 3) decreased functional impairment. Because the majority of patients with chronic daily headache have a migraine component to their illness, trials of medications with proven efficacy in migraine are reasonable. Additionally, anecdotal, open-label, and clinical trial evidence exists for some agents in the chronic daily headache population. The efficacy of prophylaxis in chronic daily headache is certainly no better than that of prophylaxis for episodic migraine, and it is possibly worse because these patients tend to be more refractory to treatment. As with that disorder, a common measure of treatment success is a 50% reduction in headache frequency or severity. Given the often refractory nature of chronic daily headache, however, many clinicians and patients are pleased with lesser reduction and may choose to continue treatment despite such modest gains, particularly when other therapeutic options have been exhausted.

There are no drugs currently approved by the Food and Drug Administration specifically for the treatment of chronic daily headache. However, given the chronic nature of the disorder and the risk of MOH in patients with frequent headaches, prophylactic therapy seems warranted for most patients. Because chronic headache is a disorder of central pain processing, medications with central pain modulating effects tend to be the most effective (32). These include tricyclic antidepressants, NSAIDs, muscle relaxants, and anticonvulsants. Beta-blockers and calcium channel blockers, which are effective preventives for episodic migraine, tend to be less effective agents for the daily headache component of chronic migraine.

Preventive therapies for chronic daily headache can be categorized into first- and second-line therapies (Table 7-6). First-line therapies generally include medications with relatively low side-effect profiles such as tricyclic antidepressants, NSAIDs, and muscle relaxants. Second-line therapies include anticonvulsants, which generally have more significant side effects (some lead to teratogenic side effects in women of childbearing age). First-line

Table 7-6   First-Line and Second-Line Preventive Therapies for Chronic Daily Headache

Type	Therapy
First-line*	Tricyclic antidepressants, NSAIDs, muscle relaxers
Second-line†	Anticonvulsants (e.g., divalproex sodium, gabapentin, topiramate)

* First-line preventives can be used for chronic daily headache in patients with tension-type, migraine, or mixed headache disorders (migraine and tension-type headaches coexist in the same patient).
† Second-line preventives are primarily used in patients with chronic migraine or mixed headache disorders.

therapies can be used for chronic migraine or tension-type headaches; second-line therapies have been primarily studied in those with chronic migraine headache. Dosages and side effects of the various preventives are shown in Table 7-7.

TRICYCLIC ANTIDEPRESSANTS

Tricyclic antidepressants are the drugs of choice for chronic tension-type headache, and several of these agents are also effective in migraine prophylaxis. The antidepressants that have been tested in double-blind placebo-controlled studies of patients with chronic tension-type headache include amitriptyline, doxepin, and maprotiline (33). Other tricyclic antidepressants may also be effective, as suggested by clinical experience, although they have not been studied in this population.

Amitriptyline reduced the number of headache days or the duration of headache by approximately 50% in about one third of patients in some studies (34-36), although another study found it to be no better than placebo (37). The usual starting dose of amitriptyline (or a similar drug) is 10 mg at bedtime. The dosage can be increased every few days until a therapeutic result is obtained or side effects become intolerable. Antidepressants usually take 4 to 6 weeks to show beneficial effects.

The selective serotonin reuptake inhibitors (SSRIs) fluoxetine, paroxetine, and citalopram have not shown efficacy in controlled studies (38-40); however, they are sometimes used to treat depression (common in many chronic headache patients) because they have a lower incidence of side effects compared with tricyclic antidepressants. Because the efficacy of SSRIs in headache prophylaxis is less well documented, they should be primarily considered for the treatment of depression in patients who cannot tolerate, or who fail, tricyclic therapy.

MUSCLE RELAXANTS

Baclofen is a GABA analogue and has been used to treat a number of chronic pain conditions including chronic daily headache. One open study in patients with MOH found decreased headache frequency and severity and decreased daily analgesic use with baclofen taken at doses of 15-50 mg/day (41).

Tizanidine, an alpha-adrenergic blocker, was reported to be effective for chronic tension-type headache in a single placebo-controlled study (42). A randomized controlled study in chronic daily headache patients demonstrated a reduction in the headache index, mean headache days, headache severity, and headache duration in the tizanidine group (43). The dosage was titrated from 2 mg at bedtime to 24 mg per day, divided into three doses. Sedation is the most common adverse effect of this agent.

Cyclobenzaprine is a muscle relaxant that is related structurally to amitriptyline. In a 1972 double-blind study (44), 10 of 20 patients receiving

Table 7-7   Dosages and Side Effects of Common Preventives

Preventive	Dosage	Common Side Effects
Amitryptyline	Starting dose: 10 mg PO qhs Titration: Increase by 10 mg increments as tolerated at 2-4 week intervals Maintenance dose: 10-75 mg PO qhs	Sedation, dry mouth, weight gain
Nortryptyline	Starting dose: 10 mg PO qhs Titration: Increase by 10 mg increments as tolerated at 2-4 week intervals Maintenance dose: 10-75 mg PO qhs	Sedation, dry mouth, weight gain
Ibuprofen	Starting dose: 400-800 mg tid Titration: Uncertain if necessary Maintenance dose: Same	GI side effects; avoid in renal failure
Naproxen sodium	Starting dose: 550 mg PO bid Titration: None Maintenance dose: Same	GI side effects; avoid in renal failure
Rofecoxib	Starting dose: 12.5-25 mg qd Titration: None Maintenance dose: 12.5-25 mg qd	Diarrhea; avoid in renal failure
Celecoxib	Starting dose: 100 mg qd Titration: Uncertain if necessary Maintenance dose: 100-200 bid	Rash in sulfa allergic patients; avoid in renal failure
Baclofen	Starting dose: 10 mg PO tid Titration: Increase to 20 mg PO tid at 4 weeks if tolerated. Maintenance dose: 10-20 mg PO tid	Sedation, dizziness
Tizanidine	Starting dose: 4 mg PO qhs Titration: Increase by 4 mg increments at 2-4 week intervals Maintenance dose: 4-24 mg PO qhs	Somnolence, dizziness, dry mouth, asthenia
Valproate extended release	Starting dose: 500 mg PO qhs Titration: Increase from 500 to 1000 mg at 1 month Maintenance dose: 500-1000 mg PO qhs	Weight gain, tremulousness, teratogenic side effects, hepatotoxicity, pancreatitis
Gabapentin	Starting dose: 100 mg PO tid Titration: If tolerated, increase to 300 mg PO tid for 2-4 weeks, then 400 mg PO tid for 2-4 weeks, then 600 mg PO tid for 2-4 weeks, and then 800 mg PO tid Maintenance dose: 100-800 mg PO tid	Lethargy, dizziness, teratogenic side effects
Topiramate	Starting dose: 25 mg PO qhs Titration: Increase by 25 mg increments at 2 week intervals Maintenance dose: 25-200 mg PO qhs	Weight loss, kidney stones in 1%-2%, paresthesia, short-term memory loss (not permanent), glaucoma, teratogenic side effects

cyclobenzaprine showed a 50% or greater improvement in chronic tension-type headache, whereas only 5 of 20 patients receiving placebo were improved. The usual dose of cyclobenzaprine is 10 mg at bedtime.

Nonsteroidal Anti-Inflammatory Drugs
NSAIDs are widely prescribed as abortive therapy for tension-type and migraine headache and for the prophylaxis of these headache types (16). There are no randomized controlled trials of their efficacy in the prophylaxis of chronic tension-type headache, but several NSAIDs have shown efficacy for migraine prophylaxis (16). Thus their use in chronic daily headache can be considered

Divalproex Sodium
Divalproex sodium, a GABA agonist anticonvulsant, has been evaluated for efficacy in migraine and chronic daily headache (45-47). Mathew and Ali evaluated its efficacy at a dose of 1000-2000 mg/day in 30 patients with intractable chronic daily headache (migraine without aura and chronic tension-type headaches) in an open-label trial (47). Blood levels were maintained between 75 and 100 µg/mL. By the third month of therapy, two thirds of patients had improved significantly. They reported common side effects of weight gain, tremor, hair loss, and nausea. These results have not been replicated in a randomized controlled trial.

Gabapentin
Gabapentin at doses of 400-1200 mg was found to reduce headache frequency in one randomized controlled study of chronic daily headache patients (48). Another open trial in chronic daily headache patients also demonstrated a reduction in headache frequency (49). The most common side effects include fatigue, dizziness, and weight gain. The efficacy of gabapentin for migraine is also limited.

Topiramate
Topiramate is an anticonvulsant that has been shown in two randomized controlled studies to be effective in the prevention of episodic migraine headache (50,51,51a,51b). A recent randomized placebo-controlled trial in patients with chronic migraine reported a significantly lower headache frequency per 28-day treatment period with 50 mg/day of topiramate compared with placebo (8.1 days in the opiramate group vs. 20.6 in the placebo group; $P < 0.0007$) (52). A prospective open-label study in patients with chronic migraine headaches demonstrated a reduction of headache frequency of 70% (53). Three other retrospective case series suggested that topiramate reduces both the frequency and severity of chronic migraine headache (54-56). Trials assessing this possibility are underway.

BOTULINUM TOXIN

Botulinum toxin injections into the muscles of the head and neck have been found effective for the relief of chronic tension-type headache in small series of patients (57-59). Results from small clinical trials have been mixed, and two large placebo-controlled trials are being conducted, one of which examines its use in patients with chronic daily headache. Botulinum toxin treatment is expensive and rarely covered by third-party payers for headache treatment. The risks of treatment are small, however, and some patients with refractory headaches pursue this treatment

PRIMARY CARE APPROACH TO PREVENTIVE THERAPY

It is appropriate for primary care physicians to initiate first-line preventive therapies for patients with chronic daily headache. Depending on their degree of comfort, physicians may wish to initiate some second-line therapies as well. Dosages may need to be titrated for many of the medications, and it may take 1 to 2 months to see the desired preventive effect. Therefore physicians should not give up on the medications after only a short trial at a possibly inadequate dosage. It may be necessary to prescribe more than one preventive simultaneously to see clinical improvement. It is advisable to combine preventives that have different mechanisms of action (e.g., antconvulsants with a TCA, an NSAID with a muscle relaxant) Also, any existing comorbid depression must be treated for optimal response. Because all preventives can cause side effects, the lowest dose that produces the desired clinical response should be used.

Abortive Therapy

Abortive treatment is used in conjunction with prophylactic treatment. Treatment of the daily, tension-type headache with abortive medications is difficult. Muscle relaxants such as chlorzoxazone, orphenadrine citrate, carisoprodol, and metaxalone, either alone or in combination with aspirin, acetaminophen, and/or caffeine, are commonly prescribed to patients with chronic tension-type headache, but they have not been shown to be effective for acute headache relief (32). NSAIDs may be useful as analgesics for daily headache and may lack the potential for causing medication-induced headache (27). Sumatriptan has been evaluated in several studies in tension-type headache (60,61). It was no more effective than placebo in acute attacks for patients with chronic tension-type headache, but severe episodic tension-type headaches in patients with coexisting migraine appear to be responsive (62).

Migraine-specific medications such as the triptans should be used for the migraine headache. Because some patients with chronic migraine may have daily migraines, it may be advisable to restrict triptans use to fewer than 10 doses per month for less than 2 days per week. Benzodiazepines, butalbital combinations, and opioids should be avoided, or their use carefully controlled, because of the risk of habituation and analgesic-overuse headache with frequent use.

Nonpharmacological Treatment

Many clinical studies have supported the utility of relaxation and electromyographic biofeedback therapies in the management of chronic tension-type headache (63). Averaging the results of 37 trials that used daily headache recordings to evaluate relaxation or electromyographic biofeedback therapies, each therapy or their combination yielded a 50% reduction in tension-type headache activity. Studies have not found differences between the efficacy of relaxation, biofeedback, or their combination.

Stress management therapy using cognitive behavior therapy is as effective as relaxation or biofeedback therapy in reducing tension-type headache. Cognitive therapy may be most likely to enhance the effectiveness of relaxation or biofeedback therapies when chronic stress, depression, or adjustment problems aggravate the patient's headaches (63).

The combination of nonpharmacological therapy and pharmacotherapy provides greater benefit than either therapy used alone. The addition of guided imagery to pharmacotherapy resulted in significant improvements in both health-related quality of life and headache-related disability (64). In a placebo-controlled study comparing tricyclic antidepressant medication with stress management therapy, both modalities were modestly effective by themselves in treating chronic tension-type headache, but combined therapy was better than monotherapy (65).

Nonpharmacological therapy is particularly useful for patients who are reluctant to take medications due to desire for pregnancy, previous adverse reactions to medications, or concomitant medical problems. Whereas biofeedback and stress management usually require referral to psychologists, guided imagery and relaxation therapy can be learned from audio tapes or compact discs available at many book and health stores (32).

Prognosis

The natural history of chronic daily or very frequent headache is poorly understood, and there are no controlled studies of long-term outcomes. Case-control studies suggest that 35% to 43% of sufferers were still having chronic daily headaches after 1 or 2 years of follow-up (11). In elderly patients the prognosis was even worse, with approximately two thirds of patients continuing to have chronic daily headache after 2 years (11). High analgesic use predicted a worse outcome (11).

When to Refer to a Headache Specialist

Guidelines suggest the following indications for referral to a headache specialist (66):

- The headache status remains unchanged despite the best efforts of the practitioner, initial diagnosis is in question, or there is physician and/or patient discomfort with the progress of therapy.
- Headache-related disability remains moderate to severe.
- Headache symptoms change, no longer fitting diagnostic criteria.
- Comorbid conditions (i.e., psychiatric, neurological, medical) exist or develop, requiring specialized care or complex medication regimens.
- Analgesic abuse, failed outpatient detoxification, or analgesic rebound headaches limit outpatient management.
- Other conditions exist, such as intractable cluster headache or status migrainosus, for which parenteral infusion therapy may be appropriate.

After resolving any diagnostic or acute management issues, the goal of headache consultation should be the development of a long-range plan for patient management including headache prevention, abortive approaches, and rescue therapies. Because most headache disorders are chronic conditions, long-term management will usually revert to the primary care practitioner.

Key Points

- Chronic daily headache is defined as headache occurring more than 15 days per month, lasting more than 4 hours per day.
- 4% of the population suffers from chronic daily headache.
- Chronic daily headache can evolve from several different underlying headache problems.
- The key to management is making the appropriate diagnosis, then breaking these headache types into separate components for treatment.
- There is no specific treatment for chronic daily headache, but there are specific approaches that are effective for medication overuse headache, chronic tension-type headache, and migraine.
- Hospitalization or specialty inpatient headache treatment should be considered in some cases.
- Some patients with chronic daily headache will remain intractable despite aggressive treatment. For them, a functional and rehabilitative approach to treatment is best.

REFERENCES

1. **Silberstein SD, Lipton RB, Sliwinski M.** Classification of daily and near-daily headaches: field trial of revised HIS criteria. Neurology. 1996;47:871-5.

2. **International Headache Society.** Classification and Diagnostic Criteria for Headache Disorders, Cranial Neuralgias, and Facial Pain. Cephalalgia. 1988;8(Suppl 7): 1-96.

3. **Scher AI, Stewart WF, Liberman J, Lipton RB.** Prevalence of frequent headache in a population sample. Headache. 1998;38:497-506.

4. **Castillo J, Munoz P, Guitera V, Pascual J.** Epidemiology of chronic daily headache in the general population. Headache. 1999;39:190-6.

5. **Lu SR, Fuh JL, Chen WT, et al.** Chronic daily headache in Taipei, Taiwan: prevalence, follow-up, and outcome predictors. Cephalalgia. 2001;21:980-6.

6. **Hagen K, Zwart JA, Vaten L, et al.** Prevalence of migraine and non-migrainous headache: head HUNT, a large population-based study. Cephalalgia. 2000;20:900-6.

7. **Wang SJ, Fuh JL, Lu SR, et al.** Chronic daily headache in Chinese elderly. Prevalence, risk factors, and biannual follow-up. Neurology. 2000;54:314-9.

8. **Prencipe M, Casini AR, Ferretti C, et al.** Prevalence of headache in an elderly population: attack frequency, disability, and use of medication. J Neurol Neurosurg Psychiatry. 2001;70:377-81.

9. **Scher AI.** A Case-Control Study of Chronic Daily Headache in the General Population. Baltimore: Johns Hopkins University; 2001.

10. **Newman LC, Lipton SB, Solomon S, et al.** Daily headache in a population sample: results from American Migraine Study. Headache. 1994;34:295.

11. **Scher AI.** Natural history of and risk factors for headache transformation. Paper presented to American Headache Society, 21 June 2002, Seattle.

12. **Rasmussen BK, Jensen R, Olesen J.** Epidemiology of tension-type headache in a general population. In: Olesen J, Schoenen J, eds. Tension-Type Headache: Classification, Mechanisms, and Treatment. New York: Raven Press; 1993:9-13.

13. **Karpouzis K, Spierings E.** Circumstances of onset of chronic headache in patients attending a specialty practice. Headache. 1999;39:317-20.

14. **Schoenen J.** Session IV discussion summary: central mechanisms of tension-type headache. In: Olesen J, Schoenen J, eds. Tension-Type Headache: Classification, Mechanisms, and Treatment. New York: Raven Press; 1993:207-8.

15. **Vandenheede M, Schoen J.** Central mechanisms in tension-type headache. Curr Pain Headache Rep. 2002;6:392-400.

16. **Bendtsen L.** Sensitization: its role in primary headache. Curr Opin Investig Drugs. 2002;3:449-53.

17. **Scher A, Stewart W, Ricci J, et al.** Factors associated with the onset and remission of chronic daily headache in a population-based study. Pain. 2003;106:81-9.

18. **Scher A, Lipton R, Stewart W.** Habitual snoring as a risk factor for chronic daily headache. Neurology. 2003;60:1366-8.

19. **Merikangas KR, Angst J, Isler H.** Migraine and psychopathology: results of the Zurich cohort study of young adults. Arch Gen Psychiatry. 1990;47:849-53.

20. **Breslau N, Davis GC.** Migraine, physical health and psychiatric disorders: a prospective epidemilogic study of young adults. J Psychiatr Res. 1993;27:211-21.

21. **Verri AP, Cecchini P, Galli C, et al.** Psychiatric comorbidity in chronic daily headache. Cephalalgia. 1998;18:45-9.

22. **Silberstein DS, Lipton RB.** Chronic daily headache, including transformed migraine, chronic tension-type headache, and medication overuse. In: Silberstein SD, Lipton RB, Dalessio DJ, eds. Wolff's Headache, 7th ed. New York: Oxford University Press; 2001:247-82.

23. **Breslau N.** New insights into the comorbidity of migraine. Paper presented to American Headache Society, 21 June 2002, Seattle.

24. **Bech P, Langemark M, Loidrup D, et al.** Tension-type headache: psychiatric aspects. In: Olesen J, Schoenen J, eds. Tension-Type Headache: Classification, Mechanisms, and Treatment. New York: Raven Press; 1993:143-6.

25. **Goncalves JA, Monteiro P.** Psychiatric analysis of patients with tension-type headache. In: Olesen J, Schoenen J, eds. Tension-Type Headache: Classification, Mechanisms, and Treatment. New York: Raven Press; 1993:167-72.

26. **Mathew NT.** Transformed migraine. Neurol Clinics. 1997;15:167-86.

27. **Lipton RB.** Frequent headaches: a far too frequent problem. Headache World. London; Sept. 2000.

28. **Diener HC, Dahlof CG.** Headache associated with chronic use of substances. In: Olesen J, Tfelt-Hansen P, Welch KMA, eds. The Headaches, 2nd ed. Philadelphia: Lippincott Williams and Wilkins; 2000:871-8.

29. **Von Korff M.** Chronic use of symptomatic headache medications. Pain. 1995;62: 179-86.

30. **Hering R, Steiner T.** Abrupt outpatient withdrawal from medication in analgesic-abusing migraineurs. Lancet. 1991;337:1442-3.

31. **Smith TR.** Low-dose tizanidine with non-steroidal anti-inflammatory drugs for detoxification from analgesic rebound headache. Headache. 2002;42:175-7.

32. **Solomon GD.** Tension-type headache: advice for the vice-like headache. Cleve Clin J Med. 2002;69:167-72.

33. **Mathew N, Bendtsen L.** Prophylactic pharmacotherpy of tension-type headache. In: Olesen J, Tfelt-Hansen P, Welch KMA, eds. The Headaches, 2nd ed. Philadelphia: Lippincott Williams and Wilkins; 2000:667-73.

34. **Lance J, Curran DA.** Treatment of chronic tension headache. Lancet. 1964;42:236-9.

35. **Diamond S, Baltes BJ.** Chronic tension headache treated with amitriptyline: a double-blind study. Headache. 1971;11:110-6.

36. **Gobel H, Hamouz V, Hansen C, et al.** Chronic tension-type headache: amitriptyline reduces headache duration and experimental pain sensitivity but does not alter pericranial muscle activity readings. Pain. 1994;59:241-9.

37. **Pfaffenrath V, Diener HC, Isler H, et al.** Efficacy and tolerability of amitriptylinoxide in the treatment of chronic tension-type headache: a multi-centre controlled study. Cephalalgia. 1994;14:149-55.

38. **Saper J, Silberstein S, Lake A, Winters M.** Double-blind trial of fluoxetine: chronic daily headache and migraine. Headache. 1994;34:497-502.

39. **Foster CA, Bafaloukos J.** Paroxetine on the treatment of chronic daily headache. Headache. 1994;34:587-9.

40. **Bendtsen L, Jensen R, Olesen J.** A nonselective (amitriptyline), but not a selective (citalopram), serotonin reuptake inhibitor is effective in the prophylactic treatment of chronic tension-type headache. J Neurol Neurolsurg Psychiatry. 1996; 61:285-90.

41. **Hering R.** Abrupt withdrawal of medication using baclofen in migraineurs with chronic headache [Abstract]. Cephalalgia. 1997;17:460.

42. **Fogelholm R, Murros K.** Tizanidine in chronic tension-type headache: a placebo-controlled double-blind crossover study. Headache. 1992;32:509-13.

43. **Saper J, Lake A, Cantrell D, et al.** Chronic daily headache prophylaxis with tizanidine: a double-blind, placebo-controlled, multicenter outcome study. Headache 2002;42:470-82.

44. **Lance JW, Anthony M.** Cyclobenzaprine in the treatment of chronic tension headache. Med J Aust. 1972;2:1409-11.

45. **Sorensen K.** Valproate: a new drug in migraine prophylaxis. Acta Neurol Scand. 1988;78:346-8.

46. **Hering R, Kuritzky A.** Sodium valproate in the prophylactic treatment of migraine: a double-blind study versus placebo. Cephalalgia. 1992;12:81-4.

47. **Mathew N, Ali S.** Valproate in the treatment of persistant chronic daily headache: an open-label study. Headache. 1991;31:71-4.

48. **Nicolodi M, Sicuteri F.** NMDA-negative modulation in the therapy of chronic migraine [Abstract]. Cephalalgia. 1997;17:436.

49. **Mathew N.** Gabapentin in migraine prophylaxis [Abstract]. Cephalalgia. 1996; 16:367.

50. **Silberstein S, Hulihan J, Kamin M, Karim M.** Topiramate in migraine prevention: a randomized, double-blind placebo-controlled trial [Abstract]. Headache. 2002;42:407.

51. **Storey JR, Calder CS, Hart DE, Potter DL.** Topiramate in migraine prevention: a double-blind, placebo-controlled study. Headache. 2001;41:968-75.

51a. **Brandes JL, Saper JR, Diamond M, et al.** Topiramate for migraine prevention: a randomized controlled trial. JAMA. 2004;291:965-73.

51b. **Silberstein S, Neto W, Schmitt J, Jacobs D.** Topiramate in migraine prevention: results of a large controlled trial. Arch Neurol. 2004:61:490-5.

52. **Silverestrini M, Bartolini M, Coccia M, et al.** Topiramate in the treatment of chronic migraine. Cephalagia. 2003;23:820-4.

53. **Krusz J.** Topiramate: effective prophylaxis treatment for refractory migraines and mixed headaches [Abstract]. Cephalalgia. 2001;4:371.

54. **Mathew N, Kailasam J, Fischer A.** Prophylaxis of migraine, transformed migraine and cluster headache with topiramate. Headache. 2002;42:796-803.

55. **Young W, Hopkins M, Shechter A, Silberstein S.** Topiramate: a case series study in migraine prophylaxis. Cephalalgia. 2002;22:659-63.

56. **Von Seggern R, Adelman J, Mannix L.** A retrospective chart review demonstrating the efficacy of topiramate for prophylaxis of migraine [Abstract]. Cephalalgia. 2001;4:369.

57. **Carruthers A, Langtry J, Carruthers J, Robinson G.** Improvement in tension-type headache when treating wrinkles with botulinum toxin A injections. Headache. 1999;39:662-5.

58. **Smuts J, Baker M, Smuts H, et al.** Prophylactic treatment of chronic tension-type headache using botulinum toxin type A. Eur J Neurol. 1999;6(Suppl 4):S99-S102.

59. **Rollnik JD, Tanneberger O, Schubert M, et al.** Treatment of tension-type headache with botulinum toxin type A: a double-blind, placebo-controlled study. Headache. 2000;40:300-5.

60. **Brennum J, Kjeldsen M, Olesen J.** The 5-HT 1-like agonist sumatriptan has a significant effect in chronic tension-type headache. Cephalalgia. 1992;12:375-9.

61. **Brennum J, Brinck T, Schriver L, et al.** Sumatriptan has no clinically relevant effect in the treatment of episodic tension-type headache. Eur J Neurol. 1996;3:23-8.

62. **Cady R, Gutterman D, Saiers JA, Beach ME.** Responsiveness of non-IHS migraine and tension-type headache to sumatriptan. Cephalalgia. 1997;17:588-90.

63. **Holyroid KA.** Behavioral treatment strategies. In: Olesen J, Schoenen J, eds. Tension-Type Headache: Classification, Mechanisms, and Treatment. New York: Raven Press; 1993:245-54.

64. **Mannix LK, Chandurkar RS, Rybicki LA, et al.** Effect of guided imagery on quality of life for patients with chronic tension-type headache. Headache. 1999; 39:326-34.

65. **Holroyd K, O'Donnell F, Stensland M, et al.** Management of chronic tension-type headache with tricyclic antidepressant medication, stress managemnet therapy, and their combination. JAMA. 2001;285:2208-15.

66. **Solomon GD, Cady R, Klapper J, Ryan R.** National Headache Foundation: standards of care for treating headache in primary care practice. Cleve Clin J Med. 1997;64:373-83.

8

Other Primary and Secondary
Headache Disorders

Frederick G. Freitag, DO

Elizabeth W. Loder, MD

Vincent T. Martin, MD

n addition to migraine, tension-type, and cluster headache, there are
less common primary and secondary headache disorders. They may
occur in isolation or co-exist with other headache disorders. These disorders can be encountered within primary care and must be entertained in
the differential diagnosis of the headache patient.

Other Primary Headaches

The International Headache Society (IHS) category of "Other Primary
Headaches" includes headaches whose causes are less well understood
than those of migraine, tension-type, and cluster headache, and for which
treatment is less well-defined. Their clinical presentations, too, vary consid-
erably. Several closely resemble dangerous, secondary causes of headache
and can be diagnosed only after careful evaluation has excluded structural
lesions. What these headaches have in common, though, is that they are
disorders in their own right and not due to underlying problems. Despite
the paucity of treatment options for many of these headaches, accurate
recognition is important because it can help avoid the complications of excessive or nonindicated medical evaluation or treatment.

Eight forms of other primary headaches are recognized by the IHS:

- Primary stabbing headache
- Cough headache

137

- Primary exertional headache
- Headache associated with sexual activity
- Hypnic headache
- Primary thunderclap headache
- Hemicrania continua
- New daily-persistent headache

Primary Stabbing Headache

Primary stabbing headache is often referred to as "ice-pick" or "jabs and jolts" headache because those terms are commonly used by patients in describing the quality of the pain (1,2). This headache is often found in combination with the primary headache disorders of migraine (40% of migraine patients experience this headache at some point) and cluster headache (30% of patients). Interestingly, when stabbing headache co-exists with these disorders, it is often in the same distribution as the other headache, almost always somewhere in the distribution of the first division of the trigeminal nerve. The stabs can switch from location to location within this area, though, and such alteration is reassuring of a benign origin for the pain, although frequently confusing for patients. The pain itself is intense and excruciating but lasts only a few seconds. (The single published descriptive study concluded that 80% of stabs last 3 seconds or less.) This headache is unaccompanied by other symptoms (e.g., nausea, photophobia, phonophobia) and can occur as an isolated jab or a series of jabs ranging from one to many per day.

Primary stabbing headache is more common in females than males. If stabs occur only on occasion, reassurance is often the only treatment indicated. If more frequent occurrence is troublesome, this headache is often responsive to indomethacin. Because these headaches are so short and unpredictable, treatment must be on a scheduled basis; a common regimen is indomethacin 25 mg PO tid (1).

Primary Cough Headache

Primary cough headache is precipitated by coughing, straining (often at toilet), or other forms of exertion that cause sudden elevations in venous pressure. The headache comes on suddenly and lasts from only a second up to 30 minutes. This form of headache is due to serious underlying problems in about 40% of cases, and evaluation should be thorough. MRI is indicated to rule out secondary causes of headache in all patients who have posterior fossa signs or do not respond to attempts at symptomatic treatment with indomethacin. The most common secondary causes of headache include posterior fossa abnormalities such as meningiomas, Arnold-Chiari malformation, acoustic neuromas, and other brain tumors. Benign cough headache is generally shorter than exertional headache and is more often found in older patients; in one series, the oldest patient with benign exertional headache was 48 years of age. Benign cough headache may respond to treatment with indomethacin, but a response to this medication has also been reported in secondary cough headache, so a good response to treatment cannot be taken as evidence of the underlying cause (3).

Primary Exertional Headache

Often termed "benign exertional" to distinguish it from the "symptomatic exertional" headache that may herald subarachnoid hemorrhage or posterior fossa lesions such as Arnold-Chiari malformation, this headache has many characteristics in common with its dangerous counterpart. *Thus any patient with exertional headache must be carefully evaluated for the possibility of subarachnoid hemorrhage or other intracranial abnormalities* (see Chapter 3). Primary exertional headache can be precipitated by any form of exertion; most often it is sustained, rather than short-term. Weight-lifting is such a common precipitant that the term "weight-lifters'" headache is occasionally used. Many experts, however, feel that headache caused by weight-lifting has more in common with cough headache and consider it a subtype of that disorder.

The pain of benign exertional headache most often begins *during* exertion, not immediately, a historical feature worth inquiring about but not one which can be depended upon to indicate a benign cause for the headache. The headache itself is pulsating, usually nonexplosive, in quality, with no characteristic location and no associated features such as nausea or vomiting. It lasts from 5 minutes to 48 hours, during which time the intensity of the pain may gradually diminish. Occasionally, headache occurring with exertion may be explosive and reach maximal intensity within minutes, a form that is especially worrisome for subarachnoid hemorrhage. Exertion is also a trigger and aggravating factor for migraine; in that case, the headache that results has the usual features of the sufferer's migraine attacks such as nausea, vomiting, phototobia, and phonophobia (4).

Benign exertional headache may be more likely to occur at high altitudes, in hot weather, or in other circumstances that make activities unusually strenuous. Once it has been determined that the headache is primary, and not due to some other disorder, treatment consists of alterations in the physical activity that provokes the headache, where feasible (e.g., substituting other nonprovocative activities, decreasing the intensity of a workout but increasing its length). Pharmacological treatment with indomethacin 25 mg alone or in combination with propranolol 20-40 mg an hour before the planned activity is successful in preventing the headache in many cases; pre-treatment with ergotamine is often successful as well. If attacks occur daily, at relatively low exertional intensities, preventive treatment may be necessary. Beta-blockers and NSAIDs are most commonly used, although no clinical trial evidence supports this decision (4).

Primary Headache Associated with Sexual Activity

Two types of benign headache attributable to sexual activity are recognized and can occur with either coitus or masturbation. *Preorgasmic headache* begins during sexual activity and increases with the degree of sexual excitement. This is usually described as a bilateral, dull, achy sensation in the head and neck area, and often seems to correlate with the degree of neck or jaw muscle contraction. It is improved or prevented by ceasing sexual activity. *Orgasmic headache,* in contrast, is a sudden, severe, and explosive headache that begins with orgasm. As with cough headache, this form of headache is worrisome for structural problems such as subarachnoid hemorrhage and carotid dissection, and it must be thoroughly investigated. Benign sexual and exertional headaches are associated in 50% of cases, suggesting that patients who report exertional headache should be queried about headache with sexual activity. Many patients are embarrassed to describe the circumstances of headache onset, which may be one reason for the apparent overlap. Once the benign nature of the headache has been established, treatment is similar to that for exertional headache.

Hypnic Headache

Hypnic headache is a recently recognized, rare primary headache syndrome in which attacks of dull head pain awaken the patient from sleep. Most patients are older, with a mean age at onset of 66. The disorder is more common in women. The pain is usually moderate, bilateral in two thirds of cases, and without associated autonomic symptoms. The headache typically lasts from 15 minutes to 3 hours but is occasionally longer. Nausea, photophobia, and phonophobia occasionally occur but are not characteristic.

This diagnosis can be made only when the headache occurs during sleep. Like cluster headache, attacks often occur at specific times each night, frequently correlating with rapid-eye movement sleep, and can even occur with napping. Bedtime doses of lithium carbonate 300-600 mg and caffeine have been used successfully for treatment. The cause of hypnic headache is unknown, but speculation centers on the hypothalamus because of the timing of attacks. Hypnic headache must be distinguished from cluster headache and trigeminal autonomic cephalgias (see Chapter 6); once this is done, patients can be assured that it is a benign disorder with no long-term medical implications (5,6).

Primary Thunderclap Headache

Primary thunderclap headache is a suddenly occurring, intense headache with pain that mimics that occurring with subarachnoid hemorrhage, carotid dissection, pituitary apoplexy, colloid cysts of the third ventricle, and other abrupt central nervous system vascular emergencies. Because the headache is initially indistinguishable from those occurring with more dangerous entities, it is a diagnosis that can only be made in retrospect. The search for an underlying explanation for the headache must be thorough, in most cases including appropriate imaging studies (MRI or MRA) and lumbar puncture. In fact, negative imaging and CSF studies are required by IHS criteria before the diagnosis can be made.

Head pain is severe and reaches maximum intensity in under a minute. It may be described by the patient as the "worst headache ever", words that should prompt immediate suspicion of a serious underlying cause for the headache, even in a patient with a previously existing headache disorder. Thunderclap headache can last from 1 hour to 10 days and does not occur in any regular pattern, a feature useful in distinguishing it from migraine or other primary headache disorders. The IHS comments that "the evidence that thunderclap headache exists as a primary condition is poor" but includes it because there are cases in which this headache cannot be attributed to underlying pathology even after exhaustive evaluation. Treatment is poorly defined, and empirical trials of agents typically used in migraine treatment are usually recommended (7,8).

Hemicrania Continua

Hemicrania continua is a rare and poorly understood headache disorder that is so responsive to treatment with indomethacin that is has been included in a category of headaches termed "indomethacin-responsive". Although response to indomethacin is included in the diagnostic criteria for the disorder, this response to treatment is probably not absolute. The headache of hemicrania continua is continuous, waxing and waning, and strictly unilateral. In contrast to migraine, in which headache may be unilateral but switch sides during or between attacks, the side of headache never varies, and the headache never disappears completely. Superimposed primary stabbing headache may occur. Exacerbations of pain in hemicrania continua may be associated with autonomic features of the sort seen in cluster headache and the TACs; however, this is not a short-lasting headache. The autonomic symptoms and signs can include ipsilateral tearing, ptosis, miosis, and sweating. Occasionally features of migraine, such as nausea, photophobia, or phonophobia, may be present.

Remitting and continuous forms of hemicrania continua have been recognized. In the remitting variety, the headache phases last weeks to months, with long pain-free remission periods. In the continuous variety, headaches occur daily and can be continuous for years. In some patients, the continuous variety develops from the remitting form of the disorder; in others, it is present from onset.

The rarity of this condition has made it difficult to study its epidemiology and pathophysiology. Response to indomethacin means that it is the initial treatment of choice, usually in daily doses from 50 to 150 mg. Other NSAIDs have been effective in some patients. Many patients are able to discontinue treatment after several months and remain pain-free. Others require longer therapy, in which case prevention of gastric ulceration with appropriate medications should be considered.

New Daily-Persistent Headache

This headache disorder begins abruptly and becomes daily within 3 days of onset. Patients generally have no history of a past headache disorder such as migraine or tension-type headaches. These bilateral headaches are described as pressing and tightening with a mild-to-moderate pain intensity. Patients may experience mild photophobia, phonophobia, or nausea (only one of these) (9). These headaches may resemble chronic tension-type headache but may be differentiated from the latter by their sudden onset and daily pattern from the start in a patient with no past history of headache. They tend to be refractory to treatment, but recent case reports suggest a response to anticonvulsants.

Other Secondary Headache Disorders

This section reviews other secondary headache disorders that generally have a more favorable prognosis than those described in Chapter 3. They can be divided into the following categories:

- Headaches associated with the ingestion of food or beverages
  —Alcohol-induced headaches
  —Cold stimulus headache
  —Headaches induced by food components or additives
- Headaches in the obese patient
  —Sleep apnea
  —Idiopathic intracranial hypertension
- Headaches attributed to low cerebral spinal fluid (CSF) pressure
- Headaches associated with head and neck disorders
  —Cervicogenic headaches
  —Occipital neuralgia
  —Temporomandibular joint disease
  —Headaches related to ophthalmological disorders
  —Headaches attributed to rhinosinusitis and mucosal contact points
- Headaches associated with head or neck trauma
  —Post-traumatic headaches
  —Headaches attributed to neck flexion-extension (whiplash) injury
- Headaches associated with systemic illnesses
  —Hypertension
  —Infection
  —Metabolic and endocrine diseases
  —Other systemic illnesses

Headaches Associated with the Ingestion of Food or Beverages

Alcohol-Induced Headaches

The IHS has divided alcohol-induced headaches into two groups: those with immediate and those with delayed onset (9).

Immediate Alcohol-Induced Headaches

The immediate alcohol-induced headache occurs within 3 hours after ingestion and resolves within 72 hours. It is generally located in the bilateral fronto-temporal regions and may be pulsating in nature. Alcohol may trigger a "true migraine" headache in migraineurs or may produce "migraine-like" headaches in those without a history of recurrent headache disorders. The quantity of alcohol required to induce headaches varies from patient to patient but may occur after one or two beverages. Generally these patients are not intoxicated at the start of the headache. The beverages most commonly reported to trigger immediate alcohol-induced headaches in migraineurs are beer and red wine (10).

The mechanisms through which alcoholic beverages induce immediate headache are not well known but have been best studied for red wine. Various investigators have attributed "red wine" headache to the content of phenolic flavinoids and histamine within the beverage. Phenolic flavinoids from red wine have been shown to release serotonin from the platelets of susceptible patients, which could theoretically mirror release of serotonin within the central nervous system (11). Another study reported that headaches were induced by the histamine content of the wine in those with histamine intolerance syndrome and that the headache could be blocked by pretreatment with an H1 blocker (12). Histamine could provoke headache through release of nitric oxide from the dural vasculature or within the central nervous system. Studies have not convincingly demonstrated that other substances such as tyramine and sulfites are related to the development of red wine headache.

Delayed Alcohol-Induced Headaches

Delayed alcohol-induced headaches may be experienced as part of a withdrawal syndrome after the ingestion of moderate-to-large quantities of alcoholic beverages over a short period of time. "Hangover" headaches begin when alcohol levels decline or are absent. The characteristics of the headaches are similar to those for immediate headaches given above, but they may also be associated with other hangover symptoms such as diarrhea, anorexia, tremulousness, fatigue, and nausea. The occurrence of a hangover does not predispose to the development of alcoholism. Light-to-moderate drinkers are more likely to suffer from these headaches than heavy drinkers.

Dehydration, hormonal alterations, prostaglandin release, and the other effects of alcohol may cause delayed alcohol-induced headaches. Acute treatments for the headaches include include rehydration, anti-inflammatories, and vitamin B_6. Pretreatment with NSAIDS has been shown to significantly attenuate hangover symptoms including headache (13).

Cold Stimulus Headaches

Cold stimulus headaches are typically associated with the ingestion of cold beverages or foods or the inhalation of cold air. This headache is often called "ice cream" headache when provoked by that food. The headache occurs within 15 seconds after ingestion and resolves less than 5 minutes after withdrawal of the cold stimulus. Temporary, brief freezing of the soft palate has been hypothesized to cause transient decreases in cerebral blood flow that may play a contributory role in development of these headaches (14). No specific therapy is recommended for these headaches other than avoidance of the offending stimulus.

Headaches Induced by Food Components or Additives

Food components or additives may induce headaches in susceptible patients. A number of substances have been implicated (e.g., nitrates, monosodium glutamate, aspartame, phenylethylamine, tyramine), but their role in the provocation of headaches is not firmly established. The headaches are typically described as located in the bilateral frontotemporal region and described as throbbing. The headache generally develops within 12 hours after ingestion and resolves in less than 72 hours (9).

Headaches in the Obese Patient

Obesity is a worldwide epidemic and may be a risk factor for development of chronic daily headache syndromes (15). Sleep apnea and idiopathic intracranial hypertension are commonly associated with obesity and should be considered in the differential diagnosis of recurrent headache disorders in the obese patient.

Sleep Apnea

Clinical studies have reported an increased risk of morning headache in those with obstructive sleep apnea and snoring. Morning headaches may occur in 18% to 41% of those with obstructive sleep apnea and may be correlated with the degree of sleep apnea (e.g., morning headache may be more common in those with greater nocturnal oxygen desaturations) (16-18). The headaches tend to be short-lived, lasting <30 minutes, and are present upon awakening. These bilateral headaches are described as "pressing" and have a frequency of >15 days per month (9). Treatment of the obstructive sleep apnea may eliminate or decrease the frequency of these headaches (16).

Idiopathic Intracranial Hypertension

Women in their childbearing years are most likely to develop idiopathic intracranial hypertension, which is synonymous with pseudotumor cerebri and benign intracranial hypertension. Headache, the hallmark of this disorder, is throbbing and frontal or temporal in location. The pain is generally moderate to severe, daily, and may be accompanied by cervical pain (19). Transient visual loss and pulsatile tinnitus may also be reported by the patient. Examination of the patient generally reveals papilledema, though it is not required for diagnosis (20). Some patients may also have horizontal diplopia or CN VI palsies. The patients may have visual field defects, which may be difficult to detect without formal examination by an ophthalmologist.

A strong association exists between rapid weight gain in the preceding year and development of idiopathic intracranial hypertension (21). A wide variety of pharmaceutical agents have also been linked to the secondary development of this disorder, including hormones, anti-inflammatory drugs, vitamin A, and several antibiotics. If the intracranial hypertension occurs as a result of dural venous thrombosis, it is classified under the primary disorder.

The diagnosis is made with a lumbar puncture, performed after an MRI scan rules out mass lesions or other causes of elevated pressure. An opening of >250 in an obese patient and >200 in a nonobese patient confirms the diagnosis. The CSF chemistries (e.g., protein) and cell counts must be normal. A MR venogram should also be obtained to exclude dural venous thrombosis in all patients with unexplained intracranial hypertension.

The treatment of pseudotumor cerebri is predominately medical and includes weight loss as the first line of therapy. Patients successful in losing weight are more likely to have resolution of papilledema (22). The diuretic acetazolamide is the drug of first choice for this condition. It decreases CSF production and reduces intracranial pressure. An initial dose of 250 mg twice a day is increased in stepwise fashion to an average maintenance dose of 1 to 2 g/day. An alternative treatment is the diuretic furosemide. An initial dose of 20 mg twice a day is tapered up to 40 mg three times a day if needed (23). Corticosteroids have been used with good effect and produce rapid resolution of papilledema. Steroid dose must be reduced slowly to avoid recurrence of visual loss (24). Steroids, in fact, should probably only be used in cases of impending visual loss, because of possible systemic side effects.

Periodic lumbar puncture has been used as a treatment for idiopathic intracranial hypertension. Unfortunately, CSF pressure may return to pre-treatment levels within 82 minutes (25). Therefore repeat lumbar puncture as a treatment is probably best avoided. Surgery is directed towards relieving the elevated pressure by shunting or optic nerve sheath fenestration. The procedures can be invaluable but should be reserved for patients with visual loss refractory to medical therapy.

Headaches Attributed to Low Cerebral Spinal Fluid Pressure

Headache is the most common initial symptom of low CSF pressure, which is generally suspected based on a history of positional headache but is diagnosed by lumbar puncture. Paradoxically, causes of this syndrome include persistent CSF leak following lumbar puncture or diagnostic procedures such as myelograms. Headaches following lumbar puncture occur in 15% to 30% of patients and seem to be most common in young females. The headache may begin anywhere from minutes up to 12 days after the procedure and last for 2 to 14 days, rarely months. This condition should be considered when headache occurs after epidural or spinal anesthesia. Other causes include CSF fistulas from trauma or surgery and tears of the sheaths of vertebral nerve roots. The headache is usually bilateral, worsens within 15 minutes after standing, and is improved within 30 minutes of lying down. Coughing or straining aggravates the headache (26).

Diagnosis is first suspected clinically and later confirmed with a lumbar puncture demonstrating low CSF pressures (usually <60 mm Hg) in a seated position. One must also perform other radiological tests to determine the site of the CSF leak if there is no antecedent procedure to explain the headache syndrome. A radionuclide cisterogram or myelogram may be necessary to identify a potential site in the head or spine. To identify a leak of the cribiform plate one might place intranasal pledgets and check their radioactive content after injection of a radionuclide into the subarachnoid space.

These headaches are usually refractory to pharmacological interventions but may respond to the ingestion of caffeine. Epidural blood patches and/or saline have been used to resolve these headaches.

Headaches Associated with Head and Neck Disorders

Cervicogenic Headaches
Cervicogenic headaches result from pathology of the cervical spine, with referral of pain to the head. Pain may refer to the head because afferents from C1-C3 nerve roots synapse on second-order neurons of the spinal nucleus of the trigeminal nerve, the main sensory nerve of the head. Causes of cervicogenic headaches include tumors, fractures, infection, and rheumatoid arthritis of the upper cervical spine. The role of cervical spondylosis and cervical disc disease in the provocation of cervicogenic headaches has not been elucidated by clinical studies (27).

These headaches are located in the cervical and occipital regions but may refer to the frontal or orbital areas. The intensity of the pain is moderate to severe and often nonthrobbing. Nausea, photophobia, or phonophobia may accompany the headaches but tend to occur less frequently than with migraine attacks. Certain neck movements or head positioning and palpation of the upper cervical or occipital regions often aggravate the pain. There is frequently restriction in the range of motion of the cervical spine on physical examination, and ipsilateral shoulder or arm pain may be associated with the headaches. Radiological evaluation may show movement abnormalities on flexion/extension, abnormal posture, fractures, congenital abnormalities, rheumatoid arthritis, or other cervical pathology. Anesthetic nerve blocks of the greater or lesser occipital nerves, facet joints, or cervical nerve roots provide complete or near-complete (>90% improvement) resolution of the pain for short periods of time. The headaches also resolve within 3 months after treatment of the underlying disorder (9,28).

Treatment depends on the underlying cervical disorder leading to the headaches. Sometimes anesthetic nerve blocks with or without steroids of the involved nerve or facet joint may provide long-lasting improvements. More commonly, however, the pain temporarily improves and relapses days to weeks later. Some advocate radiofrequency ablative procedures of the involved nerve in such cases, but prospective studies are lacking to demonstrate their long-term benefit. Surgical procedures such as anterior fusion of the cervical spine and laminectomy of cervical vertebrae have been reported to improve neck pain from cervical disc disease, but their specific role in the treatment of cervicogenic headache has not been well defined (27).

There are no medications approved by the Food and Drug Administration for the treatment of cervicogenic headaches. However, tricyclic antidepressants (e.g., amitryptyline, nortryptyline), anticonvulsants (e.g., gabapentin), NSAIDS (e.g., ibuprofen, naproxen sodium), and muscle relaxants (e.g., tizanidine, baclofen) have been used anecdotally for preventive treatment (27).

Occipital Neuralgia

Occipital neuralgia is categorized as a distinct entity separate from cervicogenic headaches in the 2004 IHS diagnostic criteria. The pain is paroxysmal, sharp, and located in the distribution of the greater or lesser occipital nerves or third occipital nerve. There may also be a persistent aching in the same areas between paroxysms of pain. Decreased sensation or dysesthesia of the involved nerve may be demonstrated on physical examination. The pain is improved temporarily by diagnostic nerve blocks (9).

Treatment of occipital neuralgia may include repeated anesthetic blocks of the occipital nerve (with or without steroids). Surgical therapies have included surgical liberation and decompression of the entrapped occipital nerve. One study reported short-term improvement in pain with decompression of the nerve, but 46 of 50 patients had relapsed at 3 to 4 year follow-up (29). Neurectomy of the occipital nerve has not been helpful in the treatment of occipital neuralgia (27).

Temporomandibular Joint Disorder

The temporomandibular joints (TMJs) are often thought by many, especially dentists, to be a common cause of headaches. The joints themselves are substantially different from other joints in the body because of their nonhyaline fibroconnective tissue, articular coverings, diarthroidal structure, and limitation of motion caused by the teeth. The joint may undergo remodeling processes induced by tooth loss, dental restorations, trauma, clenching, and grinding. The changes often begin with alterations in the disc mechanics but can progress to osteoarthritic changes in the joints. These processes are not typically painful, although associated musculoskeletal changes may lead to pain. Disruption in the diarthroidal disc mechanics may produce noise from the joint and is found in up to 30% of the population (30). Dental appliances and craniofacial massage may be helpful in this syndrome.

Headaches associated with the TMJs are located in the ipsilateral temporal or parietal regions. They generally are of mild-to-moderate intensity and often are daily. In order to attribute the pain to this disorder one of the following four IHS criteria (9) must be met:

1. Pain must be precipitated by jaw movements and/or chewing of hard or tough food
2. Reduced range of or irregular jaw opening
3. Noise from one or both TMJs during jaw movement
4. Tenderness of the joint capsule of one or both TMJs

The disorder may be demonstrated on X-ray, MRI, or bone scintigraphy. To confirm the diagnosis the headache must resolve or improve within 3 months after successful treatment of the disorder (9).

Myofascial pain syndromes are the most common attendant cause of pain associated with structural abnormalities of the TMJ. These pain syndromes are associated with trigger points that can produce both local and referred pain (31). The pain of these trigger points is variable in nature and may be associated with autonomic phenomena including photophobia and phonophobia (32). The referred pain may not follow neurological pathways and may be mediated by interactive pain processing occulting in the brainstem and spinal cord in a manner analogous to that which has been described for migraine (33). Treatment involves antidepressants to enhance central pain inhibition, physical therapy, exercises, trigger-point injections, and correction of underlying joint mechanics.

Headaches Related to Ophthalmological Disorders

Many patients seek care for their headaches from optometrists and ophthalmologists because they either experience visual disturbances related to their headaches or their headaches occur related to visual activities. The eye rarely plays a direct role in these headaches (2). Visual disturbances related to headache in the vast majority of cases are migraine auras or other visual disturbances related to migraine headache attacks. Refractive errors may occasionally cause tension-type headache if the refractive error is great. Disorders of eye muscle balance may cause headaches if the patient has to markedly alter head and neck positioning to alleviate diplopia.

Acute eye diseases such as acute angle-closure glaucoma, corneal erosions, and iritis will typically present with pain localized to the eye itself. Occasionally the patient may experience referral of the pain into areas of the first division of the trigeminal nerve. The headache is a secondary phenomenon compared with the localized eye findings in the vast majority of cases. Recently there have been cases of acute angle-closure glaucoma associated with the use of topiramate for migraine prevention in which the patients experience visual changes in advance of significant eye pain.

Headaches Attributed to Rhinosinusitis and Mucosal Contact Points

Certainly, acute rhinosinusitis can cause pain over the involved sinus and may even worsen existing migraine headache, but these symptoms abate with treatment of the acute infection. Chronic sinus disease has not been convincingly shown to provoke headache.

The role of anatomic abnormalities of the nose in the provocation of headache is less clear. It has been theorized that mucosal contact points between different structures within the nose could trigger afferents from the first and second divisions of the trigeminal nerve leading to facial pain. Examples of mucosal contact points include the medial turbinate contacting the nasal septum or lateral nasal wall, the inferior turbinate touching the septum, a nasal spur contacting the lateral nasal wall or superior turbinate, and an ethmoidal bulla contacting the nasal septum.

The IHS does not formally recognize mucosal contact points as causing a distinct headache disorder but has proposed criteria as a guide to future research (9):

1. A headache located in the periorbital/retro-orbital, medial canthal or temporozygomatic regions

2. Demonstration of an ipsilateral mucosal contact point on nasal endoscopy or CT

3. The headache must be relieved in 5 minutes by the intranasal administration of topical anesthetic or cocaine, or the pain is worse with recumbent positions

4. The headache must be relieved in 7 days by the surgical correction of the mucosal contact point

Case series in the otolaryngological literature have reported the improvement of headache with the surgical correction of mucosal contact points within the nose (34-37). Mucosal contact points, however, are commonly found in those with and without facial pain (38). Therefore it can be difficult to determine if a mucosal contact point is causing the facial pain or is simply found incidentally during an otolaryngological evaluation. Until definitive research is conducted, such surgery cannot be routinely recommended.

Headaches Associated with Head or Neck Trauma

Post-Traumatic Headaches

Headaches may develop after minor and major head injuries. Interestingly, impact of the head may not be necessary to provoke post-traumatic headaches. Of this type of headache, 42% are attributed to motor vehicle accidents and 25% to falls (39). The annual incidence of head injuries requiring hospitalization is 0.2 cases per 100, and 80% suffer headaches as a consequence. Concussion can lead to headache in 90% of those who sustain this injury (40).

Post-traumatic headaches do not have specific characteristics that distinguish them from other headache disorders and in fact most resemble tension-type headaches (41). The diagnosis is primarily made by the temporal relationship between the injury and the new onset of headaches or the worsening of an existing headache disorder. To meet IHS criteria (9) the headaches must arise within 7 days of the injury and be associated with one of the following:

1. Loss of consciousness

2. Memory loss

3. Glasgow Coma Scale score <13

4. Neuroimaging demonstrating an intracerebral bleed, brain contusion, subarachnoid hemorrhage, or skull fracture

Post-traumatic headaches rarely occur in isolation; patients commonly have some degree of neurocognitive impairment. Memory impairments, difficulty concentrating, absentmindedness, easy distractibility, and mood or personality changes can often be demonstrated in these patients (42). Sexual dysfunction, weight changes, vertigo, and insomnia may also be experienced (43).

Women are nearly two times more likely than men to develop a post-traumatic syndrome following minor head injury (44). Older age may portend a worse prognosis with a delay in the resolution of post-traumatic syndrome when compared with younger patients (45). The nature of the injury may influence the symptoms of post-traumatic headaches. Patients who experience rotational forces as part of the injury are more likely to develop cervical as well as cerebral complaints (46).

The relationship between the severity of the head injury and the likelihood of development of a post-traumatic syndrome remains unresolved. Some evidence even suggests an inverse correlation between the severity of injury and the occurrence of the syndrome: patients with less severe injury being more likely to develop symptoms than those with more severe injury (47,48). Initial loss of consciousness, early development of neurological signs on examination, and a high frequency of initial complaints may all adversely affect the course of the post-traumatic headache. Some evidence suggests that patients with either a history of pre-existing migraine or a positive family history of migraine are more likely to develop a post-traumatic migraine pattern (44,49). Psychological factors, including depression and personality disorders, do not appear to dramatically influence the course of the syndrome.

The mechanism by which post-traumatic headache occurs is highly controversial. Some argue that the disorder is merely related to the possibility of compensation or other elements of secondary gain, whereas others implicate axonal shearing and alteration in brain chemistry as causative factors. Diagnostic scans are most commonly performed on those patients with significant head injury. In patients with mild-to-moderate head injury, MRI may be superior to CT scan, demonstrating abnormalities at the juncture of the gray-and-white matter as well as evidence of axonal shearing (50,51). Other diagnostic tests that are commonly available, such as brainstem auditory evoked response, somatosensory evoked response, and electronystagmography (ENG), do not show significant correlations between the injury and the occurrence of positive findings. Patients with concomitant dizziness associated with their post-traumatic symptoms may have a positive ENG in about two thirds of cases (52). Neuropsychological testing is frequently positive in the immediate post-traumatic period but shows resolution for most patients within 3 months (53).

Treatment of post-traumatic headache is similar to that for primary headache disorders such as migraine. This includes both preventive and acute therapy. Additionally, physical treatments directed at the cervical spine may prove useful for some patients. Facet joint injection of zygapophyseal joints in the upper neck may produce benefit (54). Other physical modalities, including exercise and heat-and-cold applications, may also be of benefit. Behavioral approaches may be entertained, especially cognitive retraining in those with cognitive impairment.

Headaches Attributed to Whiplash Injury

"Whiplash" refers to a sequence of flexion and extension motions of the neck following motor vehicle impact, but lateral and rotatory motions may also play a role in its development. Approximately 8% of patients will develop a new headache after a whiplash injury (55). Whiplash may lead to a type of cervicogenic headache caused by injuries to the cervical spine such as facet arthropathy, cervical disc disruptions, or traction injuries of cervical nerve roots. The IHS recognizes whiplash as a cause of both acute and chronic headaches, but they must arise within 7 days of the injury (9).

These headaches are located in the occipital regions and are often associated with neck pain. Whiplash injuries in those with pre-existing migraine headache may produce more frequent migraine headaches. The treatment of whiplash injuries often includes physical therapy, anesthetic blocks of involved nerves, and medical therapies (e.g., tricyclic antidepressants, muscle relaxants, anticonvulsants). The headaches have completely resolved in >50% of patients at 1-year follow-up (55).

Headaches Associated with Systemic Illnesses

Hypertension

Arterial hypertension is an unlikely cause of headache unless the blood pressure is greater than 220/120 or rises very rapidly, as seen with an acute pressor response to an exogenous agent, or in conditions such as preeclampsia or eclampsia. In these cases, hypertensive encephalopathy may occur, with symptoms that include headache as well as nausea, vomiting, seizures, and alterations in level of consciousness. Papilledema and retinal hemorrhages may be seen on examination. Pheochromocytoma is an unusual cause of hypertensive headache that can be suspected when headache occurs in association with episodes of diaphoresis, palpitations, anxiety, and hypertension.

Systemic Infection

Headaches may arise after a variety of systemic infections including upper respiratory infections, bacterial and fungal sepsis, and viral syndromes caused by Epstein-Barr, cytomegalovirus, and HIV. Patients with a pre-existing headache disorder may be more prone to the development of headaches after a systemic infection. In most cases the headaches are self-limited and only persist for the duration of the systemic infection.

Headache may be especially likely to arise from infections that involve the central nervous system, such as meningitis, encephalitis, and brain abscesses. These infections are often suspected in those with symptoms of fever (often unexplained), nuchal rigidity, altered mental status, and other focal neurological signs or symptoms.

Metabolic and Endocrine Diseases

Metabolic and endocrine diseases such as hypoxemia, hypercapnea, anemia, hypoglycemia, dehydration, and hypothyroidism have all been associated with headache. Dialysis may also produce headache in renal failure patients; this is thought secondary to the large fluid and electrolyte shifts experienced with this procedure.

Other Systemic Illnesses

Many other disorders such as lupus erythematosus, sarcoidosis, syphilis, subacute bacterial endocarditis, and vasculitis (primary and secondary) can produce headache when these disorders affect the central nervous system. They should be suspected in patients that have headaches and other systemic signs or symptoms (e.g., arthritis, weight loss, shortness of breath, fever, unexplained or new aortic insufficiency, petechiae, splinter hemorrhages of the nail beds).

* * *

Key Points

- Primary stabbing headaches ("icepick" headaches) last for seconds, respond well to preventive treatment with indomethacin, and do not require evaluation for secondary headache disorders.

- Headaches associated with cough, exertion, and sexual activity are generally benign but may occasionally be associated with secondary headache disorders such as subarachnoid hemorrhages, Arnold-Chiari malformation, and malignancies. Neuroimaging is recommended if there is suspicion of these disorders.

- Hypnic headaches occur in older patients (>60 years of age), last for 15 minutes to 3 hours, and often awaken the patient from sleep.

- Some foods and beverages (e.g., alcohol, ice cream) and food additives may provoke headache in susceptible patients.

- Idiopathic intracranial hypertension and sleep apnea should be considered in patients with headache and obesity.

- Diagnosis of cervicogenic headache should be considered when headaches originate from the neck and radiate into the occipital or frontal regions.

- Post-traumatic headaches may occur after minor or major head traumas and begin within one week after the insult.

- Systemic illnesses should be suspected in patients with headaches and signs or symptoms characteristic of the underlying disorder.

REFERENCES

1. **Medina JL, Diamond S.** Cluster headache variant: spectrum of a new headache syndrome. Arch Neurol. 1981;38:705-9.

2. **Mathew NT.** Indomethacin responsive headache syndromes. Headache. 1981;21:147-50.

3. **Pascual J, Igessias F, Oterino A, et al.** Cough, exertional and sexual headaches: an analysis of 72 benign and symptomatic cases. Neurology. 1996;46:1520-4.

4. **Sands GH, Newman L, Lipton R.** Cough, exertional, and other miscellaneous headaches. Med Clin N Am. 1991;75:733-46.

5. **Raskin NH.** The hypnic headache syndrome. Headache. 1988;28:534-6.

6. **Newman LC, Lipton RB, Solomon S.** The hypnic headache syndrome: a benign headache disorder of the elderly. Neurology. 1990;40:1904-5.

7. **Landtblom AM, Fridriksson S, Boivie J, et al.** Sudden-onset headache: a prospective study of features, incidence and causes. Cephalalgia. 2002;22:354-60.

8. **Linn FHH, Wijdicks EF.** Causes and management of thunderclap headache: a comprehensive review. Neurologist. 2002;8:279-89.

9. **International Headache Society.** The International Classification of Headache Disorders, 2nd ed. Cephalalgia. 2004;24(Suppl 1):9-160.

10. **Martin VT, Behbehani MM.** Toward a rational understanding of migraine trigger factors. Med Clin North Am. 2001;85:911-41.

11. **Pattichis K, Louca LL, Jarman J, et al.** 5-Hydroxytryptamine release from platelets by different red wines: implications for migraine. Eur J Pharmacol. 1995;292:173-7.

12. **Wantke F, Gotz M, Jarisch R.** The red wine provocation test: intolerance to histamine as a model for food intolerance. Allergy Proc. 1994;15:27-32.

13. **Kaivola S, Parantainen J, Osterman T, et al.** Hangover headache and prostaglandins: prophylactic treatment with tolfenamic acid. Cephalalgia. 1983;3:31-6.

14. **Sleigh JW.** Ice cream headache: cerebral vasoconstriction causing decrease in arterial flow may have a role. BMJ. 1997;315:609.

15. **Scher A, Stewart W, Ricci J, et al.** Factors associated with the onset and remission of chronic daily headache in a population-based study. Pain. 2003;106:81-9.

16. **Loh N, Dinner D, Foldvary N, et al.** Do patients with obstructive sleep apnea wake up with headache? Arch Intern Med. 1999;159:1765-8.

17. **Ulfberg J, Carter N, Talback M, Edling C.** Headache, snoring and sleep apnoea. J Neurol. 1996;243:621-5.

18. **Poceta J, Dalessio D.** Identification and treatment of sleep apnea in patients with chronic headache. Headache. 1995;35:586-9.

19. **Wall M.** The headache profile of idiopathic intracranial hypertension. Cephalalgia. 1990;10:331-5.

20. **Marcelis J, Silberstein S.** Idiopathic intracranial hypertension without papilledema. Arch Neurol. 1991;48:392-9.

21. **Giuseffi V, Wall M, Siegal PZ.** Symptoms and disease associations in idiopathic intracranial hypertension (pseudotumor cerebri): a case control study. Neurology. 1991;41:239-44.

22. **Kupersmith MJ, Gamell L, Turbin R.** Effects of weight loss on the course of idiopathic intracranial hypertension in women. Neurology. 1998;50:1094-8.

23. **Corbett JJ, Mehta MP.** Cerebrospinal fluid pressure in normal and obese subjects and patients with pseudotumor cerebri. Neurology. 1983;33:1386-8.

24. **Weisberg LA.** Benign intracranial hypertension. Medicine. 1975;54:197-207.

25. **Johnston I, Paterson A.** Benign intracranial hypertension II: CSF pressure and circulation. Brain. 1974;97:301-12.

26. **Lay CL, Campbell JK, Mokri B.** Low cerebrospinal fluid pressure headache. In: Goadsby P, Silberstein SD, eds. Blue Books of Practical Neurology: Headache. Boston: Butterworth-Heinemann; 1997:355-68.

27. **Mueller L.** Cervicogenic headache: a diagnostic and therapeutic dilemma. Headache and Pain. 2003;14:29-37.

28. **Sjaastad O, Fredriksen T, Pfaffenrath, V.** Cervicogenic headaches: diagnostic criteria. Headache. 1998;38:442-5.

29. **Bovim G, Fredriksen T, Stolt-Nielsem A, et al.** Neurolysis of the greater occipital nerve in cervicogenic headache: a follow-up study. Headache. 1992;32:175-9.

30. **Solberg WK, Woo WS, Huston JB.** Prevalence of mandibular joint dysfunction in young adults. J Am Dental Assoc. 1979;98:25-34.

31. **Travell J, Simons DG.** Myofascial Pain and Dysfunction: The Trigger Point Manual. Baltimore: Williams and Wilkins; 1984.

32. **Butler JH, Golke LEA, Bandt CL.** A descriptive survey of signs and symptoms associated with myofascial pain dysfunction syndrome. J Am Dental Assoc. 1975;90:635-9.

33. **Cady R, Schreiber C, Farmer K, Sheftell F.** Primary headaches: a convergence hypothesis. Headache. 2002;42:204-16.

34. **Welge-Luessen A, Hausea R, Schmid N, et al.** Endonasal surgery from contact point headaches. Laryngoscope. 2003;113:2151-6.

35. **Goldsmith A, Zahtz G, Stegnjajic A, Shikowitz M.** Middle turbinate headache syndrome. Am J Rhinol. 1993;7:17-23.

36. **Clerico D.** Pneumatized superior turbinate as a cause of referred migraine pain. Laryngoscope. 1996;106:874-9.

37. **Gerbe R, Fry T, Fischer N.** Headache of nasal spur origin: an easily diagnosed and surgically correctable cause of facial pain. Headache. 1984;24:329-30.

38. **Abu-Bakra M, Jones N.** Prevalence of nasal mucosal contact points in patients with facial pain compared with patients without facial pain. J Laryngol Otol. 2001;115:629-32.

39. **Kraus JF, McArthur DL, Silberman TA.** Epidemiology of mild brain injury. Semin Neurol. 1994;14:1-7.

40. **Gfeller JD, Chibnall JT, Duckro PN.** Post-concussion symptoms and cognitive functioning in posttraumatic headache patients. Headache. 1994;34:503-7.

41. **Mandel S.** Minor head injury may not "minor". Postgrad Med J. 1989;85:213-5.

42. **Andrasik F, Wincze JP.** Emotional and psychological aspects of mild head injury. Semin Neurol. 1994;14:60.

43. **Evans RW.** The post-concussion syndrome and sequelae of mild head injury. Neurol Clin. 1992;10:815-47.

44. **Jenssen OK, Nielson FF.** The influence of sex and pretraumatic headache on the incidence and severity of headache after injury. Cephalalgia. 1990;10:285-93.

45. **Fenton GW.** The post-concussion syndrome reappraised. Clin Electroencephalogr. 1996;27:174-82.

46. **Mendelson G.** Not "cured by verdict". Med J Aust. 1982;2:132-4.

47. **Yamaguchi M.** Incidence of headache and severity of head injury. Headache. 1992;32:422.

48. **Barrett K, Ward AB, Boughey A, et al.** Sequelae of minor head injury: the natural consciousness and follow-up. J Accid Emerg Med. 1994;11:79.

49. **Weiss HD, Stern BJ, Goldbert J.** Post-traumatic migraine: chronic migraine precipitated by minor head or neck trauma. Headache. 1991;31:451-6.

50. **Levin HS, Amparo E, Eisenberg HM.** Magnetic resonance imaging and computed tomography in relation to the neurobehavioral sequelae of mild to moderate head injuries. J Neurosurg. 1987;66:706-13.

51. **Mittl RL Grossman RI, Hiehle JF, et al.** Prevalence of MR evidence of diffuser axonal injury in patients with mild head injury and normal head CT findings. Am J Neuroradiol. 1994;15:1583-9.

52. **Rowe MJ, Carlson C.** Brainstem auditory evoked potentials in post-concussion dizziness. Arch Neurol. 1980;37:679.

53. **Eisenberg HM.** CT and MRI finding in mild to moderate head injury. In: Levin HL, Eisenberg HM, Benton AL, eds. Mild Head Injury. New York: Oxford University Press; 1989:133.

54. **Lord SM, Barnsley L, Wallis BJ, Bogdul N.** Chronic cervical zygapophyseal joint pain after whiplash: a placebo-controlled prevalence study. Spine. 1996;21:1737-44.

55. **Drottning M, Staff P, Sjaastad O.** Cervicogenic headache after a whiplash injury. Cephalalgia. 2002;22:165-71.

9

Women's Issues in Headache

Anne H. Calhoun, MD

The high prevalence of migraine in women and its associated clinical, social, and economic burden make it a problem that all clinicians caring for women will encounter. Women comprise the majority of patients seeking medical evaluation of headache, are more likely to use prescription medications for headache, are the majority of subjects in clinical research trials of headache treatments, and are more likely than men to be severely disabled by migraine.

Epidemiology of Migraine

The prevalence of migraine in reproductive-aged women is substantial. The accepted and frequently quoted summary statistic that migraine affects 18% of women (vs. 6% of men) obscures the prominent mid-life peak, when roughly 30% of all women are affected. During these otherwise busy and productive years, the female-to-male ratio for migraine exceeds 3:1. Migraine is much less common before puberty and typically improves after menopause (1). But an examination of lifetime prevalence by age 50 shows that migraine may affect up to 41% of women (2).

Influence of Reproductive Life Events

Reproductive milestones such as menarche, pregnancy, and menopause profoundly influence the course of migraine in many women. Peak incidence of migraine in females coincides with the onset of hormonal cycling at puberty. Commonly, attacks abate during the last two trimesters of pregnancy, though they may flare at the end of the first trimester, coinciding with the fall in HCG (3). The peak impact of migraine not uncommonly occurs during the forties, as a woman is entering the perimenopause, a time of hormonal turbulence. During the perimenopause, the follicular phase of the menstrual cycle may shorten, decreasing the interval between headaches in women who experience menstrual migraines. Later, with the hormonal stability of established menopause, migraines tend to become less frequent and severe.

These hormonally caused changes in migraine activity may explain the confusing discrepancies in some published reports that examine the impact of natural menopause on migraine (4-9). Retrospective studies that rely on a patient's ability to recall accurately whether a change in headache pattern coincided with the onset of vasomotor symptoms and sleep problems, or years later when she actually attained menopause, are notoriously prone to recall bias.

Menstrually Associated and Pure Menstrual Migraine

Although "pure menstrual migraine" – attacks occurring exclusively with menses – is seen in only 10% to 15% of female migraineurs, menstrual exacerbation of migraine is common. About 60% of female migraineurs report triggering or worsening of their headaches with menses (10). Migraines that consistently occur during the "menstrual window" (two days before menses to three days after the start of menstrual bleeding) but also occur at other times throughout the month have been termed "menstrually associated migraine" (MAM). Women who are unsure of a menstrual trigger for headaches should be encouraged to keep a calendar correlating headache days and bleeding pattern.

International Headache Society Diagnostic Criteria

The International Headache Society (IHS) published its revised criteria for the diagnosis of headache disorders in 2004. While they did not formally recognize menstrual migraine as a separate diagnostic category, they did make recommendations for its classification in the appendix of the publication, which can be used to standardize future research of menstrual migraine. They referred to pure menstrual migraine as "pure menstrual migraine without aura" and MAM as "menstrually related migraine without aura". The menstrual window is defined as occurring 2 days before to 3 days after the onset of menstruation. Attacks of "pure menstrual migraine without aura" occur only during the perimenstrual window in two thirds of menstrual cycles, whereas attacks of "menstrually related migraine without aura" occur during and outside the perimenstrual period in two thirds of menstrual cycles.

Note that IHS criteria only allow for migraine without aura to be classified as menstrual migraine. This is secondary to the fact that epidemiologic studies demonstrate an increased frequency of attacks of migraine without aura during the menstrual window, but not migraine with aura attacks (10a).

Pathogenesis

Four observations explain the influence of hormones on migraine:

Observation 1: Falls in endogenous or exogenous estrogen concentrations are the provocative factor in menstrual attacks.

In the mid-1970s Somerville demonstrated experimentally that migraine attacks coincided with falls in estrogen. He measured perimenstrual estradiol concentrations in subjects with a history of menstrual migraine, then injected estradiol valerate 4 days before the anticipated menses. Estradiol rose following the injection and was sustained for about a week and a half. The injections postponed the usual "menstrual" migraine until the estradiol concentration fell, several days after the onset of menses (11).

These results explain why 70% of oral contraceptive (OC) users experience headache during the placebo week of their pill pack, when exogenous estrogen levels drop precipitously. The peak incidence of headaches occurs on the third day of the placebo week (12).

This relationship – migraine coinciding with falls in estrogen – is consistent with the clinical observation that women are more likely to experience migraine when estrogen levels abruptly decline. Such declines occur not only with the menses but also immediately after ovulation, after childbirth, after surgical oophorectomy, and during either planned or unintentional gaps in estrogen concentrations with hormone therapy.

Estradiol has several important actions in the central nervous system, which may underlie and help explain its relationship to migraine. When estrogen concentrations decline, the production of serotonin also declines, and its rate of elimination increases (through increases in monoamine oxidase). Serotonergic tone, in women, has a positive correlation to estradiol levels. In fact, the sensitivity of 5HT1 receptors – the target of the triptans – decreases with low estrogen.

Nonmigraine pain is also perceived as more intense perimenstrually (13). This probably reflects the decrease in endogenous opioid activity and pain-relieving beta-endorphins in a low-estrogen environment (14).

Observation 2: Falls in progesterone do not trigger migraine.

Somerville also experimented with progesterone supplementation. He extended luteal phase progesterone concentrations to separate the fall in progesterone from the decline in estrogen. He found that menstrual bleeding was postponed until progesterone levels declined but that the bleeding was not accompanied by headache: migraine still occurred only when estrogen fell (15).

Observation 3: Eliminating or minimizing the premenstrual decline in estrogen decreases the likelihood that menstrual migraine will occur.

Eliminating drops in estrogen levels. Sustained *high* levels of estrogen seem beneficial in migraine. Twenty-four menstrual migraine patients were treated for up to 5 years with subcutaneous estradiol implants. Cyclic progestin was administered each month to induce withdrawal bleeding (progestin supplementation had no temporal association with migraine, in agreement with Observation 2). Twenty-three of the 24 patients improved with the treatment, 20 becoming completely or almost-completely headache-free. These implants provided sustained elevation of estradiol at a mean concentration of 600 pmol/L, levels that inhibited ovulation (16).

Sustained *low* levels of estradiol are equally beneficial. Gonadotropin-releasing hormone agonists (GnRHa) have been used to suppress ovarian steroid production in women with menstrual migraine. Leuprolide acetate was administered IM for 10 months, achieving a hypogonadal state in all the subjects (estradiol averaged 15.5 pg/mL, levels commonly seen in menopause). Migraines were markedly diminished in the subjects for the duration of the treatment. It is important to note that the women in this trial had had few headaches outside the menstrual window before this treatment. Another trial found that a GNRHa-induced medical menopause did not benefit women with migraine plus chronic daily headache (17).

Sustained *physiological* levels of estradiol likewise seem beneficial. During the last six months of the leuprolide trial described above, continuous estrogen-progestin was "added back" in oral dosages typically used in postmenopausal hormone therapy, resulting in average estradiol levels of 64.0 pg/mL. This approach was equally successful in significantly diminishing the migraines (18).

Minimizing drops in estrogen levels. In the above examples, cyclic fluctuations were completely ablated. More subtle modifications of the menstrual cycle can also benefit MAM. A 1.5 mg estradiol gel (available in Europe) was moderately effective in reducing the impact of menstrual migraine (19). Applied percutaneously for 7 days perimenstrually, the gel augmented late luteal phase estradiol concentrations, thereby reducing the extent of its premenstrual decline (the "estrogen withdrawal").

With similar trials utilizing transdermal estradiol patches, both the 0.025 and 0.05 mg doses were ineffective for migraine prophylaxis when used perimenstrually. However, the 0.1 mg patch was comparable in efficacy to the gel in the study cited above (20). This dosage is known to augment estradiol levels about 75 pg/mL, similar to the increase seen in the successful gel trials. (For comparison, the 0.025 mg patch gives only a 20 pg/mL increment.) These studies likewise fit the third observation: reduction in the decline in estradiol lessens or prevents the headache.

It has been suggested that a serum estradiol level of 60-80 pg/mL is required perimenstrually to prevent menstrual migraine. A more likely explanation is that there is a threshold for the magnitude of a decline in estrogen that can be experienced by an individual migraineur without triggering an attack. In the pellet and GnRHa studies cited above, consistency in estradiol was preventive, from supraphysiological concentrations down to the trace amounts seen in ovarian failure.

Observation 4: Increasing the magnitude of the declines in estrogen will aggravate migraine.

A frequently quoted study (21) concluded that "low dose" OCs made migraines worse. The pill used in that study contained 50 µg of ethinyl estradiol (EE). In 1977 this was, indeed, considered "low dose", but it is now the highest formulation approved by the FDA. Compared with the natural cycle, this pill doubles the magnitude of the premenstrual fall in estrogen and would be predicted to worsen menstrual migraine, which it did in 70% of the subjects. Another prospective study found that more vascular headaches occurred in women using higher dose OCs than on lower dose formulations (22).

Preventive Treatments

A variety of hormonal and nonhormonal regimens can be employed to prevent estrogen-withdrawal migraine (Table 9-1). The specific – or hormonal – regimens are designed to reduce the specific trigger of estrogen withdrawal. These include oral contraceptives, perimenstrual estrogen supplementation, and gonadotropin-releasing hormone agonists. Nonhormonal preventive therapies include all of those used for nonmenstrual migraine (see Chapter 4) but also triptans, ergots, and NSAIDs.

As with prophylaxis of nonmenstrual migraine, preventive treatment of menstrual migraine is appropriate only for women with frequent, troublesome headaches that do not respond to abortive treatment alone. In some cases, prophylaxis of menstrual migraine can be limited to only a portion of the month and need not be given daily, thus minimizing exposure to treatment side effects. Many of these treatments can only be timed correctly in women with regular menstrual periods; diaries are useful in establishing this schedule (see Appendix III).

Hormonal Treatments

Oral Contraceptives
All of today's OCs are "low dose" by the 1970s definition, yet estrogen levels vary 150% from the highest to the lowest dose pills available. If the fall in

Table 9-1   Preventive Treatments for Menstrual Migraine

Hormonal Strategies	Nonhormonal Regimens

• Oral contraceptives
  —Low dose
  —Low dose with add-back estrogen
  —Continuous active pill regimens
• Perimenstrual estrogen regimens
• Tamoxifen
• Danazol
• GnRH agonists with estrogen/progestin
  add-back
	• Perimenstrual triptans
	• Perimenstrual ergots
	• Perimenstrual NSAIDS

endogenous estradiol that accompanies migraine in the natural menstrual cycle is equivalent to 20-25 µg EE, none of the currently available OCs would be expected to improve menstrual migraine. This is because no currently available OC provides less than a 20 µg decline in EE between days 21 and 22 of its pill pack.

Similarly, a 20-25 µg pill would not be expected to exacerbate or intensify MAM, because it does not increase the magnitude of the premenstrual fall in estrogen *above what is experienced physiologically.* For women with migraine who do use OCs, several things can be usefully kept in mind. In patients who are symptomatic on a 30-50 µg OC, changing to a 20-25 µg formulation (dosed at bedtime) is rational and may provide improvement.

If lowering the strength of the OC affords insufficient relief, estrogen can be added back on days 22 to 28 in place of the placebo pills, thereby decreasing the magnitude of the withdrawal gap in estrogen (23). Sample regimens include any of the following in place of the placebo pills (or, in the case of Mircette or Kariva, in place of the placebo/active pills of the fourth week):

• Conjugated equine estrogens 0.9-1.25 mg at bedtime (days 22-28)

• Esterified estrogens 1.25 mg at bedtime (days 22-28)

• 17-beta-estradiol 0.5-1 mg twice daily (days 22-28)

• Transdermal 17-beta-estradiol in matrix patches 0.075-0.1 mg, applied days 22 (A.M.) & 25 (P.M.)

Alternatively, oral contraceptives can be prescribed in a "long-cycle" regimen. The patient is instructed to take continuous active pills of a monophasic 30-35 µg formulation for 6 to 12 weeks. She then suspends active pills and applies a 0.1 mg estradiol matrix patch for 7 days before resuming therapy with the active pills. This strategy has obvious additional benefits for the woman with co-morbid dysmenorrhea or endometriosis and is increasingly preferred by others because it minimizes withdrawal bleeding. In general, use of oral contraceptives solely to treat migraine is not recommended, but manipulating the estrogen dose or adjusting the duration of treatment can be very helpful in women with migraine already using OCs for other reasons. Aura has been reported to worsen with very high concentrations of estrogen) (usually with concentrations seen in pregnancy or with OCs) (24).

Patch Contraceptives

The introduction of a 20 µg EE patch contraceptive affords another strategy for prophylaxis, although its effect on menstrual migraine has not been formally studied. Transdermal administration alters estradiol's metabolic profile and has the advantage of providing more stable serum concentrations in smokers or in those migraineurs whose concomitant medications may increase estrogen's hepatic metabolism through cytochrome p450 3A4. If add-back estrogen is needed during the placebo week, this can be conveniently given with a 0.1 mg 17-beta-estradiol matrix patch.

Perimenstrual Estrogen Regimens

Although controlled studies have shown more robust results from strategies that suppress ovulation, for the patient in whom OCs are contraindicated, some benefit can be obtained from perimenstrually targeted patch therapy (see full discussion under Observation 3, above). In lieu of daily therapy, a 0.1 mg 17-beta-estradiol patch is applied 1 or 2 days before the anticipated date of menses (or anticipated MAM) and continued for 5 to 7 days.

Gonadotropin-Releasing Hormone Agonists

For severe and refractory cases of menstrual migraine, consideration could be given to administration of a GNRH-a to induce medical menopause. Estrogen (combined with a progestogen for the woman with an intact uterus) should be added-back to prevent the complications of a hypogonadal state. When used after GNRHa treatment in female migraineurs with chronic headache, estrogen add-back therapy provided a 33% improvement over placebo, presumably because it achieves even more stable levels of estrogen in women who may be exquisitely sensitive to even minor changes in these levels (17).

Tamoxifen

Tamoxifen is a selective estrogen receptor modulator (SERM) that has agonist or antagonist activity at various estrogen receptors. It is indicated for the prevention and treatment of some breast cancers. In a small open-label study it was effective prophylaxis for menstrual migraine, administered at 10-20 mg/day for 7 to 14 days before menses; during menses the subjects took 5-10 mg for 3 days (25). Controlled studies are needed in menstrual migraine. Side effects of tamoxifen are substantial, and include hot flushes, vasomotor instability, and endometrial proliferation with prolonged use.

SERMs vary in their affinity for estrogen receptors in target organs. Raloxifene, an SERM with indications for prevention and treatment of osteoporosis in postmenopausal women, has not been studied in relation to MAM. Side effects include hot flushes and venous thrombotic events.

Danazol

Danazol is an androgen derivative that down-regulates estradiol receptors, suppressing the pituitary ovarian axis and presumably benefiting menstrual migraine through this mechanism. A single multi-phase prospective study evaluated danazol combined with dietary restriction and acetazolamide in the prophylaxis of menstrual and ovulatory migraine. The combined treatment was judged effective in just over 60% of the women (26). Side effects of danazol include hirsutism, mood swings, aggressive behavior. blood clots, fluid retention, oily skin, and flushing.

Nonhormonal Treatments

Nonsteroidal Anti-Inflammatory Drugs (NSAIDs)

Prostaglandin synthetase inhibitors can be used perimenstrually to alleviate menstrual migraine. Naproxen sodium 550 mg twice daily for 13 days (beginning 7 days before onset of menses and continued through the sixth day of flow) produced a measurable decrease in an index of headache frequency and severity (27). Side effects include gastric irritation, peptic ulcer disease, and decreases in glomerular filtration rates.

Triptans

In a randomized double-blind placebo-controlled study, naratriptan reduced the number of menstrually associated migraines. Tablets were administered twice daily for 5 days starting 2 days before the expected onset of menses. Although more patients treated with naratriptan were headache-free across all four treated cycles compared with placebo (23% versus 8%), no difference was seen in severity in the breakthrough headaches that occurred (28). In this study, only the 1 mg bid dose was found to be effective.

Another study (29) found frovatriptan to be effective in prophylaxis of menstrual migraine. A loading dose of 10 mg was administered 2 days before the anticipated start of the menstrually associated migraine and continued for 6 days at dosages of 2.5 mg qd and 2.5 mg bid. Both doses of frovatriptan reduced the frequency, duration, and functional impairment of menstrually associated migraine ($P < 0.0001$) when compared with placebo. Freedom from menstrually associated migraine occurred in 50%, 39%, and 26% of patients for the frovatriptan 2.5 mg bid, frovatritpan 2.5 mg qd, and placebo groups, respectively. Frovatritpan 2.5 mg bid was superior to frovatriptan 2.5 mg qd.

Triptans are not FDA approved for prevention of migraine, but side effects in these trials were minimal. Both trials used triptans with longer half-lives to simplify the dosing regimen and provide the continuous levels of drug that prevent headache, as opposed to short-duration triptans, which are best suited for abortive treatment.

Ergot Prophylaxis

Ergots can be administered for 5 to 7 days perimenstrually to prevent menstrual migraine. One study (30) administered ergonovine 0.2 mg four times per day beginning one day before menstruation and ending one day after its cessation. This therapy reduced the frequency, severity, and duration of menstrual migraine in 15%, 50%, and 47% of patients, respectively. The mechanism of action of ergots is similar to that of triptans, but side effects of nausea, vomiting, and vasoconstricton are more pronounced.

Bromocriptine is an ergot alkaloid with dopamine agonist properties. In a small study, three quarters of the subjects with menstrual migraine experienced at least a 25% decrease in headaches with bromocriptine 2.5 mg three times a day added to their current regimen. Continuous therapy was significantly more effective than cyclic perimenstrual usage (31).

Abortive Therapies

Abortive therapy for the acute menstrual migraine is identical to treatment given outside the menstrual window. Studies have suggested that the triptans (32,33) are efficacious in the abortive treatment of MAM. An aspirin/acetaminophen/caffeine combination (Excedrin Migraine) was also shown to be effective in the treatment of MAM in women experiencing only mild-to-moderate discomfort (34). Abortive therapies for migraine are discussed in detail in Chapter 4.

Perimenopause, Menopause, and Hormonal Therapy

Perimenopause and Migraine

Migraines reach their peak prevalence in a woman's forties. Plausible, but unsubstantiated, explanations include the onset of perimenopausal changes. During these years, women may begin to experience vasomotor instability associated with lower serum estradiol concentrations before menses. Due to these same hormonal changes, sleep architecture and physiology are adversely affected, including a five-fold increased incidence of sleep apnea in menopausal women not receiving hormonal augmentation (35).

Cycles may become erratic and more frequent with a consequent decrease in the interval between hormonal headaches. For the nonsmoking migraineur without diabetes or hypertension, low-dose OCs remain an option for cycle control in the perimenopause.

Menopause and Migraine

With advancing age, as well as with the hormonal stability of menopause, migraines may improve. Certain hormone therapy regimens may, however, negate this expectation. Published studies examining the positive (36-38) or negative (39,40) impact of postmenopausal hormone therapy must be read with an understanding of how these varying strategies would be expected to affect migraine and with consideration given to the formulation, dosage, and timing of estrogen therapy, as well as the regimen used.

Perimenopause may have an adverse impact on migraine because of erratic cycling of estrogen secondary to the administration of hormone replacement therapy. A thorough discussion of the risks and benefits of postmenopausal estrogen therapy (ET) is beyond the scope of this book, but if ET is desired for other reasons, several things can be done to lessen its impact on migraine.

The regimen of estrogen therapy is of paramount importance. Cyclic regimens with gaps in ET allow for estrogen-withdrawal migraines and should be avoided (23).

Other recommendations for rational estrogen therapy in migraineurs are as follows:

1. Short-acting oral estrogen preparations (such as oral 17-beta-estradiol) allow for daily declines in estradiol concentrations and should be avoided. These products are best replaced with longer-acting oral or transdermal products, or given 2 or 3 times daily in divided doses.

2. Oral agents should be administered at bedtime. If a major trigger of migraine in women is a falling estrogen concentration, and the lowest threshold for migraine is in the early morning, it is best to avoid a morning nadir. If oral agents wear off in the early morning hours, sleep continuity and architecture may also suffer.

3. Transdermal formulations of estradiol may be preferable to oral formulations in some women. This is particularly true for women who smoke, frequently forget to take pills, or whose concomitant medications (some antiepileptics, antidepressants, or antibiotics, among others) may induce cytochrome p450 3A4, leading to rapid degradation of their oral estrogen.

4. When using transdermal products, matrix patches provide better consistency in concentration over their intended duration than reservoir patches. Patients on patch therapy should be questioned about headache symptoms on the day preceding patch change. In rare instances, patches may need to be changed on a more frequent schedule to prevent such headaches.

5. Interrupted estrogen therapy – with days off at the end of the month – is classically associated with migraines on the "off

days". Continuous estrogen therapy – with continuous or cyclic progestogens when needed – is preferred.

6. Monthly estrogen or estrogen/testosterone injection therapy may exacerbate migraine. Supraphysiological maximum concentrations may occur in the first week (with possible aggravation of aura); the ensuing supraphysiological decline in estradiol may then trigger monthly estrogen-withdrawal migraines.

7. If estrogen worsens visual or sensory aura symptoms, reduce the dose or change to a formulation that maintains a more constant concentration. If ET is accompanied by new onset or worsening of motor aura symptoms (hemiparesis, cranial nerve abnormalities, etc.), it should be discontinued.

Some postmenopausal women clearly have a worsening of migraine headache in the absence of hormone therapy. This may in part be due to the significant adverse impact of the hypoestrogenic state on sleep (41). In these patients, the institution of stable hormone therapy is occasionally elected as a way to lessen the frequency and disability of migraine.

The Pregnant and Lactating Patient

For 55% to 90% of women, migraines improve with pregnancy, especially during the second and third trimesters. However, a woman may experience her first migraine with pregnancy, and other disorders associated with headache occur more frequently or exclusively with pregnancy. These include preeclampsia, eclampsia, stroke, cerebral venous thrombosis, subarachnoid hemorrhage, pituitary tumor, and choriocarcinoma.

Imaging During Pregnancy

Although radiation exposure to the developing fetus is of concern, the threshold for radiation doses to cause developmental anomalies or growth retardation is ≥5 rad; the exposure required to produce deformities that might warrant pregnancy termination is ≥15 rad. A standard head or cervical spine CT scan exposes the uterus to a radiation dose of <1 mrad, one five-thousandth of the threshold dose for anomalies. Skull X-rays and cervical spine films likewise carry a <1 mrad exposure to the uterus. Head CT is considered relatively safe in pregnancy and is the neurodiagnostic study of choice for head trauma or suspected intracranial bleeds (42).

For nontraumatic or nonhemorrhagic headache evaluations, MRI is preferred, but it is somewhat controversial in pregnancy. The effect of the magnetoelectric field that is generated and of the increase in core body temperature (<1°C) on the fetus is unknown.

Indications for CT or MRI during pregnancy are the same as for headaches occurring at other life stages and include "worst headache ever", abrupt ("thunderclap") onset, abnormal neurological exam, progressive or new daily persistent headache, or new onset of seizures.

Headache Treatment During Pregnancy

For the woman whose pregnancy is complicated by migraines, nonpharmacological modalities are preferred as first-line therapy. These would include, but not be limited to, mind-body techniques, biofeedback, massage, ice packs, and sleep. Acupuncture may be safely done and provide some relief. Trigger-point infiltrations and dermal applications of capsaicin or thermal products (Biofreez or Icy-Hot) actually represent drug usages in pregnancy, but they are likely to be safe.

Ideally, medications would not be taken in pregnancy, but this ideal is infrequently achieved. A World Health Organization survey of 14,778 pregnant women from 22 countries on 4 continents found that 86% took prescription medications during pregnancy (43). The women averaged 2.9 prescriptions each, with a range of one to 15 prescriptions. It is important to bear in mind that this survey reported on prescription medication use only and did not address the use of over-the-counter medications, herbals, and supplements during pregnancy.

In the United States, studies show that two thirds of pregnant women take drugs during pregnancy; 50% take them during the first trimester (44). The Food and Drug Administration maintains a use-in-pregnancy rating system that weighs the known or potential risk to the fetus against the drug's potential benefit to the patient. The ratings and their definitions are given in Table 9-2.

A review of a comprehensive list of drugs in pregnancy reveals that few drugs are assigned risk category A. This safe-in-pregnancy designation is reserved for certain vitamins and minerals in recommended allowances and thyroid hormone in proper physiological replacement doses. Even vitamins in higher than physiological doses, however, are rated categories B to X.

Risk in human pregnancies has been documented in categories D and X. No risk in human pregnancies has been documented in categories B or C, but adequate studies to exclude risk have not been carried out. For obvious ethical reasons, such studies are rarely conducted. Data are more commonly accumulated through pregnancy registries, which may record either inadvertent exposures or enroll subjects when an informed decision is made to use the medication in question.

Attention is drawn to the caveat that with some medications risk is increased with prolonged therapy, high dosage, or exposure late in pregnancy. Whereas with teratogens the primary concern is during organogenesis in the first trimester, with many headache therapies exposure in late pregnancy may be of equal or greater concern. Notably, nonsteroidal

Table 9-2   Food and Drug Administration Use-in-Pregnancy Drug Rating System

Category	Interpretation
A	CONTROLLED STUDIES SHOW NO RISK. Adequate, well-controlled studies in pregnant women have failed to demonstrate risk to the fetus in any trimester of pregnancy.
B	NO EVIDENCE OF RISK IN HUMANS. Adequate, well-controlled studies in pregnant women have not shown increased risk of fetal abnormalities despite adverse findings in animals, or, in the absence of adequate human studies, animal studies show no fetal risk. The chance of fetal harm is remote, but remains a possibility.
C	RISK CANNOT BE RULED OUT. Adequate, well-controlled human studies are lacking, and animal studies have shown a risk to the fetus or are lacking as well. There is a chance of fetal harm if the drug is administered during pregnancy, but the potential benefits may outweigh the potential risk.
D	POSITIVE EVIDENCE OF RISK. Studies in humans, or investigational or post-marketing data, have demonstrated fetal risk. For example, the drug may be acceptable if needed in a life-threatening situation or serious disease for which safer drugs cannot be used or are ineffective.
X	CONTRAINDICATED IN PREGNANCY. Studies in animals or humans, or investigational or post-marketing reports, have demonstrated positive evidence of fetal abnormalities or risk which clearly outweighs any possible benefit to the patient.

anti-inflammatory drugs can cause premature closure of the ductus arteriosus in the fetus if given at or near term.

Of the over 3000 drugs that have been tested by the FDA, only 20 are known human teratogens. The more common risks are nonteratogenic: these include growth retardation, abnormal histogenesis, effects on uterine contraction or hemostasis, and postnatal effects, either in the immediate postpartum or delayed. The FDA ratings are inclusive of these categories of risk and not simply of teratogenicity (as the TERIS ratings are) and are more appropriate for a discussion of headache therapy in pregnancy.

Medications frequently prescribed for the headache patient and their FDA use-in-pregnancy risk category can be found in Table 9-3. Many older drugs pre-date this classification system and were not rated by their manufacturer. In those instances the author has listed the classification assigned by the reference *Drugs in Pregnancy and Lactation* (45).

Headache Treatment During Lactation

A frequent reason for the cessation of breastfeeding is the need to treat the lactating mother with medication. Often it is the patient's physician who recommends the suspension due to concerns over potential risk to the

Table 9-3　Drugs Commonly Used for Headache and Their FDA Use-in-Pregnancy Risk Category

Medication	Category	Medication	Category
Acetaminophen	B	Methysergide	D
Almotriptan	C	Metoclopramide	B
Alprazolam	D	Morphine	C (D if used for prolonged periods or in high doses at term)
Amitriptyline	D		
Aspirin	C		
Atenolol	D		
Bupropion	B	Naproxen	B (D if used in third trimester)
Butalbital	C (D if used for prolonged periods or in high doses at term)		
		Naratriptan	C
		Nortriptyline	D
Butorphanol	B (D if used for prolonged periods or in high doses at term)	Oxycodone	B (D if used for prolonged periods or in high doses at term)
Caffeine	B		
Carisoprodol	C	Paroxetine	C
Chlordiazepoxide	D	Pentazocine	C (D if used for prolonged periods or in high doses at term)
Citalopram	C		
Clonazepam	D		
Codeine	C (D if used for prolonged periods or in high doses at term)		
		Phenobarbital	D
		Prednisone	B
Cyclobenzaprine	B	Prochlorperazine	C
Dexamethasone	C	Promethazine	C
Diazepam	D	Propoxyphene	C (D if used for prolonged periods)
Dihydroergotamine	X		
Dimenhydrinate	B	Propranolol	C (D if used in second or third trimesters)
Divalproex	D		
Ergotamine	X		
Fluoxetine	C	Protriptyline	C
Gabapentin	C	Pseudoephedrine	C
Hydrocodone	C (D if used for prolonged periods or in high doses at term)	Rizatriptan	C
		Sertraline	C
		Sumatriptan	C (advancement to category B was advocated in a recent critical review of the literature and pregnancy registry data) (46)
Ibuprofen	B (D if used in third trimester)		
Imipramine	C		
Isometheptene	C		
Ketoprofen	B (D if used in third trimester)		
Levetiracetam	C	Tizanidine	C
Meperidine	B (D if used for prolonged periods or in high doses at term)	Topiramate	C
		Tramadol	C
		Valproic acid	D
Methadone	B (D if used for prolonged periods or in high doses at term)	Venlafaxine	C
		Verapamil	C
		Zolmitriptan	C

nursing infant—concerns that in many cases may be unfounded. Most drugs prescribed to the lactating woman will have no effect on milk supply or the infant's well-being.

A number of factors influence the transport of drugs into breast milk. Membrane transport is achieved primarily by passive diffusion with the usual factors of concentration gradient, lipophilicity, and degree of ionization determining transport kinetics, along with protein binding. But in breastfeeding there are additional factors to consider: frequency of dosing, frequency of nursing, and the time interval between dosage and nursing. Furthermore, it is important to bear in mind that many reviews that give concentrations of drugs in breast milk report figures that are derived from a single measurement following a single dose.

The average nursing infant consumes approximately 0.15 L/kg/day of breast milk. The infant dose (in mg/kg) is calculated based on this daily consumption and expressed as a percentage of the maternal dose. For most drugs, an arbitrary cut-off of 10% has been accepted as a guide to the safe use of drugs in lactation. For drugs with greater inherent toxicity, such as cytotoxic agents, the cut-off of 10% is too high, and breastfeeding is contraindicated in their presence.

Virtually all drugs taken by the mother will be present in breast milk. Unquestionably, although very few drugs are known to be hazardous to the nursing infant, it is best to minimize exposure to them. As a general consideration, medications taken regularly, frequently, or in high concentrations are of greater concern than medications taken episodically, infrequently, or in low concentrations, because regular exposure may confer greater risk than intermittent exposure. To minimize risk to the nursing infant, medication should be limited to necessary treatments with the safest appropriate drugs. Consideration may be given to timing dosages immediately after breastfeeding or before the baby's sleep periods.

Welcome news to those treating headaches during lactation is the recent addition of sumatriptan to the medications considered compatible with breastfeeding (47). Generalization across the class of triptans is not warranted at this time. Sumatriptan is hydrophilic, whereas the other triptans are lipid-soluble, a factor influencing transport of drugs into breast milk. Information on usage of the other triptans in the lactating patient is not yet available.

The American Academy of Pediatrics (AAP) Committee on Drugs divides medication usage in lactation into seven categories:

1. Cytotoxic drugs that may interfere with cellular metabolism of the nursing infant
2. Drugs of abuse for which adverse effects on the infant during breastfeeding have been demonstrated
3. Radioactive compounds that require temporary cessation of breastfeeding

4. Drugs for which the effect on nursing infants is unknown, but may be of concern

5. Drugs that have been associated with significant effects on some nursing infants and should be given to nursing mothers with caution

6. Maternal medication usually compatible with breastfeeding

7. Food and environmental agents

Medications and their compatibility with breast feeding are listed in Table 9-4; in cases where the AAP has issued an opinion, its statement is presented (47). Recommendations about the compatibility of certain medications with breastfeeding are based on their known pharmacological effects as well as theoretical considerations.

Table 9-4   Medications and Their Compatibility with Breastfeeding (American Academy of Pediatrics Statements in Italics)

Medication	Lactation Compatibility
Acetaminophen	*Compatible with breastfeeding*
Almotriptan	Effects unknown
Alprazolam	*Effects unknown but may be of concern (of special concern when given to nursing mothers for long duration)*
Amitriptyline	*Effects unknown but may be of concern (of special concern when given to nursing mothers for long duration)*
Aspirin	*Cautious use recommended because of potential effects in the nursing infant.* A single case of metabolic acidosis has been reported.
Atenolol	*Cautious use recommended because of potential effects in the nursing infant.* Associated with bradycardia and cyanosis; a safer alternative is propranolol.
Bupropion	*Effects unknown but possibly of concern (of special concern when given to nursing mothers for long duration)*
Butalbital	Not recommended
Butorphanol	*Compatible with breastfeeding*
Caffeine	*Usual amounts of caffeinated beverages are compatible with breastfeeding; higher doses may produce irritability and poor sleeping pattern.* Drug combinations of acetaminophen, aspirin, and caffeine are not recommended with breastfeeding.
Chlorpromazine	*Effects unknown but possibly of concern.* Produces galactorrhea in mother, drowsiness and lethargy in infant, decline in developmental scores.
Citalopram	*Effects unknown but possibly of concern (of special concern when given to nursing mothers for long duration)*
Clonazepam	*Effects unknown but possibly of concern (of special concern when given to nursing mothers for long duration).* Can produce drowsiness, decreased feeding, and weight loss.

(Cont'd)

Table 9-4   Medications and Their Compatibility with Breastfeeding (American Academy of Pediatrics Statements in Italics) *(Cont'd)*

Medication	Lactation Compatibility
Codeine	*Compatible with breastfeeding*
Divalproex	Effects unknown
Eletriptan	Effects unknown
Ergotamine	*Cautious use recommended because of potential effects in the nursing infant.* Vomiting, diarrhea, and convulsions have been associated with dosages used in migraine therapy.
Estradiol	*Compatible with breastfeeding*
Fluoxetine	*Effects unknown but possibly of concern (of special concern when given to nursing mothers for long duration).* Reported effects include colic, irritability, feeding and sleep disorders, and slow weight gain.
Frovatriptan	Effects unknown
Hydrocodone	Not recommended
Ibuprophen	*Compatible with breastfeeding*
Imipramine	*Effects unknown but possibly of concern (of special concern when given to nursing mothers for long duration)*
Indomethacin	*Compatible with breastfeeding.* There has been a single reported case of seizure.
Isometheptene	No data available
Lidocaine	*Compatible with breastfeeding*
Magnesium sulfate	*Compatible with breastfeeding*
Meperidine	*Compatible with breastfeeding*
Methadone	*Compatible with breastfeeding* When mother is taking large amounts of methadone, the baby may become dependent on it.
Metoclopramide	*Effects unknown but possibly of concern.* Drug is concentrated in breast milk.
Morphine	*Compatible with breastfeeding.* Infant may have measurable blood concentration.
Naproxen	*Compatible with breastfeeding*
Naratriptan	Effects unknown
Neurontin	Effects unknown
Nortriptyline	*Effects unknown but possibly of concern (of special concern when given to nursing mothers for long duration)*
Oral contraceptives	*Compatible with breastfeeding.* Use of OCs during lactation has been associated with decreased milk production (not confirmed in several studies). An infant consuming 600 mL of breast milk daily from a mother using a 50 µg ethinyl estradiol OC (the highest dose available in the US) will receive a daily dose of ethinyl estradiol of about 10 ng, equivalent to the amount of natural estradiol received by infants of mothers not using OCs.

(Cont'd)

Table 9-4   Medications and Their Compatibility with Breastfeeding (American Academy of Pediatrics Statements in Italics) *(Cont'd)*

Medication	Lactation Compatibility
Oxycodone	Infants should be monitored for gastrointestinal effects, sedation, and changes in feeding.
Prednisone	*Compatible with breastfeeding*
Promethazine	Detection of promethazine in breast milk is difficult due to its rapid metabolism. Potential effects are unknown.
Propoxyphene	*Compatible with breastfeeding*
Propranolol	*Compatible with breast-feeding*
Pseudoephedrine	*Compatible with breastfeeding.* Drug is concentrated in breast milk.
Rizatriptan	Effects unknown
Sertraline	*Effects unknown but possibly of concern (of special concern when given to nursing mothers for long duration).* Drug is concentrated in breast milk.
Sumatriptan	*Compatible with breastfeeding*
Tramadol	Effects unknown
Trazodone	*Effects unknown but possibly of concern (of special concern when given to nursing mothers for long duration)*
Valproic acid	*Compatible with breastfeeding*
Venlafaxine	*Effects unknown but possibly of concern (of special concern when given to nursing mothers for long duration)*
Verapamil	*Compatible with breastfeeding*
Zolmitriptan	Effects unknown
Zolpidem	*Compatible with breastfeeding*

Key Points

- Migraine is three times more common in women than men; reproductive events such as menarche, pregnancy, and menopause affect its frequency, duration, and severity.

- Menstrual migraine is triggered by "estrogen withdrawal" at the time of menstruation; hormonal and nonhormonal therapies can be effective in the prevention of menstrual migraine.

- The use of exogenous hormones can improve or worsen migraine headache; strategies that minimize falls in estrogen concentration are preferable.

- Medications for migraine should be used judiciously in pregnant and lactating women.

REFERENCES

1. **Fettes I.** Migraine in the menopause. Neurology. 1999;53(Suppl 1):S29-33.

2. **Launer LJ, Terwindt GM, Ferrari MD.** The prevalence and characteristics of migraine in a population-based cohort. Neurology. 1999;53:537-42.

3. **Ratinahirana H, Darbois Y, Bousser M-G.** Migraine and pregnancy: a prospective study in 703 women after delivery [Abstract]. Neurology. 1990;40(Suppl 1):437.

4. **Hodson J, Thompson J, Al-Azzawi F.** Headache at menopause and in hormone replacement users. Climacteric. 2000;3:119-24.

5. **Granella F, Sances G, Zanferrari C, et al.** Migraine without aura and reproductive life events: a clinical epidemiological study in 1300 women. Cephalalgia. 1993;33:385-9.

6. **Whitty C, Hockaday J.** Migraine: a follow-up study of 92 patients. BMJ. 1968;1: 735-6.

7. **Culpini L, Matteis M, Troisi E, et al.** Sex-hormone-related events in migrainous females: a clinical comparative study between migraine with aura and migraine without aura. Cephalalgia. 1995;15:140-4.

8. **Neri I, Granella F, Nappi R, et al.** Characteristics of headache at menopause: a clinico-epidemiologic study. Maturitas. 1993;17:31-7.

9. **Mueller L.** Predictability of exogenous hormone effect on subgroups of migraineurs. Headache. 2000;40:189-93.

10. **MacGregor A.** Migraine associated with menstruation. Funct Neurol. 2000;15(Suppl 3): 143-53.

10a. **Stewart WF, Lipton RB, Chee E, et al.** Menstrual cycle and headache in a population sample of migraineurs. Neurology. 2000;55:1517-23.

11. **Somerville BW.** The role of estradiol withdrawal in the etiology of menstrual migraine. Neurology. 1972;22:355.

12. **Sulak PJ, Scow RD, Preece C, et al.** Hormone withdrawal symptoms in oral contraceptive users. Obstet Gynecol. 2000;95:261-6.

13. **Hellstrom B, Anderberg UM.** Pain perception across the menstrual cycle phases in women with chronic pain. Percept Mot Skills. 2003;96:201-11.

14. **D'Amico JF, Greendale GA, Lu JKH, Judd HL.** Induction of hypothalamic opioid activity with transdermal estradiol administration in postmenopausal women. Fertil Steril. 1991;55:754-8.

15. **Somerville BW.** The role of progesterone in menstrual migraine. Neurology. 1971;21:853.

16. **Magos AL, Zilkha KJ, Studd JWW.** Treatment of menstrual migraine by oestradiol implants. J Neurol Neurosurg Psychiatry. 1983;46:1044.

17. **Martin V, Wernke S, et al.** Medical oophorectomy with and without estrogen add-back therapy in the prevention of migraine headache. Headache. 2003;43:309-21.

18. **Murray SC, Muse KN.** Effective treatment of severe menstrual migraine headaches with gonadotropin-releasing hormone agonist and "add-back" therapy. Fertil Steril. 1997;67:390-3.

19. **De Lignieres B, Vincens M, Mauvais-Jarvis P.** Prevention of menstrual migraine by percutaneous oestradiol. BMJ. 1986;293:1540.

20. **Pradalier A, Vincent D, Beaulieu PH, et al.** Correlation between oestradiol plasma level and therapeutic effect on menstrual migraine. In: Rose FC, ed. New Advances in Headache Research, 4th ed. London: Smith-Gordon; 1994:129-32.

21. **Ryan RE.** A controlled study of the effect of oral contraceptives on migraine. Headache. 1978;17:250-1.

22. **Karsay, K.** The relationship between vascular headaches and low-dose oral contraceptives. Ther Hung. 1990;38:181-5.

23. **Calhoun A.** Adjusting estradiol concentrations reduces headache frequency and severity in female migraineurs. Cephalalgia. 2001;21:448-9.

24. **MacGregor A.** Estrogen replacement and migraine aura. Headache. 1999;39:674-8.

25. **O'Dea JP, Davis EH.** Tamoxifen in the treatment of menstrual migraine. Neurology. 1990;40:1470-1.

26. **Lichten E M, Bennett RS, et al.** Efficacy of danazol in the control of hormonal migraine. J Reprod Med. 1991;36:419-24.

27. **Sances G, Martignoni E, et al.** Naproxen sodium in menstrual migraine prophylaxis: a double-blind placebo-controlled study. Headache. 1990;30:705-9.

28. **Newman L, Mannix LK, et al.** Naratriptan as short-term prophylaxis of menstrually associated migraine: a randomized, double-blind, placebo-controlled study. Headache. 2001;41:248-56.

29. **Silberstein S, Elkind A, Schrieber C.** Frovatriptan, a selective 5HT 1D/1B agonist, is effective for prophylaxis of menstrually associated migraine [Abstract]. Neurology. 2003;60:A94.

30. **Gallagher M.** Menstrual migraine and intermittent ergonovine therapy. Headache 1989;29:366-7.

31. **Herzog AG.** Continuous bromocriptine therapy in menstrual migraine. Neurology. 1997;48:101-2.

32. **Solbach P, Waymer R.** Treatment of menstruation-associated migraine headache with subcutaneous sumatriptan. Obstet Gynecol. 1993;82:769-72.

33. **Silberstein S, Massiou G, Le Jeunne C, et al.** Rizatriptan in the treatment of menstrual migraine. Obstet Gynecol. 2000;96:237-42.

34. **Silberstein S, Armellino J, Hoffman H, et al.** Treatment of menstruation-associated migraine with nonprescription combination of acetaminophen, aspirin and caffeine: results from three randomized, placebo-controlled studies. Clin Ther. 1999;21:1-17.

35. **Bixler EO, Vgontzas AN, et al.** Prevalence of sleep-disordered breathing in women: effects of gender. Am J Respir Crit Care Med. 2001;163(3 Pt 1):608-13.

36. **Campbell S, Whitehead M.** Oestrogen therapy and the menopausal syndrome. Clin Obstet Gynecol. 1977;4:31-47.

37. **Martin PL, Burnier AM, Segre EJ, Huix FJ.** Graded sequential therapy in the menopause: a double-blind study. Am J Obstet Gynecol. 1971;111:178-86.

38. **Greenblatt RB, Bruneteau DW.** Menopausal headaches: psychogenic or metabolic? J Am Geriatr Soc. 1974;22:186-90.

39. **Kudrow L.** The relationship of headache frequency to hormone use in migraine. Headache. 1975;15:36-40.

40. **Facchinetti F, Nappi RE, Tirelli A, et al.** hormone supplementation differently affects migraine in postmenopausal women. Headache. 2002;42:924-9.

41. **Antonijevic IA, Stalla GK, et al.** Modulation of the sleep electroencephalogram by estrogen replacement in postmenopausal women. Am J Obstet Gynecol. 2000;182:277-82.

42. **Schwartz RB.** Neurodiagnostic imaging of the pregnant patient. In: Devinsky O, Feldmann E, Hainline B, eds. Neurologic Complications of Pregnancy. New York: Raven Press; 1994:243-8.

43. Collaborative Group on Drug Use in Pregnancy. An international survey on drug utilization during pregnancy. Int J Risk Safety Med. 1991;1:1.

44. **Pitkin RM.** Drug treatment of the pregnant woman: the state of the art [Abstract]. In: Proceedings from the Food and Drug Administration Conference on Regulated Products and Pregnant Women; November 1995.

45. **Briggs GC, Freeman RK, Yaffe SJ.** Drugs in Pregnancy and Lactation, 5th ed. Baltimore: Williams & Wilkins; 1998.

46. **Loder E.** The safety of sumatriptan in pregnancy: a review of the data so far. CNS Drugs. 2003;17:1-7.

47. American Academy of Pediatrics, Committee on Drugs. Transfer of drugs and other chemicals into human milk. Pediatrics. 2001;Sept:776-81.

10

* * *

Headache in Children and Adolescents

Eric M. Pearlman, MD, PhD

Although primary headache is a well-recognized phenomenon in adults, it is often overlooked or minimized in children and adolescents. Headache is a common complaint in children, and migraine in particular often begins during the first two decades of life. Recognition and appropriate treatment improves quality of life for young sufferers as well as their caregivers, and may decrease long-term disability from headache.

The prevalence of headache in children varies with age. Few data are available regarding headache in infancy. Difficulty in obtaining the historical information necessary to classify headaches as well as lack of consensus about child headache classification make prevalence statistics on headache in children somewhat unreliable. There are few well-defined features that allow accurate recognition and classification of head pain in infants and young children. The data that do exist suggest that in preschool children headache prevalence increases with age. By age 3 years, headache has occurred in 3% to 8% of children (1-3), while 19% of 5-year-olds and 37% to 51% of 7-year-olds report suffering from headache (4-6). By age 15, headache prevalence reaches adult levels, occurring in up to 82% of children over a 1-year period (7). The prevalence of headache subtypes such as migraine is more difficult to ascertain, because identification depends on the specific definition used.

Tension-Type Headache

Tension-type headache is the most common form of primary headache in adults, but relatively little is known about its prevalence in children in the general population. This lack of study is likely due to the fact that tension-type headache is not widely viewed as a serious or disabling medical problem.

The International Headache Society (IHS) criteria for the diagnosis of tension-type headache in children are the same as those in adults. It is a mild or moderate headache with few associated symptoms. As in adults, tension-type headache can be subdivided into episodic and chronic forms of the disorder, and associated or unassociated with muscle tenderness on palpation. One study found a 1-year prevalence of tension-type headache of 73% in 10- to 18-year-olds. A Swedish study using strict IHS criteria found a prevalence of 10% in children between the ages of 7 to 16 years, a finding very similar to that of a study done in Brazil, which showed a prevalence of 12% in 12-year-olds (8,9). Studies from headache clinics show that tension-type headache can be diagnosed in around 35% of children who seek treatment. Not unexpectedly, the percentage of children who have chronic forms of the disorder is high, around 15% to 20%.

There are no population-based studies of the usefulness of these criteria in distinguishing this form of headache from migraine in children. Several clinic-based studies suggest that many children do not completely fulfill all of these criteria. In general, the problem is that the criteria are very sensitive (i.e., a high probability of a positive test result in those that have the disease) but not very specific (i.e., a low probability of a negative test result in those without the disease). Mild intensity of pain and the absence of nausea and vomiting were the features most useful in accurately ruling in tension-type headache as opposed to migraine (10,11).

The prognosis of tension-type headache in children appears to be favorable. One Italian study showed significant rates of improvement over an 8-year follow-up period: 36.1% of children with headache at baseline were headache-free at follow-up, and 44.4% had headache less than once per month. Only 2.7% had experienced worsening. In general, this study showed that the prognosis for tension-type headache was significantly better than that for migraine. Prognosis was poorer for girls than for boys (12).

Cluster Headache

There are no studies of the incidence or prevalence of cluster headache in children, but it certainly exists, as established by convincing case reports and series (13). The case reports suggest that childhood cluster headache is similar to the adult form in location, duration, and associated autonomic symptoms. Treatment options for children are the same as for adults, but with the added complication of adjusting dosages and monitoring response based on differing pharmacokinetics and drug properties in children. As in adults, most treatment for cluster headache will be unapproved, "off-label" uses of drugs.

Migraine

Diagnosis and Classification

The criteria for migraine in children have undergone several revisions during the last 50 years. Early definitions by Vahlquist (14) and Bille (4) described migraine in children as recurrent headache with symptom-free intervals and at least two associated features: nausea or vomiting, unilateral pain, visual aura, and positive family history. In 1988, the IHS (15) developed a definition of migraine for adults. Modification of the criteria for children less than 15 years of age was suggested, and the 2004 revisions of the IHS criteria have incorporated these suggestions (Table 10-1) (16).

Diagnostic criteria for migraine in children differ somewhat from those used for adults. The most important difference is recognition of the shorter duration of headache in children: for individuals less than 15 years of age, migraine duration can be from 1 to 72 hours instead of the 4 to 72 hours required in those over 15 years of age. The IHS also recognizes that migraine is more commonly bilateral in children than in adults. The remainder of the criteria for migraine in children are similar to the adult criteria. These include at least five attacks with either photophobia or phonophobia, nausea or vomiting, and two of the following symptoms: bilateral or unilateral pain, throbbing or pulsatile pain, moderate-to-severe pain intensity, and pain exacerbation by routine activity or causing avoidance of routine physical

Table 10-1   International Headache Society Criteria for Adolescent and Pediatric Migraine with and without Aura

Pediatric Migraine without Aura	*Pediatric Migraine with Aura*
A. At least 5 distinct attacks B. Headache attack lasting 1-72 hr C. Headache has at least 2 of the following: 　1. Bilateral (frontal/temporal) or unilateral location 　2. Pulsating quality 　3. Moderate-to-severe pain intensity 　4. Aggravation by routine physical activity D. During headache, at least one of the following: 　1. Nausea and/or vomiting 　2. Photophobia and/or phonophobia (may be inferred from child's behavior)	A. Fulfills criteria for migraine without aura B. At least 3 of the following: 　1. One or more fully reversible aura symptoms indicating focal cortical and/or brainstem dysfunction 　2. At least one aura developing gradually over more than 4 min or two or more symptoms occurring in succession 　3. No aura lasting more than 60 min 　4. Headache follows in less than 60 min

From International Headache Society. The International Classification of Headache Disorders, 2nd ed. Cephalalgia. 2004;24(Suppl 1):9-160; with permission.

activity. The revised criteria allow photophobia and phonophobia in children to be inferred rather than directly reported.

Some features of headache in children are not specifically recognized by the IHS classification but are commonly noted clinically (Table 10-2). For example, the quality of the pain is often described as constant or squeezing rather than throbbing. Children are also much more likely to report bilateral, bifrontal, or a nondescript location rather than unilateral pain. Adults with migraine with aura typically have onset and resolution of their aura before the onset of head pain. In contrast, when aura occurs in children, it may overlap with the actual headache but should resolve before the headache phase ends. Onset of head pain may be dramatic in children, with peak pain intensity occurring within 15 minutes. Pain generally resolves quickly and completely, sometimes within 2 to 4 hours, usually without the lingering post-dromal symptoms seen in many adult migraineurs. Many children may require only a short period of sleep to achieve headache resolution; not infrequently, children prefer sleep to the use of medication.

By age 7, the prevalence of migraine ranges from 1.2% to 3.2% (1,4,17). From ages 7 to 15, the prevalence is estimated at between 4% to 11% (1,4,17). Migraine prevalence is higher in boys from ages 3 to 7 years, equal in boys and girls aged 7 to 11 years, and higher in girls over age 11 years (17). Migraine clearly affects children and families and is associated with significant disability (18).

Migraine can be as disabling in children as it is in adults. Children and adolescents with migraine miss days from school and miss hours at school while in the nurse's or principal's office. Young migraineurs also miss out on after-school and social activities; in the case of older adolescents and teenagers, they may even miss work. Some children may be able to get

Table 10-2   Differential Features of Pediatric and Adult Migraine

	Pediatric Migraine	*Adult Migraine*
Duration	1-72 hr	4-72 hr
Quality	May or not be described as throbbing	Throbbing/pulsatile
Location	Unilateral, bilateral, whole head	Unilateral; bilateral less likely
Aura	May overlap with head pain	Resolves prior to head pain
Resolution	More likely to be rapid and complete; resolves with rest or brief sleep	Resolves with longer sleep; lingering post-dromal symptoms common
Associated features	Nausea/vomiting, photophobia or phonophobia – may be less prominent	Nausea/vomiting, photophobia or phonophobia – necessary for diagnosis

through the school day but be unable to finish homework because of headache. In addition, caregivers may need to miss work if they have a child who needs to stay home from school due to headache.

There are usually significant anxieties regarding the possibility of ominous causes of headache in children. Both parents and children may worry that headaches signal a more dangerous condition. As in adults, the time course, features, and associated symptoms of the headache are useful in distinguishing between recurrent benign headache (migraine, episodic tension, cluster) and secondary headache.

The primary headache disorders of migraine, episodic tension-type headache, and cluster headache are characterized by attacks of pain and associated symptoms with intervals of normal functioning between headaches. Other patterns should prompt consideration of a secondary cause of headache. The first attack always deserves special attention, because there is no pre-existing pattern that is reassuring of a primary headache disorder. A severe and disabling first attack may provoke an evaluation for causes of secondary headache. Chronic headache that gets progressively worse over time, or headache that is associated with abnormal physical or neurological examination findings, requires further investigation (19-21).

Migraine Variants

Occasionally, migraine in children is associated with unusual symptoms. These may include dramatic transient neurological changes. These variants often engender worry about an underlying dangerous cause of headache; again, family history, time course, and normal interictal status are reassuring indications of a benign condition. The biological basis of these variants is likely the same for migraine with and without aura. The fact that many of the migraine variants occur in children implies a developmental or maturational susceptibility to these associated symptoms in the cortical and brainstem areas.

Basilar-Type Migraine

Basilar-type migraine, also known as "Bickerstaff's", "basilar artery", or "vertebrobasilar" migraine, is the most common migraine variant, representing 3% to 19% of all attacks (20,22). "Basilar-type" has replaced the term "basilar" in the 2004 IHS criteria. The change reflects the absence of evidence that the basilar artery is involved in this syndrome; rather, the symptoms appear to reflect brainstem dysfunction. This syndrome is probably more accurately characterized as complicated migraine because of the unusual neurological symptoms. This diagnostic subcategory of migraine is likely to be eliminated altogether in the next iteration of the IHS classification system. In any case, the mean age of onset of the attacks is 7 years of age. Attacks are characterized by intense vertigo, dizziness, ataxia, and diplopia. These features last from minutes to an hour and are followed by the headache phase. The headache may be located occipitally and thus trigger consideration of posterior fossa pathology. The differential diagnosis includes vascular malformations such as arteriovenous malformations (AVMs) and cavernous angioma; vertebral artery dissection; Chiari malformation or Dandy-Walker variants; brainstem tumors including medulloblastoma, ependymoma, and glioma; positional vertigo; complex partial seizures; intoxications; and, rarely, inborn errors of metabolism.

Ophthalmoplegic Migraine

Ophthalmoplegic migraine is probably better considered a cranial neuropathy rather than a variant of migraine, and the new version of the IHS criteria have reclassified it as such. It is a disorder characterized by head or retro-orbital pain and ophthalmoparesis. The ophthalmoparesis can be complete or partial, with skew deviation and adductor paresis being the most frequent deficits. Ptosis is also frequently present and may be unilateral or bilateral. The clinical presentation is often pain followed by the paresis and ptosis; the neurological deficits may persist for days to weeks even after the headache resolves. Repeated bouts can also lead to permanent deficits. Acute treatment with corticosteroids can lead to a more rapid resolution of the deficits. Neuroimaging has shown enhancement and thickening of the occulomotor cranial nerve (23,24), suggesting inflammatory pathology. The steroid responsiveness and inflammatory changes on imaging suggest that this condition may an inflammatory disorder, similar to Tolosa-Hunt syndrome, rather than a migraine variant.

Confusional Migraine

Confusional migraine occurs in children and early teenagers. These episodes consist of acute onset of confusion, agitation, language difficulties, and amnesia for the event. Once the confusion resolves, a typical migraine-like headache will occur, with throbbing pain, nausea, vomiting, photophobia, and phonophobia. A family history of migraine is usually present. These events can be precipitated by minor head trauma. There may be overlap symptoms with basilar or hemiplegic migraine such as vertigo, vision loss, and sensory loss. Hemiparesis may accompany episodes of confusion. Confusional migraine is probably best considered a diagnosis of exclusion, after evaluation for intoxication, complex partial seizure, encephalitis, and metabolic encephalopathy has been completed.

Familial Hemiplegic Migraine

Familial hemiplegic migraine is an uncommon autosomal dominant headache syndrome in which the aura includes hemiparesis. The attack begins with aura that precedes headache, but instead of resolving prior to the onset of pain, the aura can continue for hours to days. The hemiparesis can be dense and persist for so long that it resembles stroke. Attacks may also be accompanied by visual, sensory, or bulbar dysfunction. Genetic loci associated with this migraine variant have been identified on chromosomes 1 and 19; they appear to encode neuronal P/Q-type voltage-gated calcium channel (25,26). Mutations on chromosome 19 are associated with hemiplegic migraine as well as episodic ataxia, suggesting a link between these two disorders.

Alternating Hemiplegia: A Migraine Variant?

Alternating hemiplegia of childhood is sometimes considered a variant of familial hemiplegic migraine, although evidence of such a link is felt by most authorities to be weak. The disorder begins in early childhood, usually before 18 months of age, and is characterized by attacks of motor impairment, which vary from attack to attack. Alternating hemiplegia can manifest as hemiparesis, monoparesis, diparesis, ophthalmoparesis, and bulbar impairment. If there is significant bulbar involvement, respiratory impairment can occur. In addition, movement abnormalities such as chorea, dystonia, and athetosis can occur. The motor impairment can resolve quickly or last for days. There is a high prevalence of migraine in family members but no clear Mendelian inheritance such as seen in familial hemiplegic migraine. Flunarizine, a neuronal calcium channel blocker not available in the United States, is very effective in preventing attacks of alternating hemiplegia, further evidence that this disorder may represent a calcium channelopathy (26a).

When a child presents with either familial hemiplegic migraine or alternating hemiplegia, evaluation for other paroxysmal conditions such as stroke, seizure, mitochondrial disorders, or inborn errors of metabolism is warranted.

Other Paroxysmal Disorders of Childhood

Other recurrent paroxysmal disorders of childhood include benign paroxysmal torticollis, benign paroxysmal vertigo, cyclic vomiting syndrome, and abdominal migraine. All are considered variants or equivalents of migraine because of neuroanatomic similarities, tendency to develop typical migraine attacks later in life, strong family history of migraine, or similarity in clinical symptoms.

BENIGN PAROXYSMAL TORTICOLLIS

Benign paroxysmal torticollis is characterized by recurrent episodes of head tilt, vomiting, and truncal ataxia. This occurs at a young age, usually in infants between 2 and 8 months of age. An episode may last hours to days, and between attacks there is no dystonia, abnormal posturing, or cerebellar dysfunction. Several lines of evidence suggest that this unusual disorder of infancy is linked to migraine: first, affected infants frequently develop migraine with or without aura later in life; second, there is usually a strong family history of migraine; third, there is evidence that the same mutation in the P/Q calcium channel that leads to hemiplegic migraine is present in infants with paroxysmal torticollis from the same kindred (27). The differential diagnosis includes idiopathic torsion dystonia, posterior fossa and cervicomedullary junction pathology, labyrinthine dysfunction, cerebellar dysfunction, occulomotor abnormalities such as trochlear nerve lesions, and skew deviation.

BENIGN PAROXYSMAL VERTIGO

Benign paroxysmal vertigo occurs in a slightly older population, usually in toddlers between 9 months and 2 years of age. This disorder consists of episodes of unsteadiness, which comes on suddenly and lasts for several minutes. During an attack, the child will grab onto a parent or nearby object and will refuse to walk. Vomiting may occur and be quite intense, and nystagmus may be present. The acute attack is often followed by sleep. When the toddler awakens, he/she is back to normal. This disorder is quite common, but the exact incidence is not known. It may go unrecognized unless attacks are severe or occur with some regularity. There is often a family history of migraine, and these toddlers are prone to develop migraine later in life (28).

CYCLIC VOMITING SYNDROME AND ABDOMINAL MIGRAINE

Cyclic vomiting syndrome and abdominal migraine are two other episodic disorders usually considered to be migraine variants. The episodes are stereotyped and consist of repeated vomiting in cyclic vomiting syndrome and abdominal pain, nausea, vomiting, and occasionally diarrhea in abdominal migraine. The abdominal pain may be described as sharp or cramping. The diagnosis is usually considered only after an extensive gastrointestinal workup is unrevealing. Cyclic vomiting syndrome is distinguished from abdominal migraine by the intensity of the vomiting. Attacks are characterized by episodes of nearly constant emesis (at least 4 per hour), and dehydration may be a risk in selected patients. Episodes occur generally less than twice a week. In both abdominal migraine and cyclic vomiting syndrome, the absence of headache is characteristic.

Treatment

The treatment of migraine and other episodic headaches in children and adolescents consists of the same interventions used in adults, including lifestyle modification, trigger avoidance, nonpharmacological treatments, acute treatment, rescue treatment and, where appropriate, preventive treatment. The threshold for use of medication in children with mild headache is often higher than it is in adults. Nevertheless, children with unrelieved pain and suffering deserve the same aggressive treatment usually offered to adults. General principles of management as identified by the US Headache Consortium Guidelines (19) are

1. Establish a diagnosis
2. Educate patients about their condition and its treatment
3. Establish realistic expectations
4. Encourage patients to participate in their own management
5. Develop an individualized management plan

It is especially important to establish the diagnosis of migraine and convey this clearly to the patient and parents. Many parents are concerned that there is an underlying organic cause for their child's headache and, unless these fears are dispelled, treatment plans will meet with limited success. Patients and parents are much more likely to accept a treatment plan if they believe the diagnosis. Therefore it is important to spend time with the patient and the parents explaining the diagnosis and the disorder. This needs to be done at a level that the child and parents can understand. Reading materials, booklets, brochures, diaries, and videos can help teach the patient and their families about their disorder, how to recognize an attack, and convey reasonable expectations of treatment benefit.

Ongoing education should be part of every office visit, with an emphasis on lifestyle modification, trigger avoidance, and treatment strategies. Patient participation is essential for treatment plan success, especially for teenagers, who are unlikely to comply with a treatment plan that they do not agree with. Adolescents and teenagers should be included in the decision-making process and can be offered choices about medication formulations, routes of administration, or types of medication. Finally, it is necessary for the patient and parents to have realistic expectations about what the treatment plan can achieve. As with adults, treatment is generally only effective at decreasing attack frequency and severity; "cure" is unlikely. A reasonable goal is a reduction of 50% in the frequency of attacks.

Nonpharmacological Therapies and Lifestyle Modification
Nonpharmacological therapies are well received by younger patients, including adolescents. Basic lifestyle modifications, such as regular and adequate amounts of sleep, need to be reviewed with children, particularly adolescents, because sleep deprivation is a common trigger in child and adolescent migraineurs. Consistent sleep routines can often reduce attack frequency. Regular meals and routine exercise are other reasonable lifestyle changes that can improve adolescent and childhood headaches. Caffeine elimination or reduction to minimal levels can be helpful in some cases; other dietary modifications are not recommended because of lack of evidence that they are helpful and because of the danger of promoting unnecessary anxiety about food.

As with adult migraine, emotional and psychological stress is frequently an aggravating factor in adolescent or child migraine. The causes of stress in children differ from those in adults. School stress can include anxiety about workload, grades, and relationships with peers. In addition, some children are overextended with extracurricular activities and may not have adequate time to complete school work, relax, or enjoy social or leisure activities. For some children, reducing the number and frequency of after-school activities allows them to focus on school work, perform well, sleep regularly, and participate in leisure activities. (Additional information on migraine triggers is given in Chapter 4.)

Other nonpharmacological therapies, such as biofeedback, acupuncture, physical therapy, massage, and cognitive imagery, that are helpful in adults (see Chapter 12) (19) may also prove helpful in children and adolescents (but have not been studied in this group). These approaches generally reduce the frequency of attacks but do not eliminate them.

Pharmacological Therapy

Medications used in the acute treatment of migraine attacks can be divided into two major categories: migraine-specific and migraine nonspecific therapies. Common nonspecific acute medications are listed in Table 10-3, and migraine-specific therapies with their formulations and available doses are given in Table 10-4. Nonspecific medications such as NSAIDS should be used as first-line treatment, with migraine-specific medications such as triptans reserved for children with more severe, disabling headaches. The goals of abortive treatment are to minimize or eliminate pain quickly, generally within 2 hours, and to allow return to normal activities. Doses of NSAIDs should not exceed safe limits (15 mg/kg/dose up to 1000 mg maximum for acetaminophen; 10 mg/kg/dose up to 800 mg for ibuprofen). Combining an NSAID and a triptan is a common and successful clinical strategy for attacks that do not respond well to use of a single medication.

Migraine Nonspecific Medications

Several studies of nonspecific treatments in children exist. One compared acetaminophen, ibuprofen, and placebo in a double-blind crossover study (29). Eighty-eight children aged 4 to 15 years were enrolled. Children were randomized to treat headaches with acetaminophen (15 mg/kg/dose),

Table 10-3   Nonspecific Medications for Acute Migraine Therapy

	Suggested Dose	*Reference*
Acetaminophen	15 mg/kg up to 1000 mg	29
Nonsteroidal anti-inflammatory drugs (NSAIDs)		
Ibuprofen	10 mg/kg up to 800 mg	29, 30
Naproxen sodium	10 mg/kg up to 400 mg	
Opioids		
Codeine	0.5-1 mg/kg up to 60 mg	

ibuprofen (10 mg/kg/dose), or placebo. Acetaminophen and ibuprofen were statistically significantly more efficacious than placebo, and ibuprofen was more efficacious than acetaminophen. Another study compared ibuprofen suspension (7.5 mg/kg/dose) to placebo in a double-blind parallel-group trial in children aged 6 to 12 years (30). There were 45 children in the ibuprofen arm and 39 children in the placebo arm. Headache response at 2 hours was significantly higher in the ibuprofen arm (76% of attacks) than the placebo arm (53% of attacks; $P = 0.006$). Pain-free response was 44% for ibuprofen compared with 25% for placebo ($P < 0.07$). Only one child in the ibuprofen arm required rescue medication compared with 15 children in the placebo arm ($P < 0.001$). These studies suggest that ibuprofen is an effective acute therapy in doses from 7.5 to 10 mg/kg.

MIGRAINE-SPECIFIC MEDICATIONS

Several studies have examined the efficacy and tolerability of sumatriptan in children under 12 years of age. In an open (unblinded) study, 17 children aged 6 to 16 years were treated with subcutaneous sumatriptan for acute migraine attacks (31). Fifteen of the 17 children received a 6 mg dose and two received a 3 mg dose. Six had headache relief within 1 hour, and five others had relief by 2 hours. The two children who received a 3 mg dose were headache-free by 2 hours. In another study, 50 patients aged 6 to 18 years were treated with subcutaneous sumatriptan at a dose of 0.06 mg/kg for acute migraine. The headache response (improvement in severity from

Table 10-4	Migraine-Specific Acute Therapies for Children*		
	Dosage and Formulation		*References*
Sumatriptan	Injection:	6 mg	31, 32
	Nasal spray:	5 mg, 20 mg	33-35
	Tablet:	25 mg, 50 mg, 100 mg	36, 37
Zolmitriptan	Tablet:	2.5 mg, 5 mg	N/A
	ODT:	2.5 mg, 5 mg	
Rizatriptan	Tablet:	5 mg, 10 mg	38
	ODT:	5 mg, 10 mg	
Naratriptan	Tablet:	1.25 mg, 2.5 mg	N/A
Almotriptan	Tablet:	6.25 mg, 12.5 mg	N/A
Frovatriptan	Tablet:	2.5 mg	N/A
Eletriptan	Tablet:	20 mg, 40 mg	N/A
Ergotamine (DHE 45)	Injection Nasal spray		N/A

*All medications are currently approved for adults 18 years of age and older by the FDA; N/A= data not available.

moderate or severe to mild or no headache) was 78% at 2 hours; 26% of children responded within 30 minutes, and 46% responded within 1 hour (32). The recurrence rate (return or worsening of headache within 24 hours of dosing) was only 6%. In both studies, sumatriptan injection was well tolerated, with 84% of children in the second study rating the treatment good to excellent.

An open-label retrospective study assessed the efficacy and tolerability of sumatriptan nasal spray 5 or 20 mg in children aged 5 to 12 years (33). Out of 10 patients assessed, one had no response, two had a 50% response, and six had a 100% response, with 47 of 52 attacks (83%) responding to medication. In a randomized, double-blind, placebo-controlled crossover trial of 14 children aged 6.4 to 9.8 years, the efficacy and tolerability of sumatriptan nasal spray 20 mg dose was assessed (34). In this study, 12 of 14 children reported a decrease in pain intensity after sumatriptan compared with 6 of 14 after placebo (P = 0.031). Complete headache relief was reported by 9 of 14 children after sumatriptan nasal spray versus 2 of 14 after placebo (P = 0.016). In a large, randomized, double-blind, placebo-controlled study of sumatriptan nasal spray 5 mg, 10 mg, and 20 mg versus placebo, investigators required that subjects had headaches lasting longer than 4 hours in addition to meeting IHS criteria for migraine with or without aura (35). Subjects were required to self-administer study medication at home under the supervision of their parents; 507 patients were enrolled. The primary endpoint was headache response at 2 hours. Results are shown in Figure 10-1. Only the 5 mg dose was found to be statistically significantly

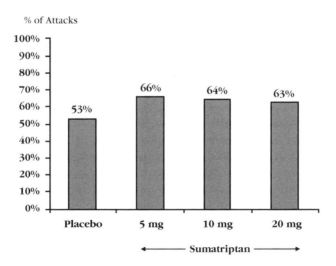

Figure 10-1   Two-hour headache response to sumatriptan nasal spray in adolescents. (Data from Winner P, Rothner AD, Saper J, et al. A randomized, double-blind, placebo-controlled study of sumatriptan nasal spray in the treatment of acute migraine in adolescents. Pediatrics. 2000;106:989-97.)

superior to placebo ($P < 0.05$). The 10 and 20 mg doses did not statistically differ from placebo, although there is a numerical trend favoring active treatment. This study differs from adult trials in that no dose-response curve was demonstrated. Collectively, however, these studies suggest that sumatriptan given subcutaneously (0.06 mg/kg) or intranasally (20 mg) is effective in treating migraine in children aged 6 to 12 years.

Studies of oral triptan use in children have shown no problems with tolerability but have had difficulty demonstrating efficacy of the treatment, largely because of very high placebo responses. These may be related to the short duration of childhood headaches as compared with adult headache, with the result that it is very difficult to distinguish active treatments from natural resolution of the headache. In one study, 23 children aged 8.3 to 16.4 years were treated with oral sumatriptan 25 mg in a double-blind placebo-controlled crossover trial (36). No statistically significant difference between sumatriptan and placebo was reported for the primary endpoint of >50% reduction in pain intensity (7 of 23 for sumatriptan and 5 of 23 for placebo) or for pain-free response (5 of 23 for sumatriptan and 2 of 23 for placebo). However, when asked which treatment they preferred, 13 of the 23 preferred sumatriptan, while only 2 chose placebo.

There is a growing body of clinical evidence from large multicenter randomized double-blind placebo-controlled parallel-group trials studying the efficacy of triptans in adolescents over 12 years of age. In a study of 302 patients comparing sumatriptan 25 mg, 50 mg, and 100 mg tablets to placebo, the primary endpoint was 2 hour headache response. Active treatment results could not be statistically distinguished from placebo (49%, 50%, 51% response for 25 mg, 50 mg, 100 mg doses versus placebo response of 42%) (37). All three doses of sumatriptan were statistically significant compared with placebo at 3 (65%, 64%, 69% versus 45%) and 4 hours (73%, 73%, 74% versus 53%). The 50 mg dose was significantly superior to placebo at 90 minutes (47% versus 30%), whereas the 25 mg (38%) and 100 mg (38%) doses were not. It is important to note that most of the placebo rates in this trial were high compared with those normally observed (% in the 30's) in most adult triptan trials. As with other studies of triptans in children, this study failed to demonstrate a dose-response curve.

A large study of rizatriptan used similar inclusion criteria as the sumatriptan nasal spray study reviewed previously (38). In addition, patients were instructed to take study medication within 30 minutes of onset of a moderate/severe attack. The primary endpoint of 2 hour pain relief was achieved in 66% of subjects treating with rizatriptan 5 mg compared with 56% for placebo, a result that was not statistically significant. Post-hoc analysis of results found that for those attacks treated on weekdays the response rate was 66% for rizatriptan and 61% for placebo. However, for those attacks treated on weekends the response rates were 65% and 36% respectively. Thus the response rates for weekday compared with weekend administration were essentially the same for rizatriptan, but a strikingly lower placebo response (consistent with that seen in adult clinical trials) was observed with weekend administration.

Adverse events did not differ significantly between active drug and placebo, with the exception of more taste disturbances with sumatriptan nasal spray. Overall, these medications are extremely well tolerated in younger patients and concerns about safety should not preclude their use. Only one serious adverse event (facial nerve ischemia, with an unclear relationship to study medication) occurred in the sumatriptan nasal spray open-label extension phase (39).

In sum, there have been over 1650 subjects between 12 and 18 years involved in clinical trials published thus far, with an excellent tolerability and safety record. It thus seems reasonable that the use of migraine-specific medications such as triptans should be considered early in the course of treatment when children have disabling headaches that do not respond to acetaminophen and ibuprofen as first-line acute therapy.

Preventive Therapy

The decision to use migraine preventive medication in children should be considered after an adequate trial of acute treatment if frequent or disabling attacks persist. As in adults, the choice of medication should be based on co-existing conditions and tolerability profiles of specific medications. Unfortunately, recommendations regarding preventive medications in children and adolescents are based on adult information and clinical experience, because there are almost no data from controlled clinical trials. The optimal duration of treatment is also unclear, and based on clinical judgment.

In children under 9 years of age, cyproheptadine in doses of 2 to 8 mg a day, given once daily at bedtime or divided twice a day, is effective and well-tolerated. In older children, adolescents, and adults, adverse events limit its use. These consist primarily of sedation and weight gain. If sleep disturbance is a significant co-existing condition, however, then cyproheptadine is an appropriate choice. Other preventives that can help with sleep are the tricyclic antidepressants amitriptyline and imipramine. Doses of 10 to 50 mg given once daily at night are usually well tolerated. These would also be appropriate choices if hyperactivity or enuresis is present. Common side effects are sedation, weight gain, and dry mouth. Beta-blockers such as propranolol are often used in doses of 20 to 80 mg divided twice a day, although many teenagers do not tolerate the fatigue and exercise intolerance that may occur. Calcium channel blockers and anticonvulsants may be used as well. Divalproex sodium is an effective migraine preventive in adults and is often used to treat epilepsy in children or adolescents. However, its adverse event profile, which includes weight gain, hair loss, tremor, and risk of birth defects, makes divalproex sodium less desirable as a migraine preventive in this population. Topiramate is being investigated as a preventive in children and adolescents. There is recently published evidence for its efficacy in adults, and it is indicated for epilepsy in children down to age 2. Dosing for migraine prevention ranges from 50 to 200 mg daily in divided doses. Side effects include paresthesia, increased risk of renal calculi, appetite suppression and weight loss, and rare cases of acute angle-closure glaucoma.

Conclusion

Migraine and tension-type headache are common disorders within pediatric populations. Unfortunately there is scant research involving the diagnosis and treatment of pediatric tension-type headache. Diagnostic criteria for pediatric migraine have undergone recent revisions by the IHS. Attacks of pediatric migraine are of shorter duration, more often bilateral, and have less prominent associated symptoms than adult attacks.

Limited evidence from controlled clinical trials exists on which to base treatment decisions about abortive or preventive migraine therapy for children and adolescents. In general, most acute medications appear to be safe and well-tolerated, but evidence of efficacy has been marred by very high placebo response rates. Clinical experience strongly suggests that these medications are effective in children, and most experts believe the evidence base to date is hampered by clinical trial methodology. The shorter duration of headache in children makes it more difficult to distinguish active treatment effects from the natural history of headache resolution. If the headache has already started to resolve at the time of treatment, then any intervention, including placebo, will appear to be successful. Adolescents and children are also highly suggestible, another reason that placebo response rates are often high in studies on pain in adolescents. In addition, the natural desire of children to please the investigator by reporting treatment benefit appears to be more pronounced than it is in adult subjects.

The combination of clinical experience, expert opinion, and clinical trial evidence thus supports use of ibuprofen, acetaminophen, and triptans for acute treatment of migraine in children and adolescents. Less evidence exists to guide the use of preventive treatment, but clinical experience suggests that nonpharmacological approaches be tried first, followed by cyproheptadine or other traditional preventive drugs, with choice depending upon co-morbid conditions and side effect profile. Recognition and treatment of migraine in children improves quality of life and may delay or minimize the development of lifelong disabling headache and subsequent disability.

Key Points

- Migraine and tension-type headache are common in children and adolescents.

- Pediatric migraine attacks differ from those experienced by adults. They are of shorter duration (often 1 to 4 hours), more likely to be bilateral, and more likely to have gastrointestinal symptoms.

- Migraine variants in children may present with a constellation of neurological and gastrointestinal symptoms that must be distinguished from secondary headache disorders.

- Appropriate treatment for pediatric migraine patients includes life modifications and abortive medications. Preventive medications are indicated for frequent attacks.

REFERENCES

1. **Sillanpaa M.** Prevalence of migraine and other headache in Finnish children starting school. Headache.1976;15:288-90.
2. **Sillanpaa M.** Headache in children. In: Olesen J, ed. Headache Classification and Epidemiology. New York: Raven Press; 1994:273-81.
3. **Zuckerman B, Stevenson J, Bailey V.** Stomachaches and headaches in a community sample of preschool children. Pediatrics. 1987;79:677-82.
4. **Bille B.** Migraine in school children. Acta Paediatr Scand. 1962;51(Suppl 136): 1-151.
5. **Sillanpaa M.** Changes in the prevalence of migraine and other headaches in the first seven school years. Headache. 1983;23:15-9.
6. **Sillanpaa M, Piekkala P, Kero P.** Prevalence of headache at preschool age in an unselected child population. Cephalalgia. 1991;11:239-42.
7. **Sillanpaa M, Piekkala P.** Prevalence of migraine and other headaches in early puberty. Scand J Prim Health Care. 1984;2:27-32.
8. **Anttila P, Metsahonkala L, Aromaa M, et al.** Epidemiology of pediatric tension-type headache. In: Proceedings of Fourth International Congress on Headache in Childhood and Adolescence; 1999.
9. **Barea LM, Tannhauser M, Rotta NT.** An epidemiologic study of headache among children and adolescents of southern Brazil. Cephalagia. 1996;16:545-9.
10. **Gallai V, Sarchielli P, Carboni F, et al.** Applicability of the 1988 IHS criteria to headache patients under the age of 18 years attending 21 Italian headache clinics. Headache. 1995;35:146-53.
11. **Wober Bingol C, Wober C, Karwautz C, et al.** Diagnosis of headache in childhood and adolescence: a study in 437 patients. Cepahlagia. 1995;15:13-21.
12. **Guidetti V, Galli F.** Evolution of headache in childhood and adolescence: an 8-year follow-up. Cephalalgia 1998;18:449-54.
13. **Maytal J, Lipton RB, Solomon S, Shinnar S.** Childhood onset of cluster headache. Headache. 1992;32:275-9.
14. **Vahlquist B.** Migraine in children. Int Arch Allergy. 1955;7:348-52.
15. Classification and diagnostic criteria for headache disorders, cranial neuralgias and facial pain. Headache Classification Committee of the International Headache Society. Cephalalgia. 1988;8(Suppl 7):1-96.

16. **International Headache Society.** The International Classification of Headache Disorders, 2nd ed. Cephalalgia. 2004;24(Suppl 1):9-160.

17. **Mortimer J, Kay J, Jaron A.** Epidemiology of headache and childhood migraine in an urban general practice using ad hoc, Valquist and IHS criteria. Dev Med Child Neurol. 1992;34:1095-1101.

18. **Powers SW, Patton SR, Hommel KA, Hershey AD.** Quality of life in childhood migraines: clinical impact and comparison to other chronic illnesses. Pediatrics. 2003;112:E1-5.

19. **Silberstein SD.** Practice parameter: evidence-based guidelines for migraine headache (an evidence-based review). Report of the Quality Standards Subcommittee of the American Academy of Neurology. Neurology. 2000;55:754-62.

20. **Bickerstaff ER..** Basilar artery migraine. Lancet. 1961;1:15-7.

21. **Lewis DW, Ashwal S, Dahl G.** Practice parameter: evaluation of children and adolescents with recurrent headaches. Report of the Quality Standards Subcommittee of the American Academy of Neurology and the Practice Committee of the Child Neurology Society. Headache. 2003;43:424-5.

22. **Barlow CF.** "Complex" and complicated migraine syndromes. Clin Develop Med. 1984;91:93-103.

23. **Lee TG, Choi WS, Chung KC.** Ophthalmoplegic migraine with reversible enhancement of intraparenchymal abducens nerve on MRI. Headache. 2002;42:140-1.

24. **Lance JW, Zagami AS.** Ophthalmoplegic migraine: a recurrent demyelinating neuropathy? Cephalalgia. 2001;21:84-9.

25. **Ducros A, Denier C, Joutel A, et al.** The clinical spectrum of familial hemiplegic migraine associated with mutations in a neuronal calcium channel. N Engl J Med. 2001;345:17-24.

26. **Kors EE, Haan J, Giffen NJ, et al.** Expanding the phenotypic spectrum of the CACNA1A gene T666M mutation: a description of 5 families with hemiplegic migraine. Arch Neurol. 2003;60:684-8.

26a. **Lewis DW, Scott D, Rendin V.** Treatment of paediatric headache. Expert Opin Pharmacother. 2002;3:1433-42.

27. **Giffin NJ, Benton S, Goadsby PJ.** Benign paroxysmal torticollis of infancy: four new cases and linkage to CACNA1A mutation. Dev Med Child Neurol. 2002;44:490-3.

28. **Lanzi G, Balottin U, Fazzi E, et al.** Benign paroxysmal vertigo of childhood: a long-term follow-up. Cephalalgia. 1994;14:458-60.

29. **Hamalainen ML, Hoppu K, Valkeila E, Santavuori P.** Ibuprofen or acetaminophen for the acute treatment of migraine in children: a double-blind, randomized, placebo-controlled, crossover study. Neurology. 1977;48:102-7.

30. **Lewis DW, Kellstein D, Dahl G, et al.** Children's ibuprofen suspension for the acute treatment of pediatric migraine. Headache. 2002;42:780-6.

31. **MacDonald J.** Treatment of juvenile migraine with subcutaneous sumatriptan. Headache. 1994;34:581-2.

32. **Linder SL.** Subcutaneous sumatriptan in the clinical setting: the first 50 consecutive patients with acute migraine in a pediatric neurology office. Headache. 1996;36:419-22.

33. **Hershey AD, Powers SW, LeCates S, Bentti AL.** Effectiveness of nasal sumatriptan in 5- to 12-year-old children. Headache. 2001;41:693-7.

34. **Ueberall MA, Wenzel D.** Intranasal sumatriptan for the acute treatment of migraine in children. Neurology. 1999;52:1507.

35. **Winner P, Rothner AD, Saper J, et al.** A randomized, double-blind, placebo-controlled study of sumatriptan nasal spray in the treatment of acute migraine in adolescents. Pediatrics. 2000;106:989-97.

36. **Hamalainen ML, Hoppu K, Santavuori P.** Sumatriptan for migraine attacks in children: a randomized placebo-controlled study. Do children with migraine respond to oral sumatriptan differently from adults? Neurology. 1997;48:1100-3.

37. **Salonen R, Ashford EA, Gibbs M, Hassani H.** Patient preference for oral sumatriptan 25 mg, 50 mg, or 100 mg in the acute treatment of migraine: a double-blind, randomized, crossover study. Sumatriptan Tablets S2CM11 Study Group. Int J Clin Pract Suppl. 1999;105:16-24.

38. **Winner P, Lewis D, Visser WH, et al.** Rizatriptan 5 mg for the acute treatment of migraine in adolescents: a randomized, double-blind, placebo-controlled study. Headache. 2002;42:49-55.

39. **Rothner AD, Winner P, Nett R, et al.** One-year tolerability and efficacy of sumatriptan nasal spray in adolescents with migraine: results of a multicenter, open-label study. Clin Ther. 2000;22:1533-46.

11

Headache in Older Patients

Robert Smith, MD

Headache, though less common in the elderly, remains a significant problem. Ten percent of women and 5% of men report significant headache at the age of 70 years (1). As the incidence of primary headaches declines with age, the incidence of secondary headaches increases (2). (Hypnic headache, a rare primary headache, is an exception in that its incidence increases with age and it occurs almost exclusively in older patients.)

Suspicion of underlying disease should always be increased when an elderly patient presents with a new-onset headache. There are many disorders (e.g., systemic disease, Parkinson's disease) for which headache is but one symptom. Table 11-1 lists some of these disorders. In other disorders, however, headache is the primary symptom (e.g., subdural hematoma, cervicogenic headache, subarachnoid hemorrhage), and it is these disorders that are discussed herein.

Secondary Causes of Headache

Brain Tumor

Brain tumor is a rare cause of headache. Although only a remote possibility, brain tumor should always be considered a possible cause of a new-onset headache in the elderly (3). Metastatic tumors, most frequently arising from cancer of the lung and breast, occur in about 25% of these patients with brain tumors (4).

Headache occurs in 36% to 86% of patients with brain tumor. The headaches from brain tumor meet the diagnostic criteria for tension-type headache in 77% and migraine headache in 9% (5). The pain is usually intermittent and lasts for several hours. The pain is unilateral in 25% to 30%; unilaterality

---

Table 11-1   Systemic Diseases Associated with Headache

- Viral and bacterial infections (including upper respiratory infections, sinus infections, meningitis, encephalitis, brain abscess)
- Acute (but not chronic) hypertension
- Hypercalcemia (hyperparathyroidism, myeloma, vitamin D overmedication, thiazide diuresis, immobilization in osteoporosis)
- Hypoxia or hypercarbia (pulmonary disease, sleep apnea)
- Angina may present as exertional headache without thoracic pain
- Thyroid disease (hypothyroidism and hyperthyroidism)

---

generally predicts an ipsilateral malignancy. The clinical features of headache commonly thought to be associated with brain tumor occur infrequently: worse with bending (32%), worse with valsalva (23%), worse in the morning (36%), interference with sleep (32%), worse with straining (18%), and worse with movement (7%). Thus the absence of these symptoms does not provide reassurance that one is *not* dealing with a brain tumor (4).

Increased intracranial pressure, infratentorial and leptomeningeal carcinomatosis, a midline shift, increasing size of the tumor, and a past history of headache make it more likely that a headache may be experienced with brain tumor (6). Headache may not occur until a late stage of the disease, when it is often mistaken for tension-type headache (7). Headache may antedate neurological findings, which justifies a need for early neuroimaging in all puzzling headaches in the aged (5).

Chronic Subdural Hematoma

The elderly are more prone to subdural hematoma because of their greater risk of falls and head trauma. An intracranial bleed may occur even after a minor blow to the head. Brain atrophy decreases support of smaller bridging veins, which then tear and bleed more easily. The hematoma may create an intracranial mass effect and, acting like a tumor, produce similar headache symptoms. Focal neurological signs are less likely because brain tissue damage may be absent. Headache secondary to a subdural hematoma may not be detected until long after the injury because the latter has been forgotten. Sixty-two percent of patients with subdural hematoma have headache, and 96% have a history of past head trauma.

There are no characteristics of headache unique to subdural hematoma. The headaches are often unilateral and ipsilateral to the hematoma. They resemble those of any "space occupying" lesion and can be intermittent or constant. The headache intensity can be described as mild to moderate (8). The insidious nature of the problem should be kept in mind in patients presenting with headache and increasing confusion or fluctuating level of consciousness (9).

Giant Cell Arteritis (Temporal Arteritis)

Epidemiology and Symptoms

Giant cell arteritis (GCA) is a systemic arteritis affecting medium-sized vessels. It is rare before 50 years of age (10) and is three times more common in women. Headache is present in 70% to 90% of patients and is variable. Pain may be intermittent or constant, mild or severe, aching or throbbing, and is located over one or both temples or other scalp areas. Local pressure, such as wearing a hat or the head on a pillow, draws attention to the pain. Polymyalgia rheumatica is present in 25% of patients with GCA. Monocular visual loss due to ischemic optic neuropathy may also occur and can result in permanent blindness. Visual loss occurs in nearly 40% of untreated cases (11).

Giant cell arteritis is commonly associated with symptoms such as jaw claudication, weight loss, night sweats, fatigue, diplopia, depression, fever, and visual loss. The presence of jaw claudication and diplopia were found to be very predictive of temporal arteritis, with positive-likelihood ratios of 4.2 and 3.4 respectively (12). The absence of any of the above symptoms, however, does not exclude a diagnosis of temporal arteritis.

Physical findings encountered in GCA include scalp tenderness, optic atrophy, fundoscopic changes, visual loss, and temporal artery abnormalities. The temporal artery abnormalities include beading, tenderness, or enlargement of the artery or absence of its pulse. The presence of any temporal artery abnormality significantly increases the likelihood of GCA (12). As with the associated symptoms, the absence of these physical findings does not exclude the diagnosis.

Diagnosis

An elevated ESR is common in GCA, as are an elevated C-reactive protein, anemia, and liver abnormalities. An ESR of 50 mm/hr or above with the appropriate symptoms of GCA should arouse suspicion in older patients. Conversely, the presence of a normal ESR makes temporal arteritis very unlikely, although rare cases have been reported with a normal ESR (12a). An ESR > 100 is moderately predictive of GCA, with a positive likelihood ratio of 1.9 (12). The ESR may be normal or suppressed in patients with GCA taking aspirin, NSAIDs, or steroids.

Diagnosis can only be established with certainty by biopsy of an adequate length of temporal artery showing the presence of giant cells. Past retrospective studies have reported that biopsies must be performed within 1 to 2 weeks of the institution of steroid therapy (13). However, a recent prospective study suggests that biopsies could still be positive for up to 4 weeks after the start of steroids (14). Bilateral temporal artery biopsies may increase the yield of a positive result by 2% to 3% (15).

The American College of Rheumatology has developed five criteria for the diagnosis of temporal arteritis (Table 11-2) (10). Presence of more than

Table 11-2   American College of Rheumatology Criteria for the Diagnosis of Giant Cell Arteritis (Temporal Arteritis)*

- Age >50 years
- New onset of localized headache
- Sedimentation rate (Westergren) > 50
- Biopsy of temporal artery characterized by predominance of mononuclear cell infiltrates or a granulomatous process with multinucleated giant cells
- Temporal artery tenderness or decreased temporal artery pulse

*The presence of more than three of these criteria conferred a sensitivity and specificity of 93.5% and 91.2% respectively for the diagnosis of GCA.

three of the five conferred a sensitivity of 93.5% and a specificity of 91% for the diagnosis of GCA.

Treatment

Prompt treatment of GCA is essential to avoid sudden irreversible visual loss. Treatment with prednisone 60-80 mg daily should be initiated while waiting for the biopsy result. Headache and other systemic symptoms usually subside within 48 hours. The dose of prednisone should be maintained for 4 to 6 weeks, then gradually reduced. A maintenance dose is usually required for 6 to 12 months, during which time steroid side effects will require monitoring. Visual fields and visual acuity require periodic monitoring.

The addition of adjunctive therapies such as methotrexate to existing corticosteroid therapy has not been shown to reduce the frequency of relapse, which occurs in up to one third of patients upon withdrawal of the steroids (16,17). Case reports have suggested efficacy of infliximab, an anti-TNF-alpha antibody, in the treatment of GCA (18,19).

Trigeminal Neuralgia

Epidemiology and Symptoms

Trigeminal neuralgia, a disorder of the trigeminal nerve causing episodes of intense electric shock-like or shooting pain, occurs twice as often in women than in men, with an average age of onset of 50 years (20). In younger patients, vascular compression of the trigeminal nerve root has been implicated as a cause, as has multiple sclerosis (21). In older patients neuroimaging to exclude mass lesions compressing the nerve root at its exit foramen is indicated. However, diagnostic studies are usually normal, and the diagnosis is usually made on clinical grounds.

Trigeminal neuralgia is characterized by paroxysmal severe stabbing or burning facial or frontal pain lasting seconds to 2 minutes. The pain is distributed along one or more divisions of the trigeminal nerve (usually maxillary or mandibular). Trigger zones may be found around the nares.

The pain may therefore be easily triggered by activities as routine and triv-ial as eating, brushing teeth, washing face, or shaving. Neurological exami-nation is usually normal. Typically the patient experiences recurrent bouts of pain throughout the course of the day over periods that can last months. Pain-free periods may spontaneously occur and can last for up to a year.

Treatment

Medical therapy is the first line of treatment for the majority of patients with trigeminal neuralgia. In the absence of structural disease the treatment of choice is carbamazepine. The usual starting dose is 100 to 300 mg twice daily, increasing by 200 mg every three or four days until pain free or limited by side effects. The dose should not exceed a total of 1200 mg/day. The re-sponse is often speedy. Ninety-four percent of patients have relief of their pain within 48 hours with carbamazepine, although many will relapse over time. Drug side effects, more likely in the aged, are gastrointestinal discom-fort, drowsiness, and ataxia. A pretreatment CBC and hepatic profile should be obtained as a base line because of possible adverse hematological and hepatic reactions. After 6 to 8 pain-free weeks, the drug may be discontinued.

Phenytoin is a second-line agent for this disorder. A 200 mg/day start-ing dose is escalated to 300 to 500 mg/day based on response. Like carba-mazepine, the onset of relief is relatively rapid and can occur within days but effects tend to diminish with time. Carbamazepine and phenytoin are given together in resistant cases. However, close monitoring of laboratory studies, including blood levels, is needed because carbamazepine can in-crease phenytoin levels and phenytoin can decrease carbamazepine levels.

Baclofen is a non anti-epileptic drug that is helpful for trigeminal neu-ralgia. The initial dose is 5 mg three times a day. It can be titrated up in split doses as high as 80 mg/day. The drug should be slowly tapered at a rate not to exceed 10 mg/week to avoid withdrawal effects including hallu-cinations. The combination of baclofen with either carbamazepine or phenytoin enhances their analgesic effects in this disorder; therefore lower doses of both of these agents should be used when given in combination with baclofen. A host of other agents have been tried in this condition, but none have the proven efficacy of these three agents.

Many surgical methods have been introduced in attempts to provide pain relief for intractable trigeminal neuralgia. The most common treatments in-volve the gasserian ganglion. The radiofrequency approach is the most often performed and has been successful in upwards of 90% of patients, with up to 65% having some recurrence based on the length of time after the proce-dure. Complications can include dysesthesia, loss of corneal sensation, and anesthesia dolorosa. These can be minimized by providing the patient with only partial sensory loss rather than complete ablation of the pain.

Glycerol injections can be beneficial in up to 90% of patients but are slower to produce results than radiofrequency procedures. Additionally, recurrence is much more common, with half of patients having recurrence within 2 years. Peripheral trigeminal alcohol injections give poor results. Better results have been obtained with ganglion injections, but corneal anesthesia and poor long-term cure rates are common. In a small number of patients, facial dysesthesia is more distressing than the original pain.

Side effects are less common with radiofrequency procedures, and general anesthesia is not needed. Radiofrequency gangliolysis can be performed without a general anesthetic, which is an important consideration in elderly frail patients. Recent promising results have been reported using ionization radiation of the trigeminal nerve root as it enters the pons (Gamma Knife radiosurgery) (20a).

The definitive surgical procedure for trigeminal neuralgia is suboccipital retromastoid craniotomy with microvascular decompression of the trigeminal root by an arterial vascular loop. Patients with evidence of a vascular loop on MRI in the region of the trigeminal root entry zone are most likely to benefit from microvascular decompression surgery. The procedure has come to be known as the Jannetta procedure, honoring Peter Joseph Jannetta's work on refining the process. This major surgical procedure has a very high success rate: over 80% of patients have immediate and complete relief and an additional 7.6% have partial relief. Recurrence rates are less than 6% within the first 2 years. But serious complications and death can occur. Hearing and other sensory loss can occur in up 30% of patients. Patients with higher risk for recurrence are women, those with venous versus arterial compression, those with trigeminal neuralgia for over 8 years, and those who lack immediate post-operative pain relief.

Glossopharyngeal Neuralgia

Like trigeminal neuralgia, the less common glossopharyngeal neuralgia usually presents in older patients. It produces stabbing intense unilateral pain at the base of the tongue and tonsillar area, radiating to the ear and angle of the jaw. This is triggered by swallowing, talking, and coughing. Multiple attacks may occur during the day or night (22). The pain is generally severe, transient, and often described as "stabbing". It may continue for months with periods of remission much like trigeminal neuralgia. It may also be accompanied by a feeling of a foreign body in the throat. Treatment is similar to trigeminal neuralgia, and surgery of the glossopharyngeal nerve has been performed. Glossopharyngeal and trigeminal neuralgias may occur together.

Postherpetic Neuralgia

Seventy-five percent of patients over the age of 70 with acute zoster involving ophthalmic or maxillary divisions of the trigeminal nerve subsequently develop postherpetic neuralgia compared with 5% of patients less than 40 years old. Postherpetic neuralgia is more likely to follow acute attacks involving the ophthalmic nerve and occur in diabetic and immunologically compromised patients. The condition gradually subsides; over 50% of patients are pain free in 3 years (23). Tricyclic antidepressants help to relieve symptoms but must be used with caution in older patients. The substance P depleter capsaicin applied locally is reported to be beneficial, but some patients find it difficult to tolerate the burning sensation it may produce (24). Gabapentin may also reduce the pain severity of postherpetic neuralgia (25). Topical 5% lidocaine patches are also used but can be difficult to apply to the face.

Cervicogenic Headache

Degenerative disease of the cervical spine is an almost universal radiological finding in older patients. Cervical spine abnormalities have been found to be similar in age-matched control patients without pain complaints (26). However, the role of such abnormalities as a cause of headache is controversial; many patients given a diagnosis of cervicogenic headache may have symptoms that meet the criteria for migraine or tension-type headache.

Compression of the upper cervical nerve roots (C1 or C2) or the greater occipital nerve may result in neck pain and unilateral headache. Posterior scalp tingling and sensory loss over the distribution of the greater occipital nerve is confirmatory evidence of root pressure. Aggravation of headache by pressure on the nerve as it emerges occipitally, and temporary relief of symptoms when infiltrated with 0.5 cc of 2% lidocaine, together provide evidence in support of nerve root compression.

Physiotherapy and muscle-relaxing exercises may be helpful. Long-term use of analgesics and muscle relaxants requires appropriate monitoring. Chiropractic manipulation of neck spine in older patients should be approached cautiously.

Glaucoma

The more common primary open-angle glaucoma found at routine tonometry screening does not cause headache. Treatment with miotic eyedrops such as pilocarpine may cause frontal headache. The less common acute angle-closure glaucoma causes acute radiating eye pain, red eye, corneal cloudiness, and nausea. The affected globe is hard. The attack may occur at night and, because of the unilateral headache and nausea, be mistaken for migraine (27). Tricyclics such as amitriptyline and doxepine may exacerbate glaucoma. Immediate ophthalmic referral is necessary. Laser iridotomy is curative.

Cerebrovascular Disease

Headache may occur before, during, or after stroke or transient ischemic attack (TIA). Sudden severe headache reaching peak intensity within seconds to minutes ("thunderclap") is characteristic of subarachnoid hemorrhage. When this is due to ruptured aneurysm, it may be preceded by so-called "sentinel" headaches. These are thought to be due to aneurysmal leak before rupture.

Headache is present in 80% of stroke due to intracerebral hemorrhage but is less frequent in thrombotic, embolic, and lacunar strokes. It is more likely in larger strokes. About half of stroke headaches are similar to tension-type headaches, and 25% are ipsilateral to the stroke area and resemble migraine (28). Unilateral headache may also occur following carotid endarterectomy. Subarachnoid and intracerebral hemorrhage are discussed in detail in Chapter 3.

Transient ischemic attacks produce headaches less frequently than strokes. Headaches are episodic, lasting about 2 hours, and of mild-to-moderate intensity (26). The neurological symptoms of TIAs must be distinguished from migraine aura. The development of motor and sensory symptoms is usually much more rapid in TIAs; scintillating scotoma is rare. Although migraine may emerge at any age, in older patients with migrainous symptoms who have had no previous history of migraine, ischemic cerebrovascular disease should be ruled out before migraine is considered.

Parkinson's Disease

Early morning headache is reported in nearly half of patients with Parkinsonism (29). The cause is uncertain but may be due to the contraction of head and neck muscles and depression often associated with the disease. Headaches improve with levodopa treatment.

Medications Causing Headache

Because older patients commonly use mediations that cause headaches (30,31), drug-induced headaches should be considered in patients without a previous history of headaches, and all medications should be elicited during the clinical interview. Drugs may initiate a new headache or re-activate an existing headache disorder. In addition, withdrawal from some medications may cause headache. ("Medication overuse" headaches are discussed in Chapter 7.) Common headache triggers in the elderly are alcohol and nitroglycerine. Hormonal replacement therapy, monosodium glutamate, and caffeine (in previous migraine patients) (32) may all increase headache frequency (Table 11-3).

Primary Causes of Headache

Hypnic Headache

The only primary headache found almost exclusively in older patients is hypnic or "alarm clock" headache, so called because of its occurrence

Table 11-3   Medications Causing Headaches

Medication Class	Examples
Antihypertensives	Hydralazine, nifedipine
Psychiatric medications	SSRIs, MAO inhibitors, phenothiazines
Hormonal therapies	Estrogens, progestins, tamoxifen
NSAIDs	Indomethacin
Immunosuppressive agents	Cyclophosphamide, cyclosporin, corticosteroids
Antibiotics	Tetracycline, sulfa drugs
Antianginals	Nitrates
Lipid lowering agents	Nicotinic acid
Anti-Parkinson agents	L-DOPA, amantidine
Miscellaneous	Caffeine-containing medications, ranitidine, cimetidine, ethanol, dipyridamole

mainly at night, when it awakens the patient from sleep. (A small number of patients report similar headaches after daytime napping.) Headaches occur at least 15 times per month for at least one month. Pain, which is moderate to severe, may be bilateral or unilateral and is not associated with autonomic features. The duration of attacks is 5 to 60 minutes.

A rapid response to 300 mg lithium at bedtime is usual. Verapamil 240 mg per day may be helpful if lithium is not tolerated, the patient is receiving diuretics, or there is existing renal disease. Combination analgesics containing caffeine have also proved useful (33).

Migraine

Migraine usually remits with age, and new onset of migraine in patients older than 60 is rare. Migraine with aura occurs more commonly than without aura. Previous migraine with aura may continue as aura alone, known as "late-life migraine accompaniment". Migraine may convert into chronic daily headache with or without medication overuse (34). Co-morbid depression and chronic anxiety may be aggravating factors in older patients.

Specific migraine treatments (triptans, ergot preparations) are effective in the aged, but because of their vasoconstrictive action should be used with caution. They may exacerbate controlled pre-existing hypertension or latent vascular diseases. Other drugs used in treating migraine in younger patients must also be used cautiously in older persons. NSAIDs more readily cause peptic ulcer disease; anti-emetics may cause tardive dyskinesia; barbiturates may cause excessive sedation. Emphasis on nonpharmacological approaches is important. These include elimination of trigger factors, balanced regular meals and sleep, and avoidance of excess caffeine.

(Relaxation therapy and biofeedback, however, appear to be of lesser value in older patients.)

Tension-Type Headache

The prevalence of tension-type headache, like migraine, declines with age. Only 10% of true tension-type headache starts after age 50. Careful exclusion of secondary headache is required. The differential includes brain tumor, cervicogenic headache, stroke headaches, mass lesions, temporal arteritis, visual acuity problems, and chronic daily headache evolving from migraine (35).

Combination analgesics with sedatives or caffeine should be limited because of dependence and greater likelihood of side effects in these patients. Control is often best achieved with preventive antidepressants. SSRIs, rather than the tricyclics, are the medications of choice.

Cluster Headache

New-onset cluster headache has been reported occurring as late as the eighth decade (36). Previous quiescent cluster may recur as a result of use of sublingual or transdermal nitroglycerine use. Triptan and ergot preparations must be used with caution in the elderly given the higher likelihood of existing unrecognized coronary and cerebrovascular disease. Likewise, verapamil for prophylactic treatment and anti-seizure medications (divalproex sodium and gabapentin) should be used cautiously because they are more likely to cause side effects in the elderly. Oxygen inhalation may be the safest and most effective abortive treatment in patients with good pulmonary function.

Key Points

- When an elderly patient presents with a new-onset headache, it is important to search for an underlying cause.
- If secondary headache is excluded, a specific primary headache disorder should be diagnosed.
- With age, the prevalence of secondary headache increases and that of primary headache diminishes.
- Hypnic headache is the one primary headache found almost exclusively in the elderly.
- Many drugs widely used by older patients are known to be associated with headaches.

REFERENCES

1. **Stewart WF, Lipton RB , Celentano DD, Reed ML.** Prevalence of migraine headache in the United States. JAMA. 1992;267:64-9.

2. **Newman LC, Lipton RB, Solomon S.** The hypnic headache syndrome. Neurology. 1990;40:1904-5.

3. **Schoenberg B.** Nervous system. In: Schotterfeld D, Joseph F, eds. Cancer Epidemiology and Prevention. Philadelphia: WB Saunders; 1982:969-83.

4. **Pickren JE, Lopez G, et al.** Brain metastasis: an autopsy study. Cancer Treatment Symposium. 1983;2:295-313.

5. **Forsyth PA, Posner JB.** Headaches in patients with brain tumors: a study of 111 patients. Neurology. 1993;43:1678-83.

6. **Forsyth P, Posner P.** Intracranial neoplasms. In: Olesen J, Tfelt-Hansen P, Welch KMA, eds. The Headaches, 2nd ed. Philadelphia: Lippincott Williams and Wilkins; 2000:849-57.

7. **Lipton RB, Pfeffer D, Newman L, Solomon S.** Headaches in the elderly. J Pain Symp Mgt. 1993;8:87-97.

8. **Jensen TS, Gorelick.** Headache associated with ischemic stroke and intracranial hematoma. In: Olesen J, Tfelt-Hansen P, Welch KMA, eds. The Headaches, 2nd ed. Philadelphia: Lippincott Williams and Wilkins; 2000:781-7.

9. **Silbersten S, Lipton R, et al.** Geriatric headache. In: Headache in Clinical Practice. New York: Oxford University Press; 1988;17:201-2.

10. **Hunder G, Bloch D, Michel B, et al.** The American College of Rheumatology 1990 criteria for the classification of giant cell arteritis. Arthritis Rheum. 1990;33:1122-9.

11. **Goodman BS.** Temporal arteritis. Am J Med. 1979;67:839-52.

12. **Smetana GW, Shmerling RH.** Does this patient have temporal arteritis? JAMA. 2002;287:92-101.

12a. **Wong RL, Korn JH.** Temporal arteritis without an elevated erythrocyte sedimentation rate. Am J Med. 1986;80:959-64.

13. **Allison M, Gallagher P.** Temporal artery biopsy and corticosteroid treatment. Ann Rheum Dis. 1984;43:416-7.

14. **Ray-Chandhuri N, Kine D, Tigani S, et al.** Effects of prior steroid treatment on temporal artery biopsy findings in giant cell arteritis. Br J Opthamol. 2002;86:530-2.

15. **Bayev L, Miller N, Green W.** Efficacy of unilateral versus bilateral temporal artery biopsies for the diagnosis of giant cell arteritis. Am J Opthalmol. 1999;128;211-5.

16. **Hoffman G, Cid M, Hellmann D, et al.** A multicenter, randomized, double-blind, placebo-controlled trial of adjuvant methotrexate treatment for giant cell artheritis. Arthritis Rheum. 2002;46:1309-18.

17. **Jover J. Hernandez-Garcia C, Morado IC, et al.** Combined treatment of giant call arteritis with methotrexate and prednisone: a randomized, double-blind, placebo-controlled trial. Ann Int Med. 2001;134:104-14.

18. **Airo P, Antonioli A, Vianelli M, Toniati P.** Anti-tumor necrosis factor treatment of inflixamide in a case of giant cell arteritis resistant to steroid and immunosuppressive drugs. Rheumatology. 2002;41:347-9.

19. **Cantini F, Niccoli L, Salvarani C, et al.** Treatment of longstanding giant cell arteritis with infliximab: report of four cases. Arthritis Rheum. 2001;44:2933-5.

20. **Penman J.** Trigeminal neuralgia. In: Vinken PJ, Bruyn GW, eds. Handbook of Clinical Neurology, vol 5. Amsterdam: North Holland; 1968:296-322.

20a. **Young RF, Vermeulen SS, Grimm P, et al.** Gamma Knife radiosurgery for treatment of trigeminal neuralgia: idiopathic and tumor related. Neurology. 1997;48: 608-14.

21. **Jensen TS, Rasmussen P, Reske-Nelsen E.** Association of trigeminal neuralgia and multiple sclerosis: clinical and pathological features. Acta Neurol Scan. 1982; 65:182-9.

22. **Dalessio DJ, Silberstein S.** Diagnosis and classification of headache. In: Wolff's Headaches and Other Head Pain, 6th ed. New York: Oxford University Press; 1993:318.

23. **Kost RG, Straus SE.** Postherpetic neuralgia: pathogenesis, treatment and prevention. N Engl J Med. 1996;335:32-42.

24. **Bernstein JE, Korman NJ, Bickers DR, et al.** Topical capsaicin in chronic postherpetic neuralgia. J Am Acad Dermatol. 1989;21:265-270.

25. **Rowbotham M, Harden N, Stacey B, et al.** Gabapentin for the treatment of postherpetic neuralgia: a randomized controlled trial. JAMA. 1998;280:1837-42.

26. **Edmeads J.** Headaches and head pains associated with diseases of the cervical spine. Med Clin North Am. 1978;62:533-44.

27. **Martin TJ, Soy KAD.** Ocular causes of headache. In: The Headache, vol 2. 1993;110:747-52.

28. **Jensen TS, Gorebck PB.** Headache association with ischemic stroke and intracranial hematoma In: Olesen J, Tfelt-Hansen P, Welch KMA, eds. The Headaches, 2nd ed. Philadelphia: Lippincott Williams and Wilkins; 2000;104:781-7.

29. **Indo T, Naito A, et al.** Characteristics of headache in Parkinson's disease. Headache. 1983;23:211-2.

30. **Silberstein S, Lipton R, Goadsby P, Smith R.** Geriatric headache. In: Headache in Clinical Practice. 1998;17:201-12.

31. **Askmark H, Lundberg P, Olsson S.** Drug-related headache. Headache. 1989;29: 441-4.

32. **Gibb CM, Davies PT, Glover V, et al.** Chocolate is a migraine-provoking agent. Cephalalgia. 1991;11:93-5.

33. **Dodick DW, Mosek AC, Campbell JK.** The hypnic ("alarm clock") headache syndrome. Cephalalgia. 1998;18:152-6.

34. **Mathew NT.** Drug-induced headache. Neurol Clin. 1990;8:903-12.

35. **Baumel B, Eisner RS.** Diagnosis and treatment of headache in the elderly. Med Clin North Am. 1991;75:661-75.

36. **Raskin N.** Headache, 2nd ed. New York: Churchill Livingstone; 1988:229-30.

12

■ ■ ■

Complementary and Nonpharmacological Therapies

Timothy R. Smith, MD, RPh

lternative and nonpharmacological therapies have become increasingly popular among patients for the treatment of all types of pain. Eighty-five percent of all headache sufferers have used alternative medical therapies for relief of their headache symptoms, and up to 60% perceived a benefit, according to one study. Almost all patients surveyed were familiar with one or more alternative treatments for headache (1). Patient motives for pursuing complementary or nonpharmacological therapy vary. Some patients may have a philosophical desire to avoid pharmacologically based treatments, while others may be dissatisfied with the effectiveness and costs of traditional treatments or concerned about their risks and possible side effects. Some pregnant patients, for example, may wish to avoid pharmacological treatments even when the risk of teratogenicity has been shown to be low for a particular medication.

Perhaps because of the upsurge of patient interest in the subject, physicians and other health professionals are becoming increasingly interested in such treatments as well. Regardless of an individual physician's views on alternative and complementary medicine, a working knowledge of those in common use is essential. Knowledgeable physicians are in a better condition to steer patients away from dangerous or useless interventions and towards those that offer potential benefit and are reasonably safe (2).

The evidence base for alternative and complementary headache treatments is thin. The kind of randomized controlled trials necessary to provide convincing scientific evidence of benefit have not been performed for many of these treatments, and serious methodological problems mar many of the studies that do exist. The anecdotal evidence often cited in support of these therapies is difficult to interpret for both abortive and prophylactic therapies. Patient expectation of benefit, placebo effects, and the natural tendency for headache to wax and wane may all contribute to a sincere belief that a particular treatment is helpful, but only comparison of such treatment with placebo, sham treatment, or a no-treatment group can clearly distinguish any specific benefit of a particular therapy. For many alternative therapies, however, comparison with a placebo or sham treatments is not even possible. This chapter summarizes current knowledge of a variety of the most popular alternative and complementary treatments for headache.

Herbal Treatments

Feverfew

Feverfew (*Tanacetum parthenium*) is an herbal remedy that consists of the dried leaves of the plant; parthenolide is the putative active ingredient (3). Feverfew inhibits the synthesis of prostaglandins, affects the release of serotonin from platelets, and may possess nonspecific antagonist properties against norepinephrine, bradykinin, and acetylcholine. It is generally well tolerated. The most common adverse events are oral ulcerations, oral inflammation, and loss of taste (4).

Daily doses ranging from 50 to 82 mg have been tested for the prevention of migraine in four placebo-controlled randomized trials (5-8). Unfortunately, trial results have been inconsistent. A systematic review of early trials indicated a trend toward efficacy of feverfew over placebo, but the trials included in the review were of varying quality (9). A recent high-quality trial evaluated three doses of a highly purified extract of *T. parthenium* and placebo for migraine prevention. No dose-response curve was observed, and no statistical difference was demonstrated between any of the doses and placebo. However, a subset of patients with more frequent headache attacks seemed to benefit, leading the researchers to suggest that further study is needed (10).

The benefit of feverfew has not been clearly established, but there is little evidence that it is harmful. Because the strength and potency of the herb varies depending on the source and methods of manufacture, patients wishing to try it should be instructed to choose a single brand of feverfew and follow the instructions on the package regarding dosing. As with all preventive medications, a minimum of 2 to 3 months is likely to be necessary to determine any benefit. Of great concern is a recent Canadian study showing that dramatic variations in strength existed in 27 tested brands of feverfew. The amount of active ingredient found on analysis often varied, in some cases by up to 400%, from the package label (10a). Because of its anti-prostaglandin activity, feverfew is contraindicated in patients with active peptic ulcer disease, bleeding disorders, and those on coumadin. No evidence exists regarding its safety in pregnancy.

Butterbur Extract

Butterbur extract (*Petasites hybridus*) is an herbal remedy whose use for a variety of purposes dates back to medieval times. Three German studies performed since the mid-80s have investigated its daily use for the prevention of headache (11-13). Its active components, petasine and inopetasine, appear to inhibit leukotriene synthesis and thus exert an anti-inflammatory effect (14). In one randomized placebo-controlled double-blind study composed of 60 patients, the mean number of migraine attacks in a 4-week period decreased from 2.9 to 1.7 days after treatment for 12 weeks. This compares to a decrease from 2.9 to 2.6 days per 4-week period after 12 weeks of placebo. This difference was statistically significant, although its clinical importance is open to question (15).

A larger placebo-controlled study of 230 patients showed a 51% reduction in headache attack frequency after 4 months for the group receiving *Petasites* 75 mg bid compared with a 32% reduction for placebo for the same length of time (16). These results translate into a therapeutic gain of 19% and a number needed to treat (NNT) of roughly 5. Naturally occurring *Petasites* contains alkaloids that may be harmful to the liver or be carcinogenic. Commercial producers of this herb report that they are able to eliminate these substances, but because herbs and supplements are not subject to the same regulatory requirements as prescription pharmaceutical products, considerable caution should be exercised until more information is available. Use during pregnancy should be avoided.

Vitamins, Minerals, and Supplements

Riboflavin

Riboflavin (vitamin B_2) has been studied in one prospective randomized placebo-controlled study for the prevention of migraine attacks. Fifty-nine percent of 55 patients treated for 3 months with 400 mg daily of riboflavin experienced a decrease in headache frequency of 50% or more. In contrast, only 15% of placebo-treated patients experienced such an improvement. This difference was statistically significant. Only three adverse events were experienced, none of which was serious (17). The maximum therapeutic effect was achieved at 3 months. The effect of riboflavin may stem from its role in mitochondrial energy metabolism in the central nervous system. Mitochondrial dysfunction with subsequent impairment of oxygen metabolism is suspected by some of involvement in the pathogenesis of migraine. Riboflavin supplementation may improve the efficiency of flavoenzymes in the electron transport chain. Because of its apparent efficacy, low safety risks, and relative low cost, riboflavin appears to be a reasonable alternative for migraine prophylaxis, although further trials to confirm its role in treatment are warranted. Use during pregnancy has not been studied.

Hydroxocobalamin

Another vitamin, hydroxocobalamin, has been tested in an open pilot study for the prophylaxis of migraine. Hydroxocobalamin acts as a scavenger of nitric oxide, a vasodilating substance implicated in migraine pathogenesis. Ten of 19 study patients who received intranasal hydroxocobalamin 1 mg daily for 4 months experienced a reduction of 50% or more in migraine frequency. Side effects were mild. Further evidence from placebo-controlled trials is necessary before this treatment can be recommended. Use during pregnancy has not been studied (18).

Coenzyme Q10

The nutritional supplement coenzyme Q10 is involved in the mitochondrial electron transport chain and has been used to treat mitochondrial disorders. When used for these problems, it appears to have very few adverse effects. Recent interest in migraine as a mitochondrial disease led to speculation that coenzyme Q10 might be useful in prophylaxis of migraine. A recent open-label trial studied a 150 mg daily dose. Side effects were largely gastrointestinal in nature and included decreased appetite, nausea, diarrhea, and heartburn. When compared with baseline assessment, 61% of subjects achieved at least a 50% reduction in headache frequency over the course of the 4-month trial (19). Enthusiasm for these results should be tempered by the fact that this was an open-label study.

A recent double-blind, placebo-controlled trial was reported comparing coenzyme Q 100 mg PO tid with placebo in the prevention of migraine headache (19a). There were significant reductions in attack frequency, headache days, and days with nausea in the treatment group. In addition, 47.6% of the coenzyme Q group had a 50% or greater reduction in migraine attacks compared with 14.3% of the placebo group ($P = 0.02$). Use during pregnancy has not been studied.

Magnesium

Magnesium is a mineral and intracellular electrolyte that functions as a catalyst in many physiological processes. Several studies have shown low serum and tissue magnesium levels in patients with migraine (20-22). Emotional and physical stress result in magnesium depletion; this may provide a partial explanation for the mechanism by which stress triggers migraine attacks (1). Magnesium has been studied for both abortive and prophylactic treatment of migraine, and interest is growing in its role in the pathogenesis of the disorder. Twenty-one of 40 patients treated with intravenous magnesium sulfate as acute migraine abortive therapy showed significant and sustained relief of pain (23). Oral elemental magnesium 400-800 mg/day has been tested as migraine prophylaxis in four double-blind trials. The treatment showed benefit in three trials and lack of effect in one (24-27). In the latter study, a poorly absorbable salt of magnesium may have contributed to the negative result. Except for mild diarrhea, which occurred in about 20% of patients, no side effects were reported.

In addition, intravenous magnesium sulfate is a reasonable option for the abortive therapy of individual migraine attacks in the clinic or emergency department setting. The clinical benefit of magnesium for prophylaxis of migraine attacks remains unclear, but it is well tolerated and has few contraindications (other than renal failure) to its use. Interested patients can be instructed to use 600 mg of trimagnesium dicitrate per day for 2 to 3 months, at which time the benefits of therapy can be assessed. Use during pregnancy may be reasonable; magnesium has been widely used for other disorders of pregnancy and is generally well tolerated.

L-Hydroxytryptophan

The amino acid L-hydroxytryptophan has been compared with placebo for the prophylaxis of chronic daily headache (28). This single study did not demonstrate a statistically significant benefit for the active treatment and had a high placebo response rate of 30%. Patients in the active treatment group did show a trend toward improvement, with decreased analgesic use and a reduction in headache days (28).

Melatonin

Melatonin is a hormone released by the pineal gland under hypothalamic control, and lower-than-normal levels of melatonin have been found in migraine patients (29-31). It has been hypothesized that pineal circadian irregularity is responsible for some primary headache disorders and that these disorders might respond to melatonin administration. Headache and insomnia related to delayed sleep phase syndrome, or "jet lag", may be particularly responsive to melatonin therapy (32).

The best evidence for melatonin in headache disorders is for cluster headache. In a small trial, 10 patients with cluster headache took 10 mg of melatonin at bedtime; half of the subjects experienced a decrease in headache frequency within 5 days, with no further headaches occurring until the melatonin was discontinued (33). Another small study provided support for these results (34). Better studies are needed to confirm these findings and to further define the role of melatonin in the treatment of other primary headaches. In the meantime, it appears reasonable to consider a trial of melatonin as suppressive therapy for cluster headache that does not respond to traditional treatment options, given its apparent safety and relative low cost. Use of this supplement during pregnancy has not been studied.

Physical Therapy and Manipulative Treatments

Abnormalities of posture have been reported in 83% of migraine patients, and myofascial trigger points in 79% (35). Physical therapy has not been demonstrated to be effective first-line therapy in migraine, but does appear beneficial in patients who fail an initial course of relaxation biofeedback (36). No well-done studies support the use of chiropractic treatment for headache. Although chiropractic treatment is often perceived to be safe, over 100 cases of serious complications, including stroke, have been reported following its use, most involving the kind of cervical manipulation likely to be used in headache treatment (37). In one controlled study of cervicogenic headache, cervical manipulation, which involves taking the neck to the limit of passive range of motion and then "popping" or "cracking" the facet joint, gave relief, but so did simple deep massage. Studies of this type generally suffer from methodological problems due to the difficulty of blinding patients and investigators to the active treatment or devising a realistic placebo.

An unblinded study evaluated the use of therapeutic exercise, manipulative therapy, and a combination of the two regimens versus no treatment for cervicogenic headache. Patients in the active treatment groups had statistically significant improvements in many headache parameters after treatment and at 12-month follow-up compared with patients in the no-treatment control group. No benefit of combined therapy over either therapy alone was demonstrable, however, suggesting a nonspecific treatment benefit. Comparison of such treatment to a sham treatment group would help clarify the mechanism of improvement (38). Although the benefits of physical therapy in headache treatment are unclear, its use is unlikely to be harmful. In particular, it is among a handful of therapies likely to be safe for use during pregnancy. Massage, deep heat, ice packs, and other physical methods are safe, inexpensive, and probably helpful, and their use may be encouraged, especially for patients with a high degree of musculoskeletal symptomatology or those who are pregnant and have few other treatment options.

Acupuncture

A 1997 National Institutes of Health consensus panel identified headache pain as a problem that may respond to acupuncture but felt that further evidence was needed before its use could be recommended (39). Animal studies suggest that the analgesic effect of acupuncture may stem from release of endorphins and serotonin (40). Uncontrolled studies show headache improvement in approximately 50% of patients undergoing acupuncture (41).

Double-blind studies of acupuncture have been challenging to conduct because of the difficulty of blinding patients to needle insertion. It has also been suggested that even sham acupuncture may have a weak therapeutic effect. However, improved techniques for masking needle insertion have been developed, and trials comparing real with sham acupuncture are now possible. In addition, the term "acupuncture" is used to describe a wide variety of treatment practices, making comparisons between studies difficult (42).

A trend favoring the use of acupuncture has been demonstrated in many trials but is unconvincing for the reasons mentioned above. However, acupuncture is unlikely to be harmful for most patients and, depending on patient preference, can be considered for those who have not benefited from traditional treatment. Individual acupuncture practitioners differ in their willingness to treat pregnant patients; no studies exist to demonstrate or refute the safety of acupuncture treatment of headache during pregnancy.

Homeopathy

Homeopathy uses minute doses of substances that provoke symptoms similar to those of the condition being treated. These substances are mixed with water, which is subsequently diluted to levels at which the treatment substances are essentially undetectable. The resulting solution is believed to stimulate self-healing mechanisms (43). Although credible scientific evidence in support of this mechanism is lacking, homeopathy is increasing in popularity; it is certainly unlikely to be medically harmful, although the disillusionment associated with ineffective therapy and the costs of therapy might be considered important drawbacks. A review of four randomized controlled trials evaluating homeopathic treatment of headache concluded that the data do not suggest an effect of active treatment greater than placebo for migraine or tension-type headache (44). Medical recommendations for use of this treatment thus are not warranted but, given the low risk of harm involved, patients determined to try homeopathy need not be actively discouraged.

Biofeedback

Biofeedback is a technique that combines breathing techniques and imagery to elicit physiological states associated with relaxation. Stress, tension, and pain produce increased muscle tension and peripheral vasoconstriction through activation of the sympathetic nervous system and the "fight or flight" response. In susceptible individuals, these factors can provoke or aggravate headache. In contrast, the state of relaxation is associated with normal finger temperature and relaxed muscles. Both thermal and electromyographic biofeedback techniques have been investigated in the treatment of headache. "Biofeedback" is a term used to describe any technique that gives information about a physiological process in the form of an observable display, such as an audio tone or graphic computer readout. This information is then used by the patient as he or she learns to regulate the response being monitored. The physiological process that is monitored is a surrogate marker of relaxation. Learning to produce states of relaxation allows patients more control over their response to stressful events.

Thermal biofeedback is most common because finger temperature can be easily measured using small fingertip monitors. Lower finger temperature is associated with sympathetic arousal and peripheral vasoconstriction; higher finger temperature is caused by vasodilatation and is associated with decreased sympathetic arousal. On average, migraineurs have finger temperatures of about 70°F compared with 85°F in nonmigraineurs (45). Through the process of progressive relaxation and abdominal breathing, most migraineurs can be taught to warm their fingers to normal temperatures. This process, referred to as "thermal biofeedback", helps patients gain voluntary control of sympathetically mediated vascular tone. With electromyographic biofeedback, muscle tension in the head and neck region, rather than finger temperature, is used to provide feedback to the patient about relaxation. The processes involved are otherwise similar to those used in thermal biofeedback.

Formal biofeedback training generally involves 8 to 10 weekly sessions, which typically take about 45 minutes each. Because daily practice is essential to developing habits of self-monitoring and periodic use of brief relaxation techniques, patients must be motivated to participate actively in treatment.

More than 500 published studies have assessed biofeedback and behavioral therapies for headache. Although trial methodology and quality vary, the preponderance of evidence suggests that biofeedback-assisted relaxation is helpful in headache (46). Typically, more than 50% of headache sufferers enrolled in such treatment experience at least a 50% decrease of headache frequency, intensity, duration, and medication needs (47). Recent treatment guidelines for headache released by the US Headache Consortium recommend the use of biofeedback-assisted relaxation training for headache (48). Additionally, combinations of pharmacological therapies with biofeedback produce greater improvement than either treatment alone (48). It is important to share this information with patients who may incorrectly believe that it is one or the other that will prove helpful.

Cognitive Behavioral Therapy and Stress Management

Cognitive behavioral therapy recognizes that a person's beliefs and behavior can influence treatment outcome. Incorrect or self-defeating ideas ("No doctor can help me", "If one pill helps, two are better") are identified and challenged. Patients are helped to "reframe" their ideas about their illness and to identify techniques and strategies that improve their ability to cope with and manage episodes of headache. Stress management techniques, including alterations of daily routines to incorporate rest periods, self-massage, meditation, and other self-calming strategies, are also helpful.

Dietary Restrictions

Many foods and beverages have been suggested to trigger migraine attacks, and their avoidance is commonly recommended to headache patients. The most commonly implicated include chocolate, coffee, cheese, dairy products, and tyramine-containing foods. It is hypothesized that ingestion of these foods changes central nervous system concentrations of neurotransmitters or other substances involved in the initiation or triggering of migraine attacks. Some authors report long-term success in as many as 85% of patients managed with food exclusion programs (49,50). Other studies have called this conventional wisdom into question and even flatly refuted it. Medina and Diamond compared the effect of the typical migraine restrictive diet with a diet requiring consumption of foods believed to be migraine triggers. The study showed that headache activity improved similarly in both treatment groups. This suggests it is being placed on a special diet, rather than the diet itself, that is beneficial in headache treatment. Only chocolate, alcohol, and fasting appeared to be significant headache triggers in this study (51).

Further doubt about the value of dietary restrictions comes from a study that shows eating amine-rich food does not increase levels of amines in the blood or brain (52). This calls into question the hypothesis underlying recommendations for low-tyramine diets. Another study examined the effect of chocolate on headache in a blinded fashion; this failed to demonstrate a triggering effect, even in individuals who reported that chocolate had historically been a trigger for them (53). For these reasons, there is considerable controversy about appropriate dietary recommendations for patients with migraine. At present, dietary restriction should be regarded as a minimally effective or possibly effective therapy for the prevention of migraine. The beneficial effects of dietary restriction appear to be nonspecific and are probably outweighed by the dangers of excessive preoccupation with diet and avoidance of important food groups (for example, dairy products or citrus fruits in women of childbearing age).

Nicotine Cessation

The effects of nicotine on the central nervous system include changes in mood, the development of physical dependence and addiction, and changes in central processing of pain. Chronic pain appears to be more prevalent in chronic users of nicotine, but the reason for this association is unclear (54). Smoking cessation appeared in one study to be beneficial in the management of cluster headaches (55). Well-done studies of the effects of smoking cessation on migraine are lacking. However, a positive correlation exists between the number of cigarettes smoked and headache activity, with heavier smokers experiencing both more frequent and more severe attacks (56). Because smoking cessation has many other health benefits, a medical recommendation to headache patients that they eliminate or, if that is not possible, at least attempt to reduce, nicotine use is appropriate.

Aerobic Exercise

The effect of regular aerobic exercise on headache has been examined, with results showing a 44% decrease in pain severity and a 36% decrease in headache duration in the exercise group compared with a control group of sedentary headache patients (57). Given the many established health benefits of regular aerobic exercise in addition to headache improvement, regular aerobic activity should be recommended to all headache patients who have no medical contraindications. Because physical activity can aggravate or provoke certain forms of headache, patients should be instructed to begin any exercise regimen slowly and titrate activity levels to avoid inducing headache. If exercise-induced headache cannot be avoided despite careful pacing and gradual increases in activity level, pre-emptive medication with 25 mg of indomethacin or 20 or 40 mg of propranolol 1 hour before expected activity is commonly recommended.

Education and Coping Skills

Almost three-quarters of surveyed migraine sufferers believe that education about headache causes and treatments is an important part of their therapy (58). The combination of general headache education with medication treatments has been shown to result in greater decreases in headache activity and inappropriate medication use compared with patients treated with medication only (59). Other studies have shown striking reductions in medication use among headache sufferers who have received effective headache education. Encouraging the development of adaptive methods of coping with headache is important because evidence suggests that patients with recurrent headache may develop avoidant or counterproductive behaviors that persist even when they are pain-free (60,61).

Maladaptive coping strategies and illness behaviors are a leading cause of disability and contribute to formal disability status and loss of employment. Although medical recommendations for disability status may be appropriate for some people with refractory headache disorders, there is no evidence that disability status has a positive effect on the disorder. Maintenance of usual work and social roles is important in maintaining a sense of well-being and self-worth; clinical experience suggests that the social isolation that results from giving up work or other roles has a negative, not a positive, effect on quality of life for most patients with headache. Thus, as a general rule, patients should be encouraged to remain employed and active. The focus of treatment should be management of pain and the development of constructive methods of coping with interval headaches (62,63).

Key Points

- Good-quality evidence supports treatment benefits and low potential for harm from use of biofeedback-assisted relaxation techniques, the vitamin riboflavin, alcohol avoidance, and caffeine reduction for the prevention of migraine, and melatonin for the prevention of cluster headache.

- Aerobic exercise and nicotine avoidance may have a positive effect on migraine in addition to other compelling medical benefits and should be recommended to most patients.

- The benefits of feverfew, hydroxocobalamin, L-hydroxytryptophan, melatonin, coenzyme Q10, acupuncture, and physical therapy for the prevention of migraine are uncertain, but the treatments are unlikely to be harmful.

- Homeopathy and chiropractic manipulation appear ineffective for headache; rare but serious harm may result from certain forms of spinal manipulation.

- The drawbacks of dietary restrictions outweigh benefits for most migraineurs.

- Unresolved concerns about toxic alkaloids should temper recommendations for use of the herb *Petasites* in migraine.

REFERENCES

1. **Von Peter S, Ting W, Scrivani S, et al.** Survey on the use of complementary and alternative medicine among patients with headache syndromes. Cephalalgia. 2002;22:395-400.

2. **Mauskop A.** Alternative therapies in headache: is there a role? Med Clin North Am. 2001;85:1077-84.

3. **Deweerdt C, Bootsma H, Hendriks H.** Herbal medicines in migraine prevention: randomized, double-blind, placebo-controlled crossover trial of feverfew preparation. Phytomedicine. 2003;3:225-230.

4. **Gray R, Goslin R, McCrory D.** Drug Treatments for the Prevention of Migraine Headache. Technical Review 2.3, Agency for Health Care Policy Research No. 290-94-2025, National Technical Information service accession 127853.

5. **Johnson ES, Kadam NP, Hylands DM, Hylands PJ.** Efficacy of feverfew as prophylactic treatment of migraine. BMJ. 1985;291:569-73.

6. **Murphy JJ, Heptinstall S, Mitchell JR.** Randomized double-blind placebo controlled trial of feverfew in migraine prevention. Lancet. 1988;2:189-92.

7. **Palevitch D, Earon G, Carusso R.** Feverfew (*Tanacetum parthenium*) as a prophylactic treatment for migraine: a double-blind placebo-controlled study. Phytother Res. 1997;11:508-11.

8. **Deweerdt CJ, Bootsma HP, Hendriks H.** Herbal medicines in migraine prevention: randomized double-blind placebo-controlled crossover trial of feverfew preparation. Phytomedicine. 1996;3:225-30.

9. **Vogler B, Pittler M, Ernst E.** Feverfew as a preventive treatment for migraine: a systematic review. Cephalalgia. 1998;18:704-8.

10. **Pfaffenrath V, Diener HC, Fischer M, et al.** The efficacy and safety of *Tanacetum parthenium* (feverfew) in migraine prophylaxis: a double blind, multicentre, randomized placebo-controlled dose-response study. Cephalalgia. 2002;22: 523-32.

10a. **Draves A, Walker S.** Parthenolide content of Canadian commercial feverfew preparations. Can Pharm J. 2003;136:23-30.

11. **Gruia F.** Zur biologischen Schmerzbekampfung. Erfahrungsheilkunde. 35:396-401.

12. **Seeger P.** Die therapeutischen Qualitarten von Petisites officianalis der Pestwurz. Erfahrungsheilkunde. 32:6-12.

13. **Steier L.** Petadolex - ein Spasmoanalgeticum und die muscularen Kopfschmerzen. Dtsch Z Biol Zahnmed. 6:114-116.

14. **Bickel D.** Charakterisierung und Isolierung der Leucotriensynthase-hemmenden Wirkkomponen aus *Petasites hybridus*. Dissertation, Universitat Erlangen-Nurnberg.

15. **Grossmann M, Schmidramsl H.** An extract of *Petasites hybridus* is effective in the prophylaxis of migraine. Int J Pharmacol Ther. 2003;38:430-5.

16. **Lipton R, Gobel H, Wilkes K, Mauskop A.** A special extract from *Petasites* hybrid root is effective as a preventive treatment for migraine. Paper presented to the 44th Annual Scientific Meeting of the American Headache Society; Seattle, 22 June 2002.

17. **Schoenen J, Jacquy J, Lenaerts, M.** Effectiveness of high-dose riboflavin in migraine prophylaxis. Neurology. 2003;50:466-470.

18. **Van der Kuy P-HM, Merkus FWHM, Lohman JJHM, et al.** Hydroxocobalamin, a nitric oxide scavenger, in the prophylaxis of migraine: an open, pilot study. Cephalalgia. 2002;22:513-9.

19. **Rozen T, Oshinsky M, Gebeline C, et al.** Open label trial of coenzyme Q10 as a migraine preventive. Cephalalgia. 2002;22:137-41.

19a. **Sandor P, Di Clemente L, Coppola G, et al.** Coenzyme Q for migraine prophylaxis: a randomized controlled trial [Abstract]. Cephalalgia. 2003;23:577.

20. **Schoenen J, Sianard-Gainko J, Lenaerts M.** Blood magnesium levels in migraine. Cephalalgia. 2003;11:97-9

21. **Ramadan N, Halvorson H, Vande-Linde A, et al.** Low brain magnesium in migraine. Headache. 2003;29:590-3.

22. **Sarchielli P, Costa G, Firenze C, et al.** Serum and salivary magnesium levels in migraine and tension type headache: results in a group of adult patients. Cephalalgia. 2003;12:21-7.

23. **Mauskop A, Altura BT, Cracco R, Altura BM.** Intravenous magnesium sulfate relieves acute migraine in patients with low serum ionized magnesium levels. Clin Sci. 1995;89:633-6.

24. **Facchinetti F, Sances G, Borella P, et al.** Magnesium prophylaxis of menstrual migraine: effects on intracellular magnesium. Headache. 2003;31:298-301.

25. **Peikert A, Wilimzig C, Kohne-Volland R.** Prophylaxis of migraine with oral magnesium: results from a prospective, multi-center, placebo-controlled and double-blind randomized study. Cephalalgia. 2003;16:257-63.

26. **Wang F, Van Den Eden S, Ackerson L, et al.** Oral magnesium oxide prophylaxis of frequent childhood migraine [Abstract]. Cephalalgia. 2003;20:424.

27. **Pfaffenrath V, Wessely P, Meyer C, et al.** Magnesium in the prophylaxis of migraine: a double-blind, placebo-controlled study. Cephalalgia. 2003;16:436-40.

28. **Fonte-Ribeiro C.** L-5-hydroxy tryptophan in the prophylaxis of chronic tension type headache: a double-blind randomized, placebo-controlled study [Abstract]. Cephalalgia. 2003;19:453.

29. **Perez M, del Rio M, Seabra M, et al.** Hypothalamic involvement in chronic migraine. J Neurol Neurosurg Psychiatry. 2001;71:747-51.

30. **Gagnier J.** The therapeutic potential of melatonin in migraines and other headache types. Alternative Medicine Review. 2001;6:383-9.

31. **Leone M.** Melatonin in primary headache. Cephalalgia. 1994;14:183.

32. **Nagtegaal JE, Smits MG, Swart ACW, et al.** Melatonin-responsive headache in delayed sleep phase syndrome: preliminary observations. Headache. 1998;38:303-7.

33. **Leone M, D'Amico D, Moschiano F, et al.** Melatonin versus placebo in the prophylaxis of cluster headache: a double-blind pilot study with parallel groups. Cephalalgia. 1996;16:494-6.

34. **Peres MFP, Rozen TD.** Melatonin in the preventive treatment of chronic cluster headache. Cephalalgia. 2001;21:993-5.

35. **Marcus D, Scharff L, Mercer S, Turk D.** Musculoskeletal abnormalities in chronic headache: a controlled comparison of headache diagnostic groups. Headache. 2003;39:21-7.

36. **Marcus D, Scharff L, Mercer S, Turk D.** Nonpharmacological treatment for migraine: incremental utility of physical therapy with relaxation and thermal biofeedback. Cephalalgia. 2003;18:266-72.

37. **Smith WS, Johnston SC, Skalabrin EJ, et al.** Spinal manipulative therapy is an independent risk factor for vertebral artery dissection. Neurology. 2003;60:1424-8.

38. **Jull G, Trott P, Potter H, et al.** A randomized controlled trial of exercise and manipulative therapy for cervicogenic headache. Spine. 2002;27:1835-43.

39. **Mayer D.** Acupuncture: an evidence-based review of the clinical literature. Annu Rev Med. 2003;51:49-63.

40. **Hans J, Terenius L.** Neurochemical basis of acupuncture analgesia. Annu Rev Pharmacol Toxicol. 2003;22:193-220.

41. **Baischer W.** Acupuncture in migraine: long-term outcome and predicting factors. Headache. 2003;35:472-4.

42. **Melchart D, Linde K, Fischer P, et al.** Acupuncture for recurrent headaches: a systematic review of randomized controlled trials. Cephalalgia. 2003;19:779-86.

43. **Jonas WB, Kaptchuk TJ, Linde K.** A critical overview of homeopathy. Ann Intern Med. 2003;138:393-9.

44. **Ernst E.** Classical homeopathy versus conventional treatments: a systematic review. J Pain Symptom Manage. 1999;18:353-7.

45. **Farmer K.** Biofeedback and the treatment of headache. In: Cady R, Fox A, eds. Treating the Headache Patient. New York: Marcel Dekker; 1995:288.

46. **Martin P, Marie G, Nathan P.** Behavioral research on headaches: a coded bibliography. Headache. 1987;27:515-32.

47. **Sargent J, Green E, Walters E.** The use of autogenic feedback training in a pilot study of migraine and tension headaches. Headache. 2003;12:120-5.

48. Evidence-based guidelines for migraine headache: behavioral and physical treatments. Neurology. 2000;55:754-62.

49. **Egger J, Carter C, Wilson J.** Is migraine food allergy? A double-blind trial of oligoantigenic diet treatment. Lancet. 1983;2:865-8.

50. **Monro J, Carini C, Brostoff J.** Migraine is a food allergic disease. Lancet. 1984;2:719-21.

51. **Medina J, Diamond S.** The role of diet in migraine. Headache. 1978;18:31-4.

52. **Karoum F, Nasrallah H, Potkin S.** Mass fragmentography of phenylethanolamine, m- and p-tyramine and related amines in plasma, cerebrospinal fluid, urine, and brain. J Neurochem. 1979;33:201-12.

53. **Marcus D, Scharff L, Turk D, Gourley L.** A double-blind provocative study of chocolate as a trigger for headache. Cephalalgia. 1997;17:855-62.

54. **Andersson H, Ejlertsson G, Leden I.** Widespread musculoskeletal chronic pain associated with smoking: an epidemiological study in a general rural population. Scand J Rehabil Med. 1998;30:185-91.

55. **Millac P, Akhtar N.** Cigarette smoking and cluster headache. Headache. 1985;25:220

56. **Payne T, Stetson B, Stevens V, et al.** Impact of cigarette smoking on headache activity in headache patients. Headache. 1991;31:329-32.

57. **Lockett DM, Campbell JF.** The effects of aerobic exercise on migraine. Headache. 1992;32:50-4.

58. **Lipton R, Stewart W.** Acute migraine therapy: do doctors understand what patients with migraine want from therapy? Headache. 1999;39(Suppl 2):S20-S26.

59. **Holroyd K, Cordingley G, Pingel J, et al.** Enhancing the effectiveness of abortive therapy: a controlled evaluation of self-management. Headache. 1989;29:148-53.

60. **De Bruijn-Kofman A, van de Wiel H, Groenman N, et al.** Effects of a mass media behavioral treatment for chronic headache: a pilot study. Headache. 1997;37:415-20.

61. **Marlowe N.** Pain sensitivity and headache: an examination of the central theory. J Psychosom Res. 1992;36:17-24.

62. **Lacroix R, Barbaree H.** The impact of recurrent headaches on behavior lifestyle and health. Behav Res Ther. 1990:28:235-42.

63. **Weeks R, Baskin S.** Psychological aspects of headache. In Cady R, Fox A, eds. Treating the Headache Patient. New York: Marcel Dekker; 1995:274.

13

■ ■ ■

Dealing with the Difficult Headache Patient

Timothy Wallace, PhD

T he vast majority of patients who visit primary care physicians complaining of headache will be no more difficult to handle than patients with other types of medical problems. A significant percentage of patients who present with chronic severe headache, however, will prove challenging to treat. This chapter provides a strategy for dealing with these patients more effectively.

Factors That Can Contribute to Difficulties

Comorbid Psychiatric Problems

Epidemiological studies have found an association between migraine and both anxiety disorders and mood disorders (1). The relationship appears to be bi-directional, with migraine predicting first-onset depression and depression predicting first-onset migraine (2). Depression or anxiety can play a role in precipitating or exacerbating headaches. Comorbid depression also seems to contribute to the intractability of migraine (3). Clinical studies have found similarly elevated rates of mood and anxiety disorders in patients with chronic tension-type headaches (4). In fact, psychological factors appear to play a more significant role in the transformation of migraine and the chronification of tension-type headaches than analgesic misuse (5).

Clinical experience suggests that patients with comorbid psychiatric disorders are less likely to respond favorably to drug and behavioral therapies initiated in the primary care setting than patients with no psychiatric problems, although controlled studies investigating this relationship are lacking (6). Psychiatric diagnosis also appears to be one of the best predictors of headache-related functional impairment, making it difficult to distinguish between impairment due to pain and impairment caused by psychological problems (6). Depression or anxiety that is brought on by the difficulty of living with chronic severe headaches, on the other hand, may abate once the headaches improve.

It is therefore essential that the primary care physician screen headache patients for comorbid psychiatric problems, particularly anxiety and mood disorders, and arrange for their treatment. The Primary Care Evaluation of Mental Disorders, or PRIME-MD (7), is a brief instrument designed to screen for common psychiatric disorders seen in medical settings.

Behavioral problems exhibited by patients with personality disorders can challenge the interpersonal skills of the physician and can make treating the patient's headache much more difficult and unpleasant. Because migraine has been shown to occur in patients diagnosed with borderline personality at a rate much higher than in the general population, in both men and women (8), it is important for the primary care doctor to learn to recognize this disorder and to learn techniques for dealing with the unpredictable displays of emotion and the manipulative, demanding behavior that may be encountered.

Past or Present Substance Abuse

Patients who misuse or abuse medications prescribed for headache management are among the most challenging to deal with, but they are usually not difficult to identify. Analgesics, especially barbiturate-containing medications, are the drugs most often abused. The primary care doctor should be alert to the following behaviors that, when displayed by a patient with chronic headaches, can indicate prescription drug misuse or abuse:

- Frequently runs out of medication early
- Sometimes reports medication was lost, stolen, or ruined, resulting in requests for unscheduled refills
- Evidence of falsified or duplicate prescriptions
- Multisourcing (i.e., receiving drugs from more than one doctor or from frequent emergency room visits)
- Combining medication with alcohol
- Medication-related functional impairment becomes greater than pain-related impairment
- Preoccupation with medication during office visits
- Objects to any reduction in dosage and/or displays excessive emotional reactivity to the suggestion of dose reduction
- Expresses no interest in nonpharmacological headache treatments such as biofeedback or relaxation training
- Family members express concern over patient's drug use

These behaviors should be addressed immediately and directly. Primary care physicians who prescribe potentially addictive drugs to chronic headache patients must establish and enforce clear limits regarding medications in order to avoid inadvertently enabling drug misuse or abuse. (See also the section on medication overuse headaches in Chapter 7.) It is important to distinguish between medication overuse by patients who are desperate to treat pain, and patients who overuse medication for other reasons.

Comorbid alcohol or illegal drug abuse problems can also complicate headache treatment. Patients being considered for, or treated with, potentially addictive medications should be routinely screened for substance abuse to determine whether further assessment and intervention are needed. The primary care physician should be alert to clinical evidence of substance abuse gained through urine drug screens and liver function tests, as well as information gleaned through observation and examination of the patient during office visits (e.g., dilated pupils, needle tracks, mental status changes). The doctor should always investigate further when any of the following behaviors are noted in a chronic headache patient:

- Refuses urine drug screen, blood alcohol level, or other drug test
- Family members report patient has drug or alcohol problem (even if the patient denies this)
- Exhibits several "soft signs" that suggest a substance abuse problem (appears "high", looks hung-over, smells of alcohol or marijuana, etc.)

A patient who is actively abusing alcohol or illegal drugs is a poor candidate for treatment with potentially addictive prescription analgesics or other dependency-inducing drugs. Addressing the comorbid substance abuse problem increases the chance of success of other treatments. Potential barriers to effective treatment in such a situation are numerous. Not only are there issues related to drug interaction, treatment noncompliance, and medication misuse, but behavior common in addicted patients (e.g., denial of the problem, projection of affect, manipulation, lying) can undermine the doctor-patient relationship so important to effective long-term headache management. Nonpharmacological strategies such as biofeedback may be effective in these situations and should be emphasized.

A history of alcoholism or other drug abuse does not automatically make a patient a management problem, nor does such a history preclude headache treatment with appropriate analgesic or abortive medication. Some patients with previous substance abuse may be appropriate for treatment with such medications, as long as they are screened carefully and their medication use is monitored closely. The risk of a former abuser misusing headache medication may be attenuated by several factors, including

- Length of time since the problem occurred
- Type(s) of substances abused (alcohol, prescription pain killers, heroin) and pattern of use (daily, weekly, occasionally)
- Whether patient received substance abuse treatment; number of relapses
- Available sources of support (family, friends, job, 12-step program)
- Willingness to try nonpharmacological headache treatment (relaxation, exercise, biofeedback) in addition to medication
- Compliance with urine drug screens

Should the physician decide, after carefully considering the above factors, that a patient with a remote drug or alcohol problem is a reasonable risk for treatment with potentially addictive headache drugs, he or she should establish clear guidelines regarding medication use (limited supplies, frequent office visits, random urine drug screens, involvement of family members) to prevent potential problems. The physician should *never* try to talk a patient into using drugs to manage headache if the patient feels anxious or unsure about his or her ability to regulate their use.

Past Experiences Involving Pain

A headache patient with a *history of childhood abuse or other trauma* may display challenging behaviors because headaches are interpreted in the context of the previous painful experience. A severe headache may evoke long-repressed memories of traumatic experiences such as physical, sexual, or emotional abuse, causing the individual to attach an enormous amount of affect to the headache experience. A migraine, for instance, might be perceived as another traumatic experience and elicit dormant symptoms of post-traumatic stress disorder (flashbacks, nightmares, suicidal thoughts, dissociative episodes). A patient with a history of abuse may feel overwhelmed by the pain and experience the same feelings of fear and helplessness he or she felt at the time of the abuse.

Many of these patients view themselves as repeatedly victimized during their lives. They may interpret a certain behavior of the physician, such as refusing to prescribe strong narcotics, as further mistreatment. Thus a patient who reacts in an overly dramatic, histrionic manner to a severe headache may have been traumatized at an earlier time in his or her life. Such behavior may seem like over-reaction to observers but to these patients it is a reasonable response, given their history. It is important for the doctor to recognize that, for these patients, today's headache is interpreted in the context of the negative affect it arouses because of painful experiences that occurred in the past. Some of these patients will present with coexisting psychiatric diagnoses, such as post-traumatic stress disorder, borderline personality disorder, or anxiety or depressive disorders.

Another group of patients, those with a *long history of poorly controlled headaches,* may come to the new primary care physician's office filled with frustration and anger at the way their headaches have been managed by past doctors. These patients may report that previous medical providers:

- Were not competent to treat their headaches
- Did not take their pain complaints seriously
- Minimized their distress
- Insinuated that they were exaggerating their pain because they did not "look" like they were in very much pain
- Told them that their headaches were "all in their heads" or "just due to stress"
- Labeled them "drug addicts" when they asked for refills of their prescription analgesics

Whether these incidents took place exactly as reported is irrelevant. What is important is that a patient with a history of these experiences comes to the new doctor's office with negative feelings toward medical professionals because past treatment was *perceived* in a negative way. The reality, of course, is that only a minority of these patients have been misdiagnosed, mismanaged, or otherwise mishandled due to their doctor's lack of adequate training in headache diagnosis and treatment. The negative affect, though, is likely to be transferred to the new physician unless he or she recognizes and validates the patient's feelings. *If a patient had issues with his or her former physician, there will be issues with the new one, too, unless different approaches are taken.* The savvy physician will acknowledge patient anger and frustration early in the visit and address any negative expectations about the success of future treatment efforts. In this way treatment will have the best possible chance of being effective.

Stress

Clinical evidence suggests that stress plays a role in the onset and exacerbation of migraines and other headaches, but studies of this subject yield contradictory results and indicate that the influence of stress on headache onset needs further investigation (9). It seems unlikely that stress alone can bring on a headache severe enough to necessitate medical attention. Other factors, such as hormonal changes and neurological and vascular events, appear to interact with stress in the onset of recurring headaches. Nevertheless, it is commonly identified by patients as a migraine trigger. Furthermore, stress clearly can affect an individual's quality of life and the effectiveness of his or her headache management program.

Clinical experience suggests that stress can both *contribute to* and *result from* severe persistent headaches. Stressors that may contribute to the onset of headaches include

- Chronic or severe family dysfunction, marital discord, domestic abuse
- Severe financial strain (chronic debt, poverty)
- Pressures related to work or family responsibilities
- Illness

Stressors that may be a result of recurring headaches include

- Lost time at work, missed deadlines, decreased productivity, lost wages, job jeopardy
- Medical bills, prescription costs, frequent physician visits
- Decreased ability to fulfill role expectations in the family, leading to guilt, family tension, and marital problems

Although high levels of stress are not uncommon in our culture, most people learn to cope reasonably well with the pressures of everyday life. When the burden of frequent severe headaches is added to an already stressed person's life, his or her coping skills may be taxed beyond capacity. A person who coped adequately before he or she had the added stress of chronic headaches may even occasionally become suicidal. It has been shown that chronic headache patients appraise stressful events more negatively than healthy people (10). They also employ less effective coping strategies in their attempts to deal with stress and pain. Unlike their healthy counterparts, headache patients tend to rely more on medication to deal with their problems, tend to catastrophize more about the pain, and tend to avoid physical and social sources of stress reduction (11-14).

The primary care physician will be better able to manage the chronic headache patient if he or she is aware of the stress the patient is experiencing. Taking a few minutes to talk can go a long way towards helping the patient recognize the role stress plays in the onset, exacerbation, and maintenance of headaches. If the doctor does not acknowledge that stress is a contributing factor, the patient will probably dismiss it as well and be unlikely to pursue the option of stress management. He or she is much more likely to do something about stress if the doctor emphasizes the importance of stress reduction in a comprehensive headache management program.

Personality Style

"Migraine Personality"

As long ago as 1937 there was an attempt to identify the "migraine personality" (15). Clinicians and researchers hove continued their efforts to isolate the personality characteristics of the chronic migraine patient, but there has been little agreement about which traits migraineurs have in common. There has been even less agreement about a "tension-type headache personality" or a "cluster headache personality". Carefully controlled investigations of this issue are lacking.

Because headache patients appear to be a heterogeneous group as far as personality traits are concerned, almost every physician will encounter a few patients that are difficult to deal with because they possess a personality style that the doctor finds especially trying. These are not patients with diagnosable psychiatric disturbances or personality disorders but individuals whose behavior "pushes the doctor's buttons". These are the people the physician dreads seeing in the waiting room because they are so disagreeable, unpleasant, or exhausting to deal with. These "difficult" patients have been recognized for decades and have often been viewed with disdain (16,17).

Most doctors accept that they have a harder time working with certain personality styles than others. Some of the patient types that physicians find especially taxing are listed below. The list is not exhaustive, and the categories are somewhat arbitrary; there is also a great deal of overlap between the various types listed.

- *Argumentative/Confrontational*—Challenges everything the physician says. Never agrees to anything without a struggle. May be loud, pushy, "in your face".

- *Rigid/Inflexible*—Rejects anything that does not fit into his or her rigid belief system. Resists new ways of looking at a problem.

- *Emotionally Reactive*—Responds with a dramatic display of emotion to benign situations or statements. Seems to over-react. May exaggerate or embellish pain complaints (pain level is "12 on a 0 to 10 scale").

- *Negative/Pessimistic*—Finds every reason the suggested treatment cannot possibly succeed. May report unusual side effects to medications or say that medications make headaches worse.

- *Narcissistic/Entitled*—Arrogant, patronizing, with a grandiose sense of self-importance. May show up late and expect to be seen anyway. Demands special treatment. May allude to litigation if needs are not met.

- *Passive/Dependent*—Relies excessively on the doctor for guidance. Seeks reassurance but is unwilling to take responsibility for his or her own behavior. May appear depressed.

- *Manipulative*—May use lies, distortions, flattery, or gifts to get what he or she wants. Not honest or direct.

- *Denier*—Minimizes problems. Reports that life is fine except for the headaches. May be somatically focused. Fails to acknowledge or modify lifestyle factors (smoking, diet) that may influence the headaches.

- *Overly Anxious*—May appear noticeably nervous and apprehensive. Prone to between-visit telephone calls and "urgent" visits. Much of office visit is spent calming patient down. May favor barbiturate-containing drugs (e.g., butalbital) and take them compulsively.

- *Somatizer*—Reports excessive number of headache triggers (light, noise, odors, foods). May report many other physical symptoms besides headaches. May display excessive avoidance and pain behaviors.

- *Impatient/Impulsive Pill Taker*—Cannot tolerate waiting for medication to work, so takes multiple doses over a short period of time. Uninterested in nonpharmacological treatments.

It can be stressful for the doctor to interact with a patient whose personality seems incompatible with his or her own. The patient's behavior elicits an emotional response in the doctor, and the doctor runs the risk of behaving in a nontherapeutic way if he or she is not aware of the fact that it is not just *this particular patient* that he or she finds difficult: people with this patient's type of personality style *always* make him or her angry, frustrated, defensive, nervous, or what-have-you. As a professional, the physician certainly would not want to react irrationally to the situation, so the emotions that are being aroused must be acknowledged and managed so that an automatic, knee-jerk response does not occur. In this way, the doctor can stay in control of the interaction by making a conscious choice to not allow the personality conflict to affect his or her judgment or behavior.

Identifying Difficult Patients Early

During the evaluation of the patient's headache complaint, the primary care physician can spot potentially problematic behaviors by using direct questions, observation of the patient's behavior, information gleaned from corroborating sources, and/or clinical intuition.

Ask Direct Questions

This is the most straightforward way to gather information but not always the most reliable. A patient can sabotage this technique by forgetting, distorting, denying, lying, or contaminating the data in a myriad of ways. If done correctly, however, asking direct questions is an efficient and reasonably reliable way to get the information the physician needs.

To increase the chance of getting valid information, the doctor is usually wise to avoid asking questions that a patient can answer with a simple "yes" or "no" (Table 13-1). It is also preferable to avoid leading questions that give the patient clues about how you want (or expect) them to respond.

Table 13-1   Avoiding "Yes" or "No" Questions

Poor Question	Better Question
"Do you drink alcohol?"	"What are your drinking habits?"
"Are you depressed?"	"How are you feeling emotionally about these headaches?"

Table 13-2   "Gentle Assumption" Questions

Poor Question	Better Question, Using Gentle Assumption
"Do you ever take more Percocet than you're supposed to?"	"How often do you find yourself taking more Percocet than you're supposed to?"
"Have you ever used street drugs to help your headaches?"	"Which street drugs have you tried to help your headaches?"

Table 13-3 "Symptom Amplification" Questions

Poor Question	Better Question, Using Symptom Amplification
"What is the largest number of Vicodins you've ever taken in one day?"	"What is the largest number of Vicodins you've ever taken in one day? 15? 20?"
"How many times have you struck your wife when you've had a bad headache?"	"How many times have you struck your wife when you've had a bad headache? 10? 20?"

Another useful method of questioning is "gentle assumption" (18). This technique is especially helpful when the doctor suspects that a patient may be hesitant to endorse or discuss a specific behavior. With gentle assumption the doctor literally *assumes that the behavior in question occurs,* rather than trying to ascertain *whether* it occurs. The objective is to determine the *extent to which the behavior occurs* (Table 13-2).

Another technique, "symptom amplification" (19), is based on the observation that patients often downplay or under-report the frequency or number of behaviors they are ashamed of or that they think might be viewed negatively by the doctor (e.g., the amount they drink). This distorting mechanism is bypassed by setting the upper limits of the quantity in question at such a high level that even if the patient downplays the amount, the physician still uncovers a significant problem (Table 13-3).

Observe Behavior

Careful scrutiny of the patient's behavior can yield a wealth of clinically useful information. Observing the patient, as well as listening to him or her, will greatly enhance the physician's awareness of potential problematic behaviors and improve the reliability of the information gathered through direct questions.

One particularly important type of behavior the doctor should attend to is *pain behavior,* which is defined as any observable behavior that the patient displays that indicates that he or she is experiencing pain. In addition to the more obvious verbal complaints, pain behaviors that may occur during an office visit can include facial grimaces, tearfulness, touching or rubbing the head, wearing dark glasses, and asking to have the lights dimmed or the window shades closed. Pain behavior reveals the patient's current manner of expressing the pain and provides an enormous amount of information about his or her coping skills. The physician should note inconsistencies between the patient's verbal report and their nonverbal pain behavior. For instance, a perfectly groomed patient who appears calm and happy, yet reports that the pain is currently at level "10" on a 0 to 10 scale, might be exaggerating his or her pain complaints. Another patient, who says that everything is fine yet is weepy and appears sad, may have psychological problems including, but not limited to, depression.

A high level of pain behavior does not necessarily mean someone's headache is more severe than that of a person with a lesser degree of pain behavior, but it does tend to escalate in a given individual as pain level increases. Furthermore, high levels of pain behavior are not always correlated with treatment resistance. In fact, patients with minimal displays of pain behavior can be more refractory to treatment than those with higher levels.

In addition to pain behavior, the physician should pay close attention to the following behaviors, which can be indicative of potential problems:

- *Affect*—Does the patient appear depressed, anxious, or angry? Does affect display normal range (i.e., patient is able to smile to a humorous comment despite feeling depressed)?

- *Appearance*—Does patient appear rested vs. exhausted, neatly groomed vs. disheveled? Are there any signs of substance abuse (e.g., bloodshot eyes, needle tracks, seems "high")?

- *Speech*—Is speech slurred, rambling, tangential, incoherent, or illogical? Is content of speech filled with somatization?

- *Unusual or Bizarre Behaviors*—Does patient lie down on the floor, appear in unusual clothing, or demonstrate bizarre coping strategies in the doctor's office? Such behaviors can indicate psychosis but may simply suggest a histrionic coping style.

- *General Behaviors*—Does patient avoid eye contact? Do cognition and/or memory appear impaired? Is mood stable throughout the visit?

The likelihood of favorable outcomes will be increased if the primary care physician always aspires to observe, evaluate, and treat the entire individual, not just the headache.

Consult Corroborating Sources

If the headache patient is accompanied to the doctor's office by a significant other, parent, roommate, friend, or relative, this individual can be an important source of information about the patient's coping behavior. It is helpful for this person to be present during the initial evaluation of the headache, as well as during follow-up sessions, to provide corroboration of the patient's report and furnish additional information. The patient's permission for this arrangement must be secured first, of course.

Friends and relatives can greatly enhance the reliability and validity of information gathered during an office visit. It is not unusual for a patient to tell the doctor that he or she takes medication exactly as prescribed but for the spouse to relate quite a different story. Likewise, a patient might report coping well but a roommate indicate that the patient frequently stays in bed all day, cries hysterically on a regular basis, and often talks about suicide. This is also an excellent way to find out if a significant person in the patient's life is functioning as an *enabler*, one who inadvertently facilitates poor headache management, poor coping, or an increased level of disability by being overly solicitous or otherwise reinforcing unhealthy coping behaviors.

Other important sources of supporting information are the referring physician, if any, who can often provide valuable insight into previous treatment failures and the patient's level of compliance with recommendations; mental health providers, such as psychologists or psychiatrists, who can help the primary care physician understand any emotional or behavioral issues that might affect their treatment; and other involved parties, such as case managers or social workers. Permission will usually have to be secured from the patient before these consultations can take place, but a patient's reluctance to allow consultation with other sources may be an indication of possible problems down the road. The doctor should always be wary of a patient who will not allow him or her to communicate with other treating providers or to examine previous medical records. In some cases the patient's refusal to allow access to this information may be so deleterious to proper treatment that the physician may have to terminate the relationship.

Use Intuition

Intuition is often dismissed as an unreliable method of evaluating a situation, but if it is used as an adjunct to the other methods of data collection it can increase the power of prediction. As used here, the word refers to the doctor's "gut feeling" about a particular state of affairs, based in part on his or her previous experiences in similar situations with similar patients and in part on a general "feeling" about the situation. Intuition is developed over time and includes the sum total of the physician's clinical experience as well his or her instinct, perception, insight, and psychological sophistication. The intuitive physician combines information gathered through interview, observation, and other sources and forms a *gestalt* or impression of the patient and the patient's headache problem. Obviously, some doctors have a well-developed sense of intuition, whereas others do not.

Intuition relies heavily on the physician's perceptiveness. Factors that can contribute to the impression that is formed include

- Does the physician "like" the patient?
- Does the physician feel motivated to help the patient?
- Does the patient seem sincere and "genuine"?
- Does the patient seem honest?
- Does information provided by and about the patient appear to make sense? Do the facts fit together logically?
- Does the physician trust the patient?
- What is the physician's "gut" telling him or her about this patient?

Of course, intuition should never be used by itself to make clinical decisions. Treatments should always be selected based on clinical findings and empirical evidence. Intuition can, however, assist the physician with the difficult task of matching the appropriate intervention with the presenting problem.

Techniques for Managing Difficult Patients

Start with Clear Expectations

Communicate Office Policies Clearly
If the physician does not train patients in his or her office policies, then patients will inevitably train the doctor in theirs. Develop straightforward, unambiguous policies regarding such matters as cancelled or failed appointments, "emergency" phone calls, and prescription refills. Such policies can preempt many problems with difficult patients. A brochure is a good vehicle for communicating office policies. It can be given to the patient during the first office visit or, even better, mailed to the patient beforehand, at the time the first appointment is scheduled.

Use Treatment Agreements When Necessary
When a potentially difficult patient has been identified, or when a problem behavior occurs that could adversely affect treatment outcome (e.g., noncompliance), the physician should consider the use of an individual *treatment agreement*. This is an explicit, written document, agreed to and signed by both patient and physician, that outlines expectations for treatment. Although it does not have legal force, it is useful to help clarify the conditions under which treatment will occur. For example, a contract for a

patient who has previously misused medication (or is at risk for misusing due to past behavior) might contain some or all of the following provisions:

- Analgesic medications are to be received only from the PCP.
- Prescriptions are to be filled at only one pharmacy.
- Medications are to be taken exactly as prescribed, even if the headache pain is not well controlled.
- Refills will not be granted ahead of schedule even if patient runs out of medication early.
- The PCP will be notified immediately if another doctor prescribes any drugs, *before* they are taken.
- Random urine drug screens will be requested.

A treatment agreement for a patient who is prone to temper outbursts might specify that

- Patient will refrain from yelling during office visits.
- Patient will not threaten the physician or any person on the office staff.
- Patient will not throw objects or damage property.
- Patient will take prescribed mood stabilizing medication as required.

An agreement for a depressed patient might stipulate that

- Patient will take antidepressant medication as prescribed.
- Patient will attend weekly psychotherapy sessions with a mental health professional.
- Patient will take agreed-upon action in the event of strong suicidal feelings (e.g., call psychotherapist, call 911, go to the nearest emergency department) but will not misuse medications.

The agreement should also outline what the patient can expect from the doctor, such as monthly appointments and collaboration with other treating providers, and the consequences of failure to adhere to any of the agreement's provisions, such as termination of treatment, referral to a substance abuse or mental health program, transfer to another physician, or (in the case of the violent patient) notification of security personnel. The more explicit the agreement the easier it is to enforce, so specifying exact numbers is extremely helpful (e.g., two failed urine drug screens results in treatment termination).

Document Behavior

Physicians routinely record important clinical information in the medical record. As part of a proactive strategy for managing difficult patients, it is also useful to monitor and record certain nonclinical information about the patient.

This can be done in large part by office staff, such as the receptionist or office manager, using a *patient log*. The log can be as simple as a set of file cards kept on the receptionist's desk or as elaborate as a computer database.

Each log documents data such as the date, time, and reason for each cancelled or failed appointment, any "urgent" between-visit telephone calls, routine calls for prescription refills, and other information that is important for patient management but not appropriate for the medical record. (Documentation of the doctor's telephone contact with patients will usually also be made in the patient's medical record.) In the event an office policy or contract provision must be enforced, the doctor will then have precise documentation to support his or her course of action. For example, if office policy stipulates that any patient who fails to show for two consecutive appointments will be terminated, the receptionist can inform a patient in this situation that he or she has been discharged when they call for another appointment. If the patient protests, the log and its data can be referred to and many "he said, she said" arguments can be avoided.

There is an important caveat regarding office policies and treatment agreements: Contingencies are only useful if the provisions are enforced immediately and consistently. It takes only one episode of a rule infraction not being followed by the promised consequence for a patient to learn that the policy or contract has no real meaning. Therefore the physician must be comfortable with the contingencies and feel that he or she will be able to enforce them if necessary.

Establish Limits

Primary care physicians have a crucial responsibility to set and enforce limits with patients, when appropriate. It is never easy to refuse the request of a patient in distress, but it is sometimes therapeutic to do so. In the case of the demanding headache patient, poor limit setting by the doctor can result in the dispensing of inappropriate types or amounts of medication, frequent "urgent" telephone calls from patients at all hours of the day and night, "acting out" by patients during office visits (e.g., temper tantrums, suicide threats), and a variety of other problematic situations.

Failing to Say "No": A Case in Point

Many doctors, lacking skills in setting and enforcing limits, have found themselves giving in to patient demands for antibiotics when there is no evidence of bacterial infection. This failure to say "no" has contributed to the growing problem of drug-resistant strains of bacteria.

Clear office policies and individual treatment contracts can set the stage for appropriate limit setting, but the power of limits is only realized when the doctor says "no" when "no" is called for. For example:

- "I understand that you'd prefer Percocet for your headaches, but in my opinion a triptan is the proper medication for your type of headache. I'm asking you to try that instead."

- "We will only have time to discuss three of the issues on the list you brought, so why don't you choose the three most important ones? We'll save the rest for your next visit."

- "I know you're upset that you're out of medication and aren't scheduled for a refill for another five days. But remember that in your treatment contract we agreed early refills would not be granted if you ran out of medicine ahead of schedule."

It is natural for physicians to try to do whatever they can to reduce patient suffering. Therefore it is important to understand limit setting as a therapeutic practice, not a punitive one. Saying "no" to inappropriate behavior allows the physician to affirm appropriate, healthy alternatives. Yielding to the inappropriate demands of challenging patients not only perpetuates unhealthy coping behavior, it places the doctor in the role of the enabler, inadvertently participating in the patient's dysfunctional headache management. Failure to enforce limits also leaves the physician vulnerable to feeling used and manipulated and can result in virtual loss of control over the patient's medical care.

Use Effective Techniques To Manage Difficult Patients

Five effective techniques will help the physician manage challenging patients with assurance: convey empathy, avoid defensiveness, side-step arguments, reinforce the positive, and manage countertransferance.

Convey Empathy
Patients will accept limits more readily if they believe the doctor really listens and understands how they feel. It is best to be direct in letting an individual know that his or her position was heard and is valued, and that their physician has empathy for them:

- "I know you're disappointed that I won't give you anything stronger then Tylenol, but . . . "

- "I understand you're frustrated that it is taking so long to get these headaches under control."

- "I appreciate that you are upset about that."

- "Your feelings certainly are understandable."

Avoid Defensiveness
A struggle is sure to ensue when the physician becomes defensive with an upset patient. It is important for the doctor to listen patiently to whatever the patient has to say, but it is equally important to avoid defending one's

behavior. Defensiveness almost invariably leads to escalation of the disagreement and almost never facilitates understanding. One of the "Seven Habits of Highly Effective People" in Stephen Covey's bestseller by the same name (20) is *to seek first to understand, then to be understood*. Again, the physician is wise to listen carefully to the upset patient and to try to identify and empathize with the affect (feeling) being conveyed, as discussed above. The important point is that it is neither necessary nor advisable for the doctor to defend his or her behavior in these situations. The "he said, she said" trap should be avoided at all costs:

- "No, that's *not* what I said. I said . . ."
- "I *did so* tell you about that policy."

In many cases just letting an upset patient know that his or her concerns were heard is sufficient to calm troubled waters. After listening patiently to the patient's complaint, a simple and sincere "Thank you for letting me know how you feel" is often sufficient to end the confrontation and will usually satisfy the patient. For decades, company presidents have been signing "Thank you for sharing your concerns with me" letters in response to customer complaints, with good results. The same strategy is also effective with upset patients.

Side-Step Arguments
Some clinicians unwittingly end up in verbal battles with patients, such as when a patient does not agree with a decision about treatment, because they fail to appreciate a simple principle of interpersonal conflict: It is impossible to have an argument with someone who will not argue back. This principle can help the doctor deal with difficult patients who are argumentative, manipulative, and/or demanding. The key is for the doctor to listen, but not respond, to the *content* of the patient's argument. As discussed above, it is helpful to acknowledge the feelings that are being expressed, but responding to the content with defensiveness or emotionality will usually escalate the argument. It is useless to try to reason with an argumentative patient.

The following example illustrates how responding to the content of a patient's statement can lead to trouble:

Doctor. I've decided to wean you off Fioricet and start you on a triptan drug.

Patient. But, Doctor, I can't cope with these headaches without Fioricet. I'll die of the pain! Why are you doing this to me?

Doctor. No one ever died from a migraine. I'm doing this because I think it's time you got off the Fioricet.

Patient. But I've been taking Fioricet for five years. I'll go through horrible withdrawal! I'll bet you think I'm abusing them. Do you think I'm a drug addict or something?

Doctor. I didn't call you an addict. You're the only one who knows if you've been abusing your meds. Yes, you'll go through withdrawal and it will be unpleasant, but that's what happens when you become dependent on narcotic medication.

Patient. "Dependent" is another word for addicted, isn't it? If I'm an addict, you're the person who made me one! You're the one who's been writing prescriptions for me for five years! And now you're going to make me suffer . . .

This disagreement is escalating quickly because the doctor is responding to the patient's provocative statements. The doctor would fare better by using the "broken-record" technique in which the original message is repeated almost verbatim, without responding to the baiting being done by the patient. The technique requires a fair degree of self-discipline, but if the physician refuses to become engaged in the argument, the patient will usually give up the struggle.

Consider the previous scenario again, but this time with a physician who uses the "broken-record" technique:

Doctor. I've decided to wean you off Fioricet and start you on a triptan drug.

Patient. But, Doctor, I can't cope with these headaches without Fioricet. I'll die of the pain! Why are you doing this to me?

Doctor. I understand your concern, but it will be best to wean you off Fioricet and start you on a triptan.

Patient. But I've been taking Fioricet for five years. I'll go through horrible withdrawal! I'll bet you think I'm abusing them. Do you think I'm a drug addict or something?

Doctor. I can understand how you might think that. Yes, you'll go through withdrawal and it may be unpleasant. Still, it's time to wean you off Fioricet and put you on a triptan. You'll be weaned off gradually and carefully, in a way that will minimize withdrawal symptoms. Let's discuss how we'll do it.

Patient. Well, I'm not happy about it, but it looks as if you've made up your mind. Do you really think a triptan can help my headaches?

It usually takes three or four repetitions, stated in almost exactly the same words, to avert the argument. The three keys to this technique are to

- Listen to the patient's response.
- Respond to the *feelings* conveyed but not to the *content* of the argument.
- Repeat, virtually verbatim, the original point until the patient realizes that the doctor is not going to argue.

Reinforce the Positive
In interpersonal relationships it is always important to remember one of the most fundamental principles of learning: Behavior that is reinforced increases in frequency, intensity, and/or duration, whereas behavior that is ignored decreases in the same dimensions. The primary care physician who practices the art of positive reinforcement with patients can increase positive behaviors such as treatment compliance, candor, and improved functioning, and decrease negative behaviors such as verbal complaints, excessive reliance on medication, and passivity. The physician should *always* verbally praise compliance with treatment recommendations, such

as exercising faithfully, regulating diet and sleep patterns, and controlling stress. A simple comment such as "That's great!" or "I'm so glad to hear that!" can powerfully reinforce a behavior. Words such as "good", "terrific", and "wonderful" should be used liberally by the physician to reinforce positive behaviors.

Attention is also a powerful reinforcement, but attending to the wrong behavior can inadvertently support inappropriate or problematic behavior. For example, if the doctor pays close attention to the patient while he or she talks, in detail, about how awful the headaches are but seems uninterested (as evidenced by writing chart notes) when the patient describes the satisfaction received from gardening even with a bad migraine, then pain behavior has been rewarded – and therefore reinforced – and positive coping skills have been ignored or even, from the patient's point of view, punished – and therefore decreased. The general strategy is quite simple: *Reinforce (through praise and/or attention) behaviors that are healthy, functional, and positive, and ignore or deter behaviors that are maladaptive, problematic, or unhealthy.*

Manage Countertransference

Patient behavior can sometimes elicit strong emotional responses in the physician. An angry, agitated patient may stir up similar feelings of anger in the doctor, while at another time a patient's anger may elicit fearful feelings. A noncompliant patient may make the physician feel frustrated or helpless. It is important for the primary care doctor to recognize these normal emotional responses and to manage them so they do not negatively affect treatment. While such emotions are not technically "countertransference" phenomena in the psychoanalytic sense of the word, the term is used here to emphasize that these are the *physician's* feelings, not those of the patient, and that the physician needs to recognize this.

When feelings are aroused in the doctor, it is necessary to label them correctly ("Is it anger I feel toward that patient, or am I having competency anxiety?") before they can be managed effectively. It is sometimes difficult to sort out emotions that "feel" similar at first, like anger and fear. Consultation with a colleague is often helpful in this regard (see below). For example, a physician might seek help from another physician or even psychologist when confronted with a patient seeking additional testing that the physician believes is not warranted. A physician colleague can review the symptoms and examination findings and provide a medical opinion about the need for further testing. A psychologist can discuss other explanations, such as somatization or hypochondriasis, that might be playing a role in the patient's presentation.

It is also normal for a physician to be fonder of some patients than others. It may be hard for the doctor to like, or even tolerate, a patient who reminds him of his obnoxious and lazy brother-in-law, or the kid who used to bully him in elementary school, or his ex-wife. It is easy to respond to such a patient as if he or she actually *is* that person because their behavior elicits long-repressed negative emotions. If it goes unrecognized, the countertransference reaction in a situation like this can elicit a variety of inappropriate, unhelpful, and unprofessional "acting out" behaviors on the part of the physician, ranging from avoiding the patient, to punishing the patient (e.g., by withholding drugs that might have been given to another patient with the same headache problem, or making the patient wait in the reception area for a long time), to transferring the patient to another doctor. Again, consultation with a colleague is an excellent way to become more aware of emotions that are being aroused by a particular patient, so that the relationship is based in the "here and now" and not in the past.

Managing one's emotions can be challenging. For example, the physician might find himself or herself getting angry in response to an angry or agitated patient, or perhaps fearful for his or her safety. At these times it is important to remember the professional boundary between doctor and patient: *This is not an angry relative, this is a patient who is in pain.* The doctor must respond professionally. A few deep breaths will usually help the doctor become composed enough to choose an appropriate response (perhaps one of the techniques previously discussed). By recognizing that it is normal to have strong feelings in response to some situations, the physician is less apt to react emotionally and more likely to respond rationally.

Seeking Help

The primary care physician will occasionally need assistance in managing the most complex headache patients. The requisite help can usually be obtained through the mechanisms of consultation and referral. To manage especially challenging patients, the primary care doctor may want to coordinate a team of specialists from several disciplines.

Obtain Consultation

Consultation is the best choice when the case will benefit from the opinion of an uninvolved colleague (e.g., fellow physician) or another professional (e.g., attorney, psychologist, psychiatrist) because the situation has become problematic in some way. Just as a physician might seek consultation from a trusted associate if a patient were not responding to standard medical interventions for a headache problem, consultation can also be helpful when challenging patient behavior threatens to get out of control.

Examples of situations for which consultation should be considered:

- *An angry patient threatens litigation because of something the physician allegedly did or did not do.* Consulting with another doctor is an important safeguard and helps assure that accepted standards of care have been followed. The consultant should be a trusted colleague who will honestly tell the physician if he or she behaved in a manner that might be regarded as unethical, illegal, unorthodox, careless, or negligent. The consultation should always be documented in the patient's medical record.

- *The physician feels anger toward a patient, or feels threatened or manipulated by a patient, or feels that he or she has lost control of the doctor-patient relationship.* Consultation can provide an opportunity for the doctor to express his or her feelings, as well as to obtain advice on how to proceed.

- *The physician is unsure whether a state of affairs is problematic.* For example, if a doctor suspects that a patient may be selling his or her medication on the street, or if the doctor is unsure about how to handle sensitive information disclosed by a patient during an office visit, a colleague can help sort out alternative ways of interpreting the behavior and help the physician select a proper course of action.

Refer the Patient

Referral is the best choice when the physician determines that the patient requires evaluation or intervention for a behavioral problem that is beyond his or her level of expertise to manage; it is often preceded by consultation. Referral is often indicated in cases where *psychiatric problems* or *substance abuse issues* lead to behavioral problems.

If the physician detects an untreated *psychiatric problem,* or if the patient's emotional problems are negatively affecting treatment of the headaches, referral to a mental health professional may be appropriate. Depressed patients, for instance, often respond poorly to medical interventions for their headaches unless the affective disorder is also treated. Similarly, an extremely anxious patient may respond better to headache medication if he or she receives concurrent relaxation training from a psychotherapist. A patient who appears psychotic (experiencing hallucinations and/or delusional thinking) or manic (pressured speech, flight of ideas, decreased need for sleep) also needs to be evaluated by a psychologist or psychiatrist. The primary care physician should develop a list of mental health professionals (including some psychologists who specialize in headache management) so that referrals can be made expeditiously.

A patient who expresses suicidal ideation during an office visit presents a particularly complicated dilemma for the primary care physician. What does a patient really mean when he or she says, "My headache was so bad last night I felt like blowing my brains out"? Is the patient serious or just being dramatic? Although most of these statements do not indicate any real threat of self-harm, any mention of suicide should be taken seriously and followed up with further probes. For instance:

Patient. These headaches are really getting to me. This is no way to live! I'd be better off dead!

Doctor. Are you seriously considering trying to kill yourself?

Patient. Well, I'd never really kill myself or anything, but sometimes I think these headaches will only stop when I'm dead.

Doctor. Are you saying you're *not* thinking of hurting yourself?

Patient. Oh, I'm not suicidal, Doctor. I'm just getting really depressed about these headaches.

For this patient, the expression of suicidal ideation was a way of communicating how depressed and hopeless he or she was feeling, but the patient does not appear to be at risk for suicide at this point. Referral to a psychologist or psychiatrist, however, is *probably* indicated to address the depression.

The following example presents another possible scenario:

Patient. Last night I had this killer migraine, and when I was taking my meds I thought "What's the use?" and I almost took the whole bottle.

Doctor. Are you saying you were thinking about overdosing—you know, killing yourself?

Patient. Yeah, I think about it every day. Sometimes I get out my pills and just stare at them and wonder what would happen if I took them all at one time . . . if I might just go to sleep and never wake up . . . never have to suffer through another migraine.

Doctor. Have you ever actually done anything like that?

Patient. No. I think about it a lot, but I don't think I'd ever go through with it. I've got kids. And I'm too much of a chicken.

Doctor. It sounds as if you're getting really depressed about all this. I'm concerned that you're having these types of thoughts. They're a sign that your depression is serious and needs to be addressed . . . Listen, I have a colleague, a psychologist who sees lots of people with chronic headaches like yours. Would you be willing to talk to him? He can teach you some better ways to cope with the pain.

Patient. I'm not crazy . . . I just have migraines!

Doctor. Of course you're not crazy, but living with migraines is hard. Dr Smith can help you learn to cope with them better and to feel less depressed. What do you think? I've referred a number of my patients to him and they've told me he helped them out.

Patient. Well, I guess I could give it a try if you're sure it will help.

This individual's suicidal ideation is more serious, but the patient denies that he or she intends to act upon the thoughts at any time in the immediate future. Referral for evaluation and treatment by a mental health professional is *definitely* indicated.

Another example illustrates a third possible development:

Patient. That's it! Nothing works. It's hopeless. I can't live like this . . . [Begins to sob]

Doctor. It sounds as though you're feeling extremely depressed.

Patient. It's way beyond depressed, Doctor. I'm scared. Last night I took out my ex-husband's gun and stared at it for hours, wondering if I had the guts to shoot myself. I don't know if I've got it in me to resist next time. Maybe soon . . .

Doctor. Is the gun still in the house?

Patient. I loaded it last night. Yeah, it's there.

Doctor. I'm really concerned for your safety. In your present state of mind I don't think it's a good idea for you to be at home alone right now. Let's have you seen over at the hospital. They know how to help people who are feeling despondent and thinking about hurting themselves.

Patient. I don't want to be locked up in the psycho ward!

Doctor. Well, they may decide that a few days in the hospital could be of help, but that's not the only option. But even if they do admit you, it won't be to the psycho ward. I just want to have someone evaluate the situation and make sure you are safe to be alone. I'll ask my receptionist to arrange a ride for you.

This individual appears to be in serious danger of hurting herself. The patient has significant, persistent suicidal ideation, a plan, readily available means to commit the act, and feelings of despondency, helplessness, and hopelessness. In this case, the physician wisely treated the matter as *urgent* and arranged to have the patient seen by specialists at a nearby emergency department for evaluation and possible inpatient psychiatric care.

Referral is also often called for when a physician determines that a headache patient has a problem with *substance abuse.* The first section of this chapter listed some behaviors the doctor should note in determining whether a patient is misusing or abusing prescription medications. It may be harder to detect whether a patient is abusing alcohol or street drugs. Patients tend to under-report their alcohol and drug use to their doctors; a patient who reports consuming "a glass or two of wine in the evening" may actually be drinking twice that amount. The "symptom amplification" technique of interviewing, discussed earlier, can help tease out problematic alcohol use patterns. Illegal drug use can be spotted using behavioral observation (noting dilated pupils, needle marks, agitation), urine drug screens, and reports from significant others.

Headache patients who are abusing alcohol, prescription medications, or illegal drugs should always be referred to substance abuse professionals or programs. These include

- Inpatient/outpatient detoxification programs
- Drug/alcohol rehabilitation programs
- Twelve-step recovery programs (e.g., Alcoholics Anonymous)
- Outpatient drug/alcohol counselors
- Multidisciplinary chronic pain management programs

Again, it is helpful to have a list of resources available, along with addresses and telephone numbers, so that referrals can be made quickly and easily.

Essential to the success of substance abuse referrals is willingness on the part of the patient to acknowledge that there is a problem. If the patient refuses the referral, he or she may be in denial about the drug or alcohol problem. Nevertheless, it is important for the primary care physician to render an opinion on the matter and recommend treatment if it appears to be indicated. Some leverage can be gained by making further treatment of the headaches contingent upon the patient's participation in a substance abuse program of some type. (Treatment contracts, discussed earlier, are helpful in these situations.) The doctor always has the option of refusing to prescribe drugs for a patient who is believed to be abusing substances and, if the patient continues to refuse to confront the substance abuse problem, the doctor may decide to terminate the relationship altogether.

Assemble a Multidisciplinary Team

The team approach, frequently used in hospitals and clinics, has been shown to be extremely effective in helping patients with chronic intractable headaches manage their pain more effectively. A pared-down version of this approach can help the primary care physician treat his or her most challenging and difficult headache patients more successfully in the office setting. Depending on the particular needs of the patient, the team might consist of the following specialists in addition to the PCP, the patient, and any significant other(s):

- Neurologist
- Dentist
- Physiatrist
- Psychologist
- Psychiatrist
- Physical therapist
- Occupational therapist
- Substance abuse professional
- Nutritionist
- Vocational counselor

For example, a patient with chronic daily headaches who is also significantly depressed may respond positively to a team made up of the primary care physician, a neurologist, a psychologist or psychiatrist who specializes in pain management, and possibly a physical therapist to help devise and implement an exercise and physical reconditioning program. A patient with migraines who has been abusing alcohol and has significant marital problems might be more effectively treated by a team consisting of the PCP, a substance abuse counselor, and a marriage counselor, each of whose treatment is enhanced by consultation with the other members of the team. Collaboration can be done by telephone, e-mail, or face-to-face-meetings, although conference calls and e-mail are the most practicable ways for the team members to communicate. Including family members as part of the team improves the reliability of the patient's self-reports and usually enhances compliance with treatment recommendations. This is also an excellent way for the primary care physician to ascertain whether family members are enabling some of the patient's unhealthy coping behaviors. The enabling behavior can then be addressed so that healthier and more effective coping behaviors are encouraged and reinforced at home.

Key Points

- *Understand the factors that can contribute to difficulties.* Behavior problems can result from comorbid psychiatric or substance abuse issues, previous traumatic experiences with pain, stress, or personality conflicts.

- *Identify challenging patients early.* Potential problems can be spotted during office visits by being alert to key behavioral cues.

- *Learn techniques that will help manage difficult patients successfully.* Simple behavior management skills are easily learned and very effective.

- *Seek help with the most difficult patients and situations.* Know when to obtain consultation, refer the patient, or assemble a multidisciplinary team.

REFERENCES

1. **Breslau N, Merikangas K, Bowden CL.** Comorbidity of migraine and major affective disorders. Neurology. 1994;44(Suppl 7):S17-S22.

2. **Breslau N, Schultz LR, Stewart WF, et al.** Headache and major depression: is the association specific to migraine? Neurology. 2000;54:308-13.

3. **Guidetti V, Galli F, Fabrizi P, et al.** Headache and psychiatric comorbidity: clinical aspects and outcome in an 8-year follow-up study. Cephalalgia. 1998;18:455-62.

4. **Breslau N, Davis GC.** Migraine, physical health and psychiatric disorder: a prospective epidemiologic study in young adults. J Psychiatr Res. 1993;27:211-21.

5. **Siniatchkin M, Riabus M, Hasenbring M.** Coping styles of headache sufferers. Cephalalgia. 1999;19:165-73.

6. **Holroyd KA, Martin PR.** Psychological treatments of tension-type headache. In: Olesen J, Tfelt-Hansen P, Welch KMA, eds. The Headaches. Philadelphia: Lippincott Williams and Wilkins; 2000:643-50.

7. **Spitzer AL, Williams JBW, Kroenke K, et al.** Utility of a new procedure for diagnosing mental disorders in primary care: the PRIME- MD 1000 study. JAMA. 1994; 272:1749-56.

8. **Hegarty AM.** The prevalence of migraine in borderline personality disorder. Headache. 1993;33:271.

9. **Passchier J.** A critical note on psychophysiological stress research into migraine patients. Cephalalgia. 1994;14:194-8.

10. **Holm JE, Holroyd KA, Hursey KG, Penzien DB.** The role of stress in recurrent tension headache. Headache. 1986;26:160-7.

11. **Geisser ME, Robinson ME, Keefe FJ, Weiner, ML.** Catastrophizing, depression, and the sensory, affective and evaluative aspects of chronic pain. Pain. 1994;59:79-83.

12. **Martin PR, Milech D, Nathan PR.** Towards a functional model of chronic headaches: investigation of antecedents and consequences. Headache. 1993;33:461-70.

13. **Scharff L, Turk DC, Marcus, DA.** Triggers of headache episodes and coping responses of headache diagnostic groups. Headache. 1995;35:397-403.

14. **Scharff L, Turk DC, Marcus DA.** Psychosocial and behavioural characteristics in chronic headache patients: support for a continuum and dual-diagnostic approach. Cephalalgia. 1995;15:216-23.

15. **Merikangas KR, Stevens DE.** Comorbidity of migraine and psychiatric disorders. Neurologic Clin. 1997;15:115-23.

16. **Groves JE.** Taking care of the hateful patient. N Engl J Med. 1978;298:883-7.

17. **Dalessio DJ.** Headache games: dealing with the difficult headache patient. Headache Q. 1993;4:240-4.

18. **Pomeroy WB, Flax CC, Wheeler CC.** Taking a Sex History. New York: Free Press; 1982.

19. **Shea SC.** Psychiatric Interviewing: The Art of Understanding. Philadelphia: WB Saunders; 1988.

20. **Covey SP.** The Seven Habits of Highly Effective People. New York: Fireside; 1990.

APPENDIX I

■ ■ ■

International Headache Society (IHS) 2004 Diagnostic Classification

IHS ICHD-II Code	WHO ICD-10NA Code	Diagnosis [and aetiological ICD-10 code for secondary headache disorders]
1.	**[G43]**	**Migraine**
1.1	[G43.0]	Migraine without aura
1.2	[G43.1]	Migraine with aura
1.2.1	[G43.10]	Typical aura with migraine headache
1.2.2	[G43.10]	Typical aura with non-migraine headache
1.2.3	[G43.104]	Typical aura without headache
1.2.4	[G43.105]	Familial hemiplegic migraine (FHM)
1.2.5	[G43.105]	Sporadic hemiplegic migraine
1.2.6	[G43.103]	Basilar-type migraine
1.3	[G43.82]	Childhood periodic syndromes that are commonly precursors of migraine
1.3.1	[G43.82]	Cyclical vomiting
1.3.2	[G43.820]	Abdominal migraine
1.3.3	[G43.821]	Benign paroxysmal vertigo of childhood
1.4	[G43.81]	Retinal migraine
1.5	[G43.3]	Complications of migraine
1.5.1	[G43.3]	Chronic migraine
1.5.2	[G43.2]	Status migrainosus
1.5.3	[G43.3]	Persistent aura without infarction
1.5.4	[G43.3]	Migrainous infarction
1.5.5	[G43.3] + [G40.x or G41.x]*	Migraine-triggered seizures

(Cont'd)

IHS ICHD-II Code	WHO ICD-10NA Code	Diagnosis [and aetiological ICD-10 code for secondary headache disorders]
1.6	[G43.83]	Probable migraine
1.6.1	[G43.83]	Probable migraine without aura
1.6.2	[G43.83]	Probable migraine with aura
1.6.5	[G43.83]	Probable chronic migraine
2.	**[G44.2]**	**Tension-type headache (TTH)**
2.1	[G44.2]	Infrequent episodic tension-type headache
2.1.1	[G44.20]	Infrequent episodic tension-type headache associated with pericranial tenderness
2.1.2	[G44.21]	Infrequent episodic tension-type headache not associated with pericranial tenderness
2.2	[G44.2]	Frequent episodic tension-type headache
2.2.1	[G44.20]	Frequent episodic tension-type headache associated with pericranial tenderness
2.2.2	[G44.21]	Frequent episodic tension-type headache not associated with pericranial tenderness
2.3	[G44.2]	Chronic tension-type headache
2.3.1	[G44.22]	Chronic tension-type headache associated with pericranial tenderness
2.3.2	[G44.23]	Chronic tension-type headache not associated with pericranial tenderness
2.4	[G44.28]	Probable tension-type headache
2.4.1	[G44.28]	Probable infrequent episodic tension-type headache
2.4.2	[G44.28]	Probable frequent episodic tension-type headache
2.4.3	[G44.28]	Probable chronic tension-type headache
3.	**[G44.0]**	**Cluster headache and other trigeminal autonomic cephalalgias**
3.1	[G44.0]	Cluster headache
3.1.1	[G44.01]	Episodic cluster headache
3.1.2	[G44.02]	Chronic cluster headache
3.2	[G44.03]	Paroxysmal hemicrania
3.2.1	[G44.03]	Episodic paroxysmal hemicrania
3.2.2	[G44.03]	Chronic paroxysmal hemicrania (CPH)

(Cont'd)

IHS ICHD-II Code	WHO ICD-10NA Code	Diagnosis [and aetiological ICD-10 code for secondary headache disorders]
3.3	[G44.08]	Short-lasting unilateral neuralgiform headache attacks with conjunctival injection and tearing (SUNCT)
3.4	[G44.08]	Probable trigeminal autonomic cephalalgia
3.4.1	[G44.08]	Probable cluster headache
3.4.2	[G44.08]	Probable paroxysmal hemicrania
3.4.3	[G44.08]	Probable SUNCT
4.	**[G44.80]**	**Other primary headaches**
4.1	[G44.800]	Primary stabbing headache
4.2	[G44.803]	Primary cough headache
4.3	[G44.804]	Primary exertional headache
4.4	[G44.805]	Primary headache associated with sexual activity
4.4.1	[G44.805]	Preorgasmic headache
4.4.2	[G44.805]	Orgasmic headache
4.5	[G44.80]	Hypnic headache
4.6	[G44.80]	Primary thunderclap headache
4.7	[G44.80]	Hemicrania continua
4.8	[G44.2]	New daily-persistent headache (NDPH)
5.	**[G44.88]**	**Headache attributed to head and/or neck trauma**
5.1	[G44.880]	Acute post-traumatic headache
5.1.1	[G44.880]	Acute post-traumatic headache attributed to moderate or severe head injury [S06]
5.1.2	[G44.880]	Acute post-traumatic headache attributed to mild head injury [S09.9]
5.2	[G44.3]	Chronic post-traumatic headache
5.2.1	[G44.30]	Chronic post-traumatic headache attributed to moderate or severe head injury [S06]
5.2.2	[G44.31]	Chronic post-traumatic headache attributed to mild head injury [S09.9]
5.3	[G44.841]	Acute headache attributed to whiplash injury [S13.4]
5.4	[G44.841]	Chronic headache attributed to whiplash injury [S13.4]
5.5	[G44.88]	Headache attributed to traumatic intracranial haematoma
5.5.1	[G44.88]	Headache attributed to epidural haematoma [S06.4]

(Cont'd)

IHS ICHD-II Code	WHO ICD-10NA Code	Diagnosis [and aetiological ICD-10 code for secondary headache disorders]
5.5.2	[G44.88]	Headache attributed to subdural haematoma [S06.5]
5.6	[G44.88]	Headache attributed to other head and/or neck trauma [S06]
5.6.1	[G44.88]	Acute headache attributed to other head and/or neck trauma [S06]
5.6.2	[G44.88]	Chronic headache attributed to other head and/or neck trauma [S06]
5.7	[G44.88]	Post-craniotomy headache
5.7.1	[G44.880]	Acute post-craniotomy headache
5.7.2	[G44.30]	Chronic post-craniotomy headache
6.	**[G44.81]**	**Headache attributed to cranial or cervical vascular disorder**
6.1	[G44.810]	Headache attributed to ischaemic stroke or transient ischaemic attack
6.1.1	[G44.810]	Headache attributed to ischaemic stroke (cerebral infarction) [I63]
6.1.2	[G44.810]	Headache attributed to transient ischaemic attack (TIA) [G45]
6.2	[G44.810]	Headache attributed to non-traumatic intracranial haemorrhage [I62]
6.2.1	[G44.810]	Headache attributed to intracerebral haemorrhage [I61]
6.2.2	[G44.810]	Headache attributed to subarachnoid haemorrhage (SAH) [I60]
6.3	[G44.811]	Headache attributed to unruptured vascular malformation [Q28]
6.3.1	[G44.811]	Headache attributed to saccular aneurysm [Q28.3]
6.3.2	[G44.811]	Headache attributed to arteriovenous malformation (AVM) [Q28.2]
6.3.3	[G44.811]	Headache attributed to dural arteriovenous fistula [I67.1]
6.3.4	[G44.811]	Headache attributed to cavernous angioma [D18.0]
6.3.5	[G44.811]	Headache attributed to encephalotrigeminal or leptomeningeal angiomatosis (Sturge-Weber syndrome) [Q85.8]
6.4	[G44.812]	Headache attributed to arteritis [M31]

(Cont'd)

IHS ICHD-II Code	WHO ICD-10NA Code	Diagnosis [and aetiological ICD-10 code for secondary headache disorders]
6.4.1	[G44.812]	Headache attributed to giant cell arteritis (GCA) [M31.6]
6.4.2	[G44.812]	Headache attributed to primary central nervous system (CNS) angiitis [I67.7]
6.4.3	[G44.812]	Headache attributed to secondary central nervous system (CNS) angiitis [I68.2]
6.5	[G44.810]	Carotid or vertebral artery pain [I63.0, I63.2, I65.0, I65.2 or I67.0]
6.5.1	[G44.810]	Headache or facial or neck pain attributed to arterial dissection [I67.0]
6.5.2	[G44.814]	Post-endarterectomy headache [I97.8]
6.5.3	[G44.810]	Carotid angioplasty headache
6.5.4	[G44.810]	Headache attributed to intracranial endovascular procedures
6.5.5	[G44.810]	Angiography headache
6.6	[G44.810]	Headache attributed to cerebral venous thrombosis (CVT) [I63.6]
6.7	[G44.81]	Headache attributed to other intracranial vascular disorder
6.7.1	[G44.81]	Cerebral Autosomal Dominant Arteriopathy with Subcortical Infarcts and Leukoencephalopathy (CADASIL) [I67.8]
6.7.2	[G44.81]	Mitochondrial Encephalopathy, Lactic Acidosis and Sroke-like episodes (MELAS) [G31.81]
6.7.3	[G44.81]	Headache attributed to benign angiopathy of the central nervous system [I99]
6.7.4	[G44.81]	Headache attributed to pituitary apoplexy [E23.6]
7.	**[G44.82]**	**Headache attributed to non-vascular intracranial disorder**
7.1	[G44.820]	Headache attributed to high cerebrospinal fluid pressure
7.1.1	[G44.820]	Headache attributed to idiopathic intracranial hypertension (IIH) [G93.2]
7.1.2	[G44.820]	Headache attributed to intracranial hypertension secondary to metabolic, toxic or hormonal causes

(Cont'd)

IHS ICHD-II Code	WHO ICD-10NA Code	Diagnosis [and aetiological ICD-10 code for secondary headache disorders]
7.1.3	[G44.820]	Headache attributed to intracranial hypertension secondary to hydrocephalus [G91.8]
7.2	[G44.820]	Headache attributed to low cerebrospinal fluid pressure
7.2.1	[G44.820]	Post-dural puncture headache [G97.0]
7.2.2	[G44.820]	CSF fistula headache [G96.0]
7.2.3	[G44.820]	Headache attributed to spontaneous (or idiopathic) low CSF pressure
7.3	[G44.82]	Headache attributed to non-infectious inflammatory disease
7.3.1	[G44.823]	Headache attributed to neurosarcoidosis [D86.8]
7.3.2	[G44.823]	Headache attributed to aseptic (non-infectious) meningitis [code to specify aetiology]
7.3.3	[G44.823]	Headache attributed to other non-infectious inflammatory disease [code to specify aetiology]
7.3.4	[G44.82]	Headache attributed to lymphocytic hypophysitis [E23.6]
7.4	[G44.822]	Headache attributed to intracranial neoplasm [C00-D48]
7.4.1	[G44.822]	Headache attributed to increased intracranial pressure or hydrocephalus caused by neoplasm [code to specify neoplasm]
7.4.2	[G44.822]	Headache attributed directly to neoplasm [code to specify neoplasm]
7.4.3	[G44.822]	Headache attributed to carcinomatous meningitis [C79.3]
7.4.4	[G44.822]	Headache attributed to hypothalamic or pituitary hyper- or hyposecretion [E23.0]
7.5	[G44.824]	Headache attributed to intrathecal injection [G97.8]
7.6	[G44.82]	Headache attributed to epileptic seizure [G40.x or G41.x to specify seizure type]
7.6.1	[G44.82]	Hemicrania epileptica [G40.x or G41.x to specify seizure type]
7.6.2	[G44.82]	Post-seizure headache [G40.x or G41.x to specify seizure type]
7.7	[G44.82]	Headache attributed to Chiari malformation type I (CM1) [Q07.0]

(Cont'd)

IHS ICHD-II Code	WHO ICD-10NA Code	Diagnosis [and aetiological ICD-10 code for secondary headache disorders]
7.8	[G44.82]	Syndrome of transient Headache and Neurological Deficits with cerebrospinal fluid Lymphocytosis (HaNDL)
7.9	[G44.82]	Headache attributed to other non-vascular intracranial disorder
8.	**[G44.4 or G44.83]**	**Headache attributed to a substance† or its withdrawal**
8.1	[G44.40]	Headache induced by acute substance use or exposure
8.1.1	[G44.400]	Nitric oxide (NO) donor-induced headache [X44]
8.1.1.1	[G44.400]	Immediate NO donor-induced headache [X44]
8.1.1.2	[G44.400]	Delayed NO donor-headache [X44]
8.1.2	[G44.40]	Phosphodiesterase (PDE) inhibitor-induced headache [X44]
8.1.3	[G44.402]	Carbon monoxide-induced headache [X47]
8.1.4	[G44.83]	Alcohol-induced headache [F10]
8.1.4.1	[G44.83]	Immediate alcohol-induced headache [F10]
8.1.4.2	[G44.83]	Delayed alcohol-induced headache [F10]
8.1.5	[G44.4]	Headache induced by food components and additives
8.1.5.1	[G44.401]	Monosodium glutamate-induced headache [X44]
8.1.6	[G44.83]	Cocaine-induced headache [F14]
8.1.7	[G44.83]	Cannabis-induced headache [F12]
8.1.8	[G44.40]	Histamine-induced headache [X44]
8.1.8.1	[G44.40]	Immediate histamine-induced headache [X44]
8.1.8.2	[G44.40]	Delayed histamine-induced headache [X44]
8.1.9	[G44.40]	Calcitonin gene-related peptide (CGRP)-induced headache [X44]
8.1.9.1	[G44.40]	Immediate CGRP-induced headache [X44]
8.1.9.2	[G44.40]	Delayed CGRP-induced headache [X44]
8.1.10	[G44.41]	Headache as an acute adverse event attributed to medication used for other indications [code to specify substance]
8.1.11	[G44.4 or G44.83]	Headache attributed to other acute substance use or exposure [code to specify substance]

(Cont'd)

IHS ICHD-II Code	WHO ICD-10NA Code	Diagnosis [and aetiological ICD-10 code for secondary headache disorders]
8.2	[G44.41 or G44.83]	Medication-overuse headache (MOH)
8.2.1	[G44.411]	Ergotamine-overuse headache [Y52.5]
8.2.2	[G44.41]	Triptan-overuse headache
8.2.3	[G44.410]	Analgesic-overuse headache [F55.2]
8.2.4	[G44.83]	Opioid-overuse headache [F11.2]
8.2.5	[G44.410]	Combination medication-overuse headache [F55.2]
8.2.6	[G44.410]	Headache attributed to other medication overuse [code to specify substance]
8.2.7	[G44.41 or G44.83]	Probable medication-overuse headache [code to specify substance]
8.3	[G44.4]	Headache as an adverse event attributed to chronic medication [code to specify substance]
8.3.1	[G44.418]	Exogenous hormone-induced headache [Y42.4]
8.4	[G44.83]	Headache attributed to substance withdrawal
8.4.1	[G44.83]	Caffeine-withdrawal headache [F15.3]
8.4.2	[G44.83]	Opioid-withdrawal headache [F11.3]
8.4.3	[G44.83]	Oestrogen-withdrawal headache [Y42.4]
8.4.4	[G44.83]	Headache attributed to withdrawal from chronic use of other substances [code to specify substance]
9.		**Headache attributed to infection**
9.1	[G44.821]	Headache attributed to intracranial infection [G00-G09]
9.1.1	[G44.821]	Headache attributed to bacterial meningitis [G00.9]
9.1.2	[G44.821]	Headache attributed to lymphocytic meningitis [G03.9]
9.1.3	[G44.821]	Headache attributed to encephalitis [G04.9]
9.1.4	[G44.821]	Headache attributed to brain abscess [G06.0]
9.1.5	[G44.821]	Headache attributed to subdural empyema [G06.2]
9.2	[G44.881]	Headache attributed to systemic infection [A00-B97]
9.2.1	[G44.881]	Headache attributed to systemic bacterial infection [code to specify aetiology]
9.2.2	[G44.881]	Headache attributed to systemic viral infection [code to specify aetiology]

(Cont'd)

IHS ICHD-II Code	WHO ICD-10NA Code	Diagnosis [and aetiological ICD-10 code for secondary headache disorders]
9.2.3	[G44.881]	Headache attributed to other systemic infection [code to specify aetiology]
9.3	[G44.821]	Headache attributed to HIV/AIDS [B22]
9.4	[G44.821 or G44.881]	Chronic post-infection headache [code to specify aetiology]
9.4.1	[G44.821]	Chronic post-bacterial meningitis headache [G00.9]
10.	**[G44.882]**	**Headache attributed to disorder of homoeostasis**
10.1	[G44.882]	Headache attributed to hypoxia and/or hypercapnia
10.1.1	[G44.882]	High-altitude headache [W94]
10.1.2	[G44.882]	Diving headache
10.1.3	[G44.882]	Sleep apnoea headache [G47.3]
10.2	[G44.882]	Dialysis headache [Y84.1]
10.3	[G44.813]	Headache attributed to arterial hypertension [I10]
10.3.1	[G44.813]	Headache attributed to phaeochromocytoma [D35.0 (benign) or C74.1 (malignant)]
10.3.2	[G44.813]	Headache attributed to hypertensive crisis without hypertensive encephalopathy [I10]
10.3.3	[G44.813]	Headache attributed to hypertensive encephalopathy [I67.4]
10.3.4	[G44.813]	Headache attributed to preeclampsia [O13-O14]
10.3.5	[G44.813]	Headache attributed to eclampsia [O15]
10.3.6	[G44.813]	Headache attributed to acute pressor response to an exogenous agent [code to specify aetiology]
10.4	[G44.882]	Headache attributed to hypothyroidism [E03.9]
10.5	[G44.882]	Headache attributed to fasting [T73.0]
10.6	[G44.882]	Cardiac cephalalgia [code to specify aetiology]
10.7	[G44.882]	Headache attributed to other disorder of homoeostasis [code to specify aetiology]
11.	**[G44.84]**	**Headache or facial pain attributed to disorder of cranium, neck, eyes, ears, nose, sinuses, teeth, mouth or other facial or cranial structures**
11.1	[G44.840]	Headache attributed to disorder of cranial bone [M80-M89.8]

(Cont'd)

IHS ICHD-II Code	WHO ICD-10NA Code	Diagnosis [and aetiological ICD-10 code for secondary headache disorders]
11.2	[G44.841]	Headache attributed to disorder of neck [M99]
11.2.1	[G44.841]	Cervicogenic headache [M99]
11.2.2	[G44.842]	Headache attributed to retropharyngeal tendonitis [M79.8]
11.2.3	[G44.841]	Headache attributed to craniocervical dystonia [G24]
11.3	[G44.843]	Headache attributed to disorder of eyes
11.3.1	[G44.843]	Headache attributed to acute glaucoma [H40]
11.3.2	[G44.843]	Headache attributed to refractive errors [H52]
11.3.3	[G44.843]	Headache attributed to heterophoria or heterotropia (latent or manifest squint) [H50.3-H50.5]
11.3.4	[G44.843]	Headache attributed to ocular inflammatory disorder [code to specify aetiology]
11.4	[G44.844]	Headache attributed to disorder of ears [H60-H95]
11.5	[G44.845]	Headache attributed to rhinosinusitis [J01]
11.6	[G44.846]	Headache attributed to disorder of teeth, jaws or related structures [K00-K14]
11.7	[G44.846]	Headache or facial pain attributed to temporomandibular joint (TMJ) disorder [K07.6]
11.8	[G44.84]	Headache attributed to other disorder of cranium, neck, eyes, ears, nose, sinuses, teeth, mouth or other facial or cervical structures [code to specify aetiology]
12.	**[R51]**	**Headache attributed to psychiatric disorder**
12.1	[R51]	Headache attributed to somatisation disorder [F45.0]
12.2	[R51]	Headache attributed to psychotic disorder [code to specify aetiology]
13.	**[G44.847, G44.848 or G44.85]**	**Cranial neuralgias and central causes of facial pain**
13.1	[G44.847]	Trigeminal neuralgia
13.1.1	[G44.847]	Classical trigeminal neuralgia [G50.00]
13.1.2	[G44.847]	Symptomatic trigeminal neuralgia [G53.80] + [code to specify aetiology]
13.2	[G44.847]	Glossopharyngeal neuralgia

(Cont'd)

IHS ICHD-II Code	WHO ICD-10NA Code	Diagnosis [and aetiological ICD-10 code for secondary headache disorders]
13.2.1	[G44.847]	Classical glossopharyngeal neuralgia [G52.10]
13.2.2	[G44.847]	Symptomatic glossopharyngeal neuralgia [G53.830] + [code to specify aetiology]
13.3	[G44.847]	Nervus intermedius neuralgia [G51.80]
13.4	[G44.847]	Superior laryngeal neuralgia [G52.20]
13.5	[G44.847]	Nasociliary neuralgia [G52.80]
13.6	[G44.847]	Supraorbital neuralgia [G52.80]
13.7	[G44.847]	Other terminal branch neuralgias [G52.80]
13.8	[G44.847]	Occipital neuralgia [G52.80]
13.9	[G44.851]	Neck-tongue syndrome
13.10	[G44.801]	External compression headache
13.11	[G44.802]	Cold-stimulus headache
13.11.1	[G44.8020]	Headache attributed to external application of a cold stimulus
13.11.2	[G44.8021]	Headache attributed to ingestion or inhalation of a cold stimulus
13.12	[G44.848]	Constant pain caused by compression, irritation or distortion of cranial nerves or upper cervical roots by structural lesions [G53.8] + [code to specify aetiology]
13.13	[G44.848]	Optic neuritis [H46]
13.14	[G44.848]	Ocular diabetic neuropathy [E10-E14]
13.15	[G44.881 or G44.847]	Head or facial pain attributed to herpes zoster
13.15.1	[G44.881]	Head or facial pain attributed to acute herpes zoster [B02.2]
13.15.2	[G44.847]	Post-herpetic neuralgia [B02.2]
13.16	[G44.850]	Tolosa-Hunt syndrome
13.17	[G43.80]	Ophthalmoplegic "migraine"
13.18	[G44.810 or G44.847]	Central causes of facial pain
13.18.1	[G44.847]	Anaesthesia dolorosa [G52.800] + [code to specify aetiology]
13.18.2	[G44.810]	Central post-stroke pain [G46.21]

(Cont'd)

IHS ICHD-II Code	WHO ICD-10NA Code	Diagnosis [and aetiological ICD-10 code for secondary headache disorders]
13.18.3	[G44.847]	Facial pain attributed to multiple sclerosis [G35]
13.18.4	[G44.847]	Persistent idiopathic facial pain [G50.1]
13.18.5	[G44.847]	Burning mouth syndrome [code to specify aetiology]
13.19	[G44.847]	Other cranial neuralgia or other centrally mediated facial pain [code to specify aetiology]
14.	**[R51]**	**Other headache, cranial neuralgia, central or primary facial pain**
14.1	[R51]	Headache not elsewhere classified
14.2	[R51]	Headache unspecified

From International Headache Society. The International Classification of Headache Disorders, 2nd ed. Cephalalgia. 2004;24(Suppl 1):9-160; with permission.
*The additional code specifies the type of seizure.
†In ICD-10 substances are classified according to the presence or absence of a dependence-producing property. Headaches associated with psychoactive substances (dependence-producing) are classified in G44.83 with an additional code to indicate the nature of the disorder related to the substance use – e.g., intoxication (F1x.0), dependence (F1x.2), withdrawal (F1x.3). The 3rd character can be used to indicate the specific substance involved – e.g., F10 for alcohol, F15 for caffeine. Abuse of non-dependence-producing substances is classified in F55, with a 4th character to indicate the substance – e.g., F55.2 abuse of analgesics. Headaches related to non-dependence-producing substances are classified in G44.4.

APPENDIX II

Resources and Recommended Reading

Susan Hutchinson, MD

Headache Calendars and Diaries

An accurate record of headache frequency, severity, and treatment is useful in assessing treatment needs and response. A variety of headache calendars and diaries have been devised. Of course, headache calendars are only helpful if patients use them, bring them to appointments, and review them with the physician when discussing treatment decisions. Several important points should be kept in mind:

- Choose a diary that is appropriate for the patient who is keeping it. The simplest diary that provides the needed information is best.
- Overly detailed calendars or diaries may only increase patient anxiety and attention to pain or environmental factors, without providing useful information.
- Review the headache calendar during the patient visit; doing so reinforces for the patient the importance of this tool and her role in keeping the diary.

For stable patients, any personal calendar can be used. Patients are asked to make a daily record of maximal pain intensity using a 0–10 scale. For example, if the patient has no headache, the number zero would be entered onto the calendar. If the patient awakes with a 9/10 headache that subsequently improves to 1/10 with treatment, the number nine would be entered. Patients can make notes about unusual headache features or treatment response if desired.

This method has the advantage of simplicity and ease of use and thus increases patient compliance. It provides information about frequency and maximum severity that are adequate for determining treatment decisions. Disadvantages are the loss of detail about individual attack and treatment response characteristics.

For new patients or those whose headache characteristics, triggers, and treatment response require detailed monitoring, consider the use of one of many published headache calendars. Many of these are provided by pharmaceutical companies or are available on professional society Web sites such as that of the American Headache Society (www.ahsnet.org) or the National Headache Foundation (www.headaches.org). Several sample calendars are reproduced in Appendix III.

These calendars are free, generally professionally produced, and provide extensive information about headache characteristics, triggers, and treatment response. Disadvantages exist, however. There may be inappropriate commercial bias in calendars obtained from pharmaceutical sources, especially if they are accompanied by promotional literature. Detailed calendars may encourage over-attention to details of everyday life, such as diet; some contain inaccurate information about headache causes or triggers. Furthermore, the complexity and time required to use the calendar may decrease compliance.

For patients with unusual or frequent headaches, such as cluster headache or idiopathic stabbing headache, specialized diaries may be needed that allow recording of multiple headache attacks in one day.

Assessing Disability

Patients with many other diseases are routinely monitored to detect the development of complications. In headache, a major complication in patients with severe pain is the development of personal, social, and occupational disability. A variety of scales exist that give quick, objective, and reliable measures of disability status. Disability assessment is useful in guiding treatment decisions (the more disabled patients need the more intense treatment and therefore benefit from higher-end medications). In addition, disability measures can be helpful in judging the effect of treatment. Consider using one of the following scales to assess and monitor disability in headache patients:

- The *Headache Impact Test (HIT-6)* was developed by Glaxo-SmithKline and QualityMetric. It consists of six questions answered by the patient to determine a total score. The higher the score, the more impact the headaches are having on that patient. HIT-6 can be accessed at www.headachetest.com; it is also available as a tear-off sheet. HIT-6 is reproduced in Appendix IV.

- The *Migraine Disability Assessment Scale (MIDAS)* was developed by AstraZeneca and Innovative Medical Research. It consists of five questions answered by the patient to determine a total score. The higher the score, the greater is the disability. MIDAS helps to assess disability of headache and provides a number that can be followed to monitor over a number of visits. MIDAS provides a more objective measure of treatment response than HIT-6 because it is based on functional impairment rather than the subjective symptom of pain. There are no copyright restrictions on the use of this instrument; AstraZeneca has generously released this to the public domain. MIDAS is reproduced in Appendix V. See also www.migraine-disability.net.

Resources

Patient Resources

American Council for Headache Education
19 Mantua Road
Mount Royal, NJ 08061
(856) 423-0258 (telephone)
(856) 423-0082 (fax)
www.achenet.org
achehq@talley.com

The *American Council for Headache Education* (ACHE) is a not-for-profit alliance of headache sufferers and physicians working together to improve quality of care and information for people with headache conditions. ACHE publishes brochures and a quarterly 12-page newsletter, maintains a Web site with an "Ask the Doctor" question board featuring answers from leading headache experts, and provides support groups; $20/year membership fee.

National Headache Foundation
428 West St. James Place, 2nd Floor
Chicago, IL 60614-2750
(888) NHF-5552
www.headaches.org

The *National Headache Foundation* (NHF) is a not-for-profit organization dedicated to providing education about headache to professionals and patients and to promoting research into headache causes and treatments. NHF publishes a bimonthly newsletter, has a library of headache resource materials including books and brochures, and provides support groups in many areas of the country; $20/year membership fee. (NHF resources for physicians are discussed below.)

Other non-commercial Web sites that provide reliable headache information include

1. www.amihealthy.com
2. www.connect2health.com
3. www.headachecare.com
4. www.headachequiz.com
5. www.migrainehelp.com
6. www.webMD.com

All of the above Web sites offer excellent educational information for the headache patient; many offer links to other sites. Familiarize yourself with them; pick your favorites. Tell your patients about them, and let these sites help you with the work of educating patients.

Physician Resources

American Headache Society

19 Mantua Road
Mount Royal, NJ 08061
(856) 423-0043
Ahsq@talley.com
www.ahsnet.org

The *American Headache Society* (AHS) is a professional society of health care providers dedicated to the study and treatment of headache and face pain. AHS publishes a scientific peer-reviewed journal, *Headache,* and holds one scientific and two educational symposia every year, including programs specifically geared for primary care providers. AHS has recently launched a large-scale Primary Care Migraine Partnership program to provide resources to primary care physicians. AHS also supervises the acclaimed Neurology Ambassadors Program, which provides one-day courses throughout the country aimed at teaching headache diagnosis and treatment.

National Headache Foundation

428 West St. James Place, 2nd Floor
Chicago, IL 60614-2750
(888) NHF-5552
www.headaches.org

Besides being a resource for patients, NHF provides educational and scientific materials for health care providers, including an extensive collection of brochures, books, and tapes. NHF sponsors two yearly educational continuing medical education (CME) programs for clinicians on headache management.

Primary Care Network
1230 E. Kingsley Street
Springfield, MO 65804
(417) 886-2026
www.primarycarenet.org

The *Primary Care Network* (PCN) is a non-profit organization of over 9000 health care providers. Those with a special interest in the management of headache can attend a relevant course (typically 4 to 8 hours), and there are other CME headache-related programs.

The AHS, NHF, and PCN all provide CME programs at low or no charge for clinicians wanting to learn more about headaches. These organizations also provide a way to meet other clinicians who are interested in headache and provide forums for research and scientific presentations.

Recommended Reading

Books for Patients

- **Conquering Headache.** Alan Rappaport, Fred Sheftell, and Stewart Tepper. Ontario: Empowering Press, 2001; 122 pages. *Written for the headache patient but also a great book for the primary care physician. Superb overview.*

- **Conquering Your Migraine.** Seymour Diamond, with Mary A. Franklin. New York: Simon and Schuster, 2001; 223 pages. *Designed to help migraine sufferers and their families better understand and treat migraines. Excellent book.*

Books for Health Care Professionals

Many excellent textbooks on headache exist. The following are a representative sample, chosen for usefulness and appeal to a primary care physician who does not have a special interest in headache. In addition to textbooks, physicians developing an interest in headache are urged to examine the two specialty journals: *Headache* and *Cephalalgia*.

- **Headache in Clinical Practice.** SD Silberstein, RB Lipton, PJ Goadsby, eds. Oxford: Isis Medical Media; 1998.

- **Mechanism and Management of Headache, 6th ed.** JW Lance, PJ Goadsby, eds. Oxford: Butterworth-Heinemann; 1998. *Concise textbook for the busy primary care physician. Useful reference in the office setting.*

- **Migraine: The Complete Guide.** American Council for Headache Education, with Lynn M. Constantine and Suzanne Scott. New York: Dell Publishing; 1994; 289 pages. *An excellent source of information and support for the migraine sufferer. Its major drawback is that it does not have information on the newer migraine medications.*

For those who want more detailed information, we recommend

- **Wolff's Headache and Other Head Pain, 7th ed.** Stephen D. Silberstein, Richard B. Lipton, and Donald J. Dalessio, eds. New York: Oxford University Press; 625 pages w/illustrations; 2001. *The most authoritative and exhaustive compendium, written by leading headache experts. Surprisingly readable, yet detailed and with valuable clinical "pearls". The place to find information on esoteric or uncommon headache presentations and thorough coverage of the primary headache disorders.*

APPENDIX III

■ ■ ■

Headache Calendars and Diaries

Headache Calendar							
Date & Time (start to finish)	Intensity Scale of 1-5[1]	Disability Scale of 0-3[2]	Preceding Symptoms	Triggers[3]	Menstrual Period[4]	Medi- cation and Dosage	Relief – complete – moderate – none

Courtesy of National Headache Foundation.

[1] Intensity: 1 = least severe; 5 = most severe.

[2] Disability: 0 = no effect on daily activities; 1 = able to carry out activities fairly well; 2 = difficulty with usual activities, canceled less important ones; 3 = missed work or stayed in bed part of day.

[3] Triggers: Record the numbrs of the triggers you may have been exposed to.

[4] Menstrual periods: Place an X on the days you have your period or write the day of your cycle if you know it. You can also mark the number for menses (12) in the trigger box.

Headache Diary						
Date and Time of Headache	Impact: - none - mild - severe - totally disabled	Headache Intensity: - mild - moderate - severe - very severe	Medication Taken	Dosage	Time to Relief	Triggers

Courtesy of American Council for Headache Education.

Headache Diary

Date of Attack:

Level of Pain:
☐ mild
☐ moderate
☐ severe

Duration of Pain Before
   Medication (in hours) :_____

Location of Pain:
☐ one sided: ☐ L   ☐ R
☐ both sides
☐ other _____

Type of Pain:
☐ throbbing
☐ dull
☐ other

Other Symptoms:
☐ nausea
☐ vomiting
☐ sensitivity to light, sound, smell
☐ loss of appetite
☐ visual disturbance
☐ other

Aura:
☐ yes   ☐ no

Potential Triggers:
_____
_____
_____
_____
_____

Medication Taken	Relief?	Time to Relief	Satisfied?
1. _____	☐ yes ☐ no	_____ hours(s)	☐ yes ☐ no
2. _____	☐ yes ☐ no	_____ hours(s)	☐ yes ☐ no
3. _____	☐ yes ☐ no	_____ hours(s)	☐ yes ☐ no
4. _____	☐ yes ☐ no	_____ hours(s)	☐ yes ☐ no
5. _____	☐ yes ☐ no	_____ hours(s)	☐ yes ☐ no

Notes: _____
_____
_____
_____

APPENDIX IV

■ ■ ■

Headache Impact Test

HIT-6™
(VERSION 1.1)

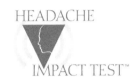

HEADACHE

IMPACT TEST™

This questionnaire was designed to help you describe and communicate the way you feel and what you cannot do because of headaches.

To complete, please circle one answer for each question.

1 When you have headaches, how often is the pain severe?

| Never | Rarely | Sometimes | Very Often | Always |

2 How often do headaches limit your ability to do usual daily activities including household work, work, school, or social activities?

| Never | Rarely | Sometimes | Very Often | Always |

3 When you have a headache, how often do you wish you could lie down?

| Never | Rarely | Sometimes | Very Often | Always |

4 In the past 4 weeks, how often have you felt too tired to do work or daily activities because of your headaches?

| Never | Rarely | Sometimes | Very Often | Always |

5 In the past 4 weeks, how often have you felt fed up or irritated because of your headaches?

| Never | Rarely | Sometimes | Very Often | Always |

6 In the past 4 weeks, how often did headaches limit your ability to concentrate on work or daily activities?

| Never | Rarely | Sometimes | Very Often | Always |

▽ +	▽ +	▽ +	▽ +	▽
COLUMN 1 (6 points each)	COLUMN 2 (8 points each)	COLUMN 3 (10 points each)	COLUMN 4 (11 points each)	COLUMN 5 (13 points each)

To score, add points for answers in each column.

Please share your HIT-6 results with your doctor.

Total Score [   ]

Higher scores indicate greater impact on your life.

Score range is 36-78.

HIT-6™ US (English) Version 1.1
©2000, 2001 QualityMetric, Inc. and GlaxoSmithKline Group of Companies

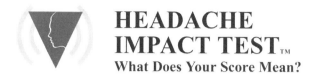

HEADACHE IMPACT TEST™
What Does Your Score Mean?

▼ If You Scored 60 or More

Your headaches are having a very severe impact on your life. You may be experiencing disabling pain and other symptoms that are more severe than those of other headache sufferers. Don't let your headaches stop you from enjoying the important things in your life, like family, work, school or social activities.

Make an appointment **today** to discuss your HIT-6 results and your headaches with your doctor.

▼ If You Scored 56 – 59

Your headaches are having a substantial impact on your life. As a result you may be experiencing severe pain and other symptoms, causing you to miss some time from family, work, school, or social activities.

Make an appointment **today** to discuss your HIT-6 results and your headaches with your doctor.

▼ If You Scored 50 – 55

Your headaches seem to be having some impact on your life. Your headaches should not make you miss time from family, work, school, or social activities.

Make sure you discuss your HIT-6 results and your headaches at your next appointment with your doctor.

▼ If You Scored 49 or Less

Your headaches seem to be having little to no impact on your life at this time. We encourage you to take HIT-6 monthly to continue to track how your headaches affect your life.

▼ If Your Score on HIT-6 is 50 or Higher

You should share the results with your doctor. Headaches that are disrupting your life could be migraine.

Take HIT-6 with you when you visit your doctor because research shows that when doctors understand exactly how badly headaches affect the lives of their patients, they are much more likely to provide a successful treatment program, which may include medication.

HIT is also available on the Internet at www.headachetest.com.

The Internet version allows you to print out a personal report of your results as well as a special detailed version for your doctor.

Don't forget to take HIT-6 again or try the Internet version to continue to monitor your progress.

▼ About HIT

The Headache Impact Test (HIT) is a tool used to measure the impact headaches have on your ability to function on the job, at school, at home and in social situations. Your score shows you the effect that headaches have on normal daily life and your ability to function. HIT was developed by an international team of headache experts from neurology and primary care medicine in collaboration with the psychometricians who developed the SF-36® health assessment tool.

HIT is not intended to offer medical advice regarding medical diagnosis or treatment. You should talk to your healthcare provider for advice specific to your situation.

SF-36® is a registered trademark of Medical Outcomes Trust and John E. Ware, Jr.

APPENDIX V

■ ■ ■

MIDAS Questionnaire

MIDAS QUESTIONNAIRE

INSTRUCTIONS: Please answer the following questions about ALL your headaches you have had over the last 3 months. Write your answer in the box next to each question. Write zero if you did not do the activity in the last 3 months.

1	On how many days in the last 3 months did you miss work or school because of your headaches?	☐	days
2	How many days in the last 3 months was your productivity at work or school reduced by half or more because of your headaches? *(Do not include days you counted in question 1 where you missed work or school)*	☐	days
3	On how many days in the last 3 months did you not do household work because of your headaches?	☐	days
4	How many days in the last 3 months was your productivity in household work reduced by half or more because of your headaches? *(Do not include days you counted in question 3 where you did not do household work)*	☐	days
5	On how many days in the last 3 months did you miss family, social or leisure activities because of your headaches?	☐	days
	TOTAL	☐	days
A	On how many days in the last 3 months did you have a headache? *(If a headache lasted more than 1 day, count each day)*	☐	days
B	On a scale of 0 10, on average how painful were these headaches? *(Where 0 = no pain at all, and 10 = pain as bad as it can be)*	☐	

Innovative Medical Research 1997

Your MIDAS score...

Grade I - Minimal or infrequent disability (score 0-5)

Grading system for the MIDAS Questionnaire:

Grade	Definition	Score
I	*Minimal or infrequent disability*	*0-5*
II	*Mild or infrequent disability*	*6-10*
III	*Moderate disability*	*11-20*
IV	*Severe disability*	*21+*

The MIDAS Questionnaire provides valuable information to help your physician recommend a suitable management strategy for your headaches. We recommend that you take the completed Questionnaire to your physician to obtain suitable treatment.

The MIDAS programme is sponsored by **AstraZeneca**

Courtesy of AstraZeneca.

273

How is the MIDAS Score Interpreted?

The MIDAS score is classified into four grades of severity that predict the patient's treatment needs. See the table below for MIDAS grade definitions, corresponding MIDAS scores and recommendations:

MIDAS Score	MIDAS Grade	Definition	Recommendations
0–5	I	Minimal or infrequent disability	MIDAS Grade I usually indicates low medical need. Simple, over-the-counter analgesics may be effective in the acute treatment of these patients. However, the impact of even a few lost days on the lifestyle of these patients should be assessed. Also, some patients with a MIDAS Grade I, such as those with infrequent, but severe migraine, may benefit from first-line treatment with specific migraine therapies (e.g. triptans). MIDAS Grade I patients who have failed to achieve effective relief with simple analgesics should also be considered for triptan therapy.
6–10	II	Mild or infrequent disability	MIDAS Grade II usually indicates moderate medical need. The patients may require an acute prescription medication. Some MIDAS Grade II patients may also qualify for first-line triptan medication if their headaches are severe. For example, a score of 10 could mean that a patient is missing ten days of school or paid work, so the headaches could be causing severe disruption in their lives. MIDAS Grade II patients should also qualify for first-line triptan medication if they have failed on simple analgesics.
11–20	III	Moderate disability	MIDAS Grade III/IV indicates a high medical need. These patients are experiencing significant disability and their migraine attacks are having a severe impact on their lives. Specific acute therapy, such as a triptan, is usually the most appropriate therapy for these patients, providing they are suitable recipients. Prophylactic treatment should also be considered. Please note that a very high MIDAS score could also indicate a high frequency of non-migraine headache, and these patients should be managed accordingly.
≥21	IV	Severe disability	

Index

Estradiol *(cont'd)*
  migraine and, 159, 160, 166
Estrogen, migraine and, 159, 160-161,
    166-167
Estrogen-receptor modulator, selective,
    163-164
Evoked potentials in migraine, 45
Evolution of headache, 82
Examination, physical and neurological,
    26-27
Exercise, aerobic, 218
Exertional headache, 139
Extraocular movement, 31
Eye
  cluster headache and, 98
  secondary headache and, 31
Eye disorder, 148-149

F
Familial migraine, 44
  in child or adolescent, 184-185
Female patient, 157-177. *See also*
    Migraine, in women
Feverfew, 210
Fluoxetine
  lactation and, 173
  for migraine, 66
  for tension-type headache, 89
Food-related headache, 144
Forme fruste version of headache, 19
Frequent headache, 113-136. *See also*
    Daily headache
Frovatriptan
  adult dosage of, 60
  lactation and, 173
  for migraine in child, 189
  for migraine in women, 164

G
Gabapentin
  for daily headache, 128, 129
  for migraine, 67
  for migraine prevention, 70
Gender, tension-type headache and, 80
Genetics
  of cluster headache, 97
  of migraine, 44
Giant cell arteritis, 199-200
Glaucoma, 203
Glossopharyngeal neuralgia, 202
Glycerol injection for trigeminal
    neuralgia, 201-202
Gonadotropin-releasing hormone, 160,
    163

H
Habituation
  detoxification from, 124
  in migraine, 45
Hand movement examination, 26
Head, palpation of, 27
Head and neck disorder, 146-149
  trauma causing, 149-151
Headache calendar, 261-262, 267-268
Headache calendar and diary, 261-262
Headache diary, 269
Headache Impact Test, 52, 53, 271-272
Heart disorder, 31
Hematoma, subdural, 37
Hemicrania
  chronic paroxysmal, 96, 108
  episodic paroxysmal, 109
Hemicrania continua, 23, 109, 114
  criteria for, 110
  differential diagnosis of, 96
  as primary headache, 141-142
Hemiplegic migraine, 184-185
Hemorrhage, subarachnoid, 35-37
  exertional headache and, 139
  orgasmic headache and, 140
Herpes encephalitis, 38
History
  in secondary headache, 30
  taking of, 14-16
Homeopathy, 215
Hormone, migraine and
  danazol and, 164
  estrogen and, 159, 160-163
  gonadotropin-releasing hormone
      agonist and, 163
  melatonin for, 213-214
  menstrually related, 158-159
  tamoxifen and, 163-164
Hospitalization for cluster headache, 107
5-HT receptor, 46
Hydrocodone, 173
Hydromorphone, 104
Hydroxocobalamin, 212
L-Hydroxytryptophan, 213
Hypertension, 151-152
  intracranial, 144-145
  secondary headache and, 30
Hypnic headache, 140, 204-205
Hypothesis, convergence, 82

I
Ibuprofen
  for daily headache, 128
  lactation and, 173